In a world reeling from the resurgence of old diseases (malaria and tuberculosis) and the emergence of new diseases (notably AIDS), the need to map the ever-changing world geography of epidemics is clear. *Deciphering Global Epidemics* shifts the focus of studies of changing disease patterns back by a century, from the present to the period from 1887 to 1912 when cities and the transport links between them were changing very rapidly. To make its maps, it draws on the unique but largely overlooked data contained in the first quarter-century of issues of the most familiar weekly journal in the epidemiological world, the *Morbidity and Mortality Weekly Report*. This was first published by the United States Public Health Service in 1878 on an irregular basis, and regularly from 1887, as weekly 'sanitary reports'. It continues to be published today by the US Centers for Disease Control and Prevention in Atlanta. In the earliest period, it included tables of weekly deaths from eleven infectious diseases for some 350 cities scattered around the world. Long before the establishment of the League of Nations Health Section and the World Health Organization, these tables provide an early global picture of what was happening to infectious diseases at a critical period in the growth of cities in six continents.

By carefully sifting through these records and discarding the most incomplete series, the authors have assembled information on six infectious diseases (diphtheria, enteric fever, measles, scarlet fever, tuberculosis, and whooping cough), for 100 world cities (mostly North American and European, but including all continents), and for more than 1,200 consecutive weeks. The authors use a variety of spatial and temporal analytical methods to paint a picture of mortality trends and cycles at the time. These are analysed at the global, the regional, and the individual city levels. To place the results in a wider time context, other data are used to look both backwards and forwards for nearly a century on either side of the 25-year time window.

Written from the viewpoint of historical geography, epidemiology, and spatial analysis, the book will also be of interest to students and scholars in demography, history of medicine, and economic history.

Cambridge Studies in Historical Geography 26

DECIPHERING GLOBAL EPIDEMICS

Cambridge Studies in Historical Geography 26

Series editors:
ALAN R. H. BAKER, RICHARD DENNIS, DERYCK HOLDSWORTH

Cambridge Studies in Historical Geography encourages exploration of the philosophies, methodologies, and techniques of historical geography and publishes the results of new research within all branches of the subject. It endeavours to secure the marriage of traditional scholarship with innovative approaches to problems and to sources, aiming in this way to provide a focus for the discipline and to contribute towards its development. The series is an international forum for publication in historical geography which also promotes contact with workers in cognate disciplines.

For a full list of titles in the series, please see end of book.

Deciphering global epidemics

Analytical approaches to the disease records of world cities, 1888–1912

ANDREW CLIFF
University of Cambridge

PETER HAGGETT
University of Bristol

MATTHEW SMALLMAN-RAYNOR
University of Nottingham

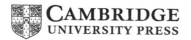
CAMBRIDGE
UNIVERSITY PRESS

PUBLISHED BY THE PRESS SYNDICATE OF THE UNIVERSITY OF CAMBRIDGE
The Pitt Building, Trumpington Street, Cambridge CB2 1RP, United Kingdom

CAMBRIDGE UNIVERSITY PRESS
The Edinburgh Building, Cambridge CB2 2RU, United Kingdom
40 West 20th Street, New York, NY 10011-4211, USA
10 Stamford Road, Oakleigh, Melbourne 3166, Australia

First published 1998

Printed in the United Kingdom at the University Press, Cambridge

Typeset in Times New Roman 10/12   [SE]

A catalogue record for this book is available from the British Library

Library of Congress cataloguing in publication data

Cliff, A. D. (Andrew David).
Deciphering global epidemics : analytical approaches to the
disease records of world cities, 1888–1912 / Andrew Cliff, Peter
Haggett, Matthew Smallman–Raynor.
    p.   cm. – (Cambridge studies in historical geography ; v. 26)
Includes bibliographical references and index.
ISBN 0 521 47266 0 (hb). – ISBN 0 521 47860 X (pb).
1. Epidemiology. 2. Mortality. 3. Urban health. I. Haggett, Peter.
II. Smallman–Raynor, Matthew. III. Title. IV. Series.
RA651.C55   1998
614.4'2–dc21   97-27050 CIP

ISBN 0 521 47266 0 hardback
ISBN 0 521 47860 X paperback

Contents

Plates

Figures

Tables

Foreword

STEPHEN B. THACKER, MD, MSC.

Assistant Surgeon General and Director of the Epidemiology Program Office, United States Centers for Disease Control and Prevention (CDC), Atlanta.

DONNA F. STROUP, PH.D, MSC.

Assistant Director for Science, Epidemiology Program Office, United States Centers for Disease Control and Prevention (CDC), Atlanta.

The public health community can trace its roots to fourteenth-century Italy, when fear of the Black Death prompted the government of Venice to exclude from their ports those ships with persons reported to have pneumonic plague. More recent epidemics of acquired immunodeficiency syndrome, vaccine-preventable diseases, and drug-resistant conditions pose imminent threats. The public health approach to such problems is fourfold: (1) define the problem; (2) identify risk factors; (3) develop and test prevention strategies; and (4) implement prevention programmes. Disease eradication, the ultimate disease control measure, is simple in concept (focusing on a single unequivocal outcome), but extraordinarily difficult in implementation.

Public health uses the sciences of geography and statistics, as well as epidemiology, the laboratory, and the behavioural and social sciences, to detect health problems in communities of people and to intervene and prevent further illness, disability, and premature death. Variations in the usual incidence of health events in different geographical areas or in different time periods may provide important clues to the aetiology of the disease or to specific risk factors for the event. A foundation of the science of epidemiology is a study of the departure of observed disease experience from the expected occurrence.

Public health surveillance provides much of the data needed for modern public health. The term surveillance is derived from the French word meaning 'to watch over' and, as applied to public health, means the close monitoring of the occurrence of selected health events in the population. Surveillance data resulting from ongoing monitoring of the occurrence of a disease or conditions provide quantitative data for deciding which public health actions are taken and whether these actions are effective.

In this book, three academic generations of British geographers offer the reader a comprehensive, analytic approach to the problem of understanding the underlying structure of epidemics in order to facilitate disease control efforts and ultimately to enable global disease eradication. The authors provide a sound taxonomy for six infectious diseases (marker diseases) and their geographical locations, and use data from public health surveillance systems to illustrate the principles of deciphering epidemics. Of particular note is the development of hypotheses for disease decline and an analytic framework for testing the hypotheses. The statistical issues underlying the methodology are explained and well illustrated. Of particular value are the comprehensive references and geographical descriptions included.

This book will be of considerable value to public health professionals involved in the continued vigilance of disease occurrence in communities. In the decision to undertake eradication campaigns, it is important to apply the methods of this book to determine when campaigns are near conclusion or when complementary implementation is effective (e.g., polio and measles), and whether one of the target diseases is confined to a limited geographical area. The prospect for global eradication of many infectious diseases during the twenty-first century is excellent. Cliff, Haggett, and Smallman-Raynor are to be commended for their timely contribution to this effort.

Preface

One of the most familiar journals in the epidemiological world is the *Morbidity and Mortality Weekly Report*. Universally abbreviated as the *MMWR*, it lands on many thousands of desks early each week with clockwork regularity (or increasingly is drawn down through an electronic web). Published by the Epidemiology Program Office of the United States Centers for Disease Control and Prevention in Atlanta, it contains a mix of invaluable information on the distribution of epidemics and plagues around the world, advice about new vaccines or protective devices, the eruption of a new influenza strain here, an outbreak of Oropouche fever there.

At its heart lie a series of tables that record the data returned by the state epidemiologist for each of the states and territories of the United States on the numbers of reported cases of fifty-two notifiable diseases. To provide perspective, the data for the current week are compared with the cumulative totals for both the current and the preceding years. The morbidity tables are supplemented by a mortality table that gives, for 121 of its great cities, from Boston to Washington, DC, the pattern of pneumonia and influenza deaths reported for the current week.

The *MMWR* is valued for its timeliness and its immediacy. As with a weather bulletin, the main interest is in the most recent readings and what they presage for the weeks and months ahead. Will a new influenza strain be sweeping the world? What progress is being made in polio vaccination? Will cholera break out in the refugee camps around Rwanda? But, again like weather records, the accumulated disease figures have a historical role. They monitor the past behaviour of epidemic diseases in the same way that weather records hint at past weather variations and even climatic changes.

This book is concerned with the historical antecedents of the *MMWR* and their importance in reconstructing a vital period of epidemiological change. The United States Public Health Service published weekly bulletins on public health from 1878 and, under various names, these bulletins have been continued up to the present day. The *Weekly Abstract of Sanitary Reports*, which forms the centrepiece of this book, appeared regularly from 1887. If we were to place a copy of the *Weekly Abstract* from the 1880s alongside the most recent copy of *MMWR* in the 1990s there would be much that was exactly the same: the same records of outbreaks, the same stress on practical public health advice, the same updating of trends and news from the battlefront with infectious diseases.

But in one respect the early tables would be strikingly different. For, from 1887 to 1912, the American weekly contained world tables for foreign cities in addition to those for cities from the United States. In this book we describe why it was that the United States Congress were persuaded to authorise the not inconsiderable cost of collecting and publishing these data and how the United States's consular service around the world was pressed, willingly or unwillingly, into acting as collectors of death statistics. For a quarter of a century, these tables give a worldwide picture of what was happening to infectious epidemic diseases. Their importance lies in the fact that they come well before the partial surveys of the League of Nations (from 1922 onwards) and the now familiar pattern of reporting by the World Health Organization (from 1946 onwards). As such they provide an epidemiological picture of disease change at a critical period in urban evolution on the global stage.

We have tried in this book to present the data culled from these weekly records in a form which gives some idea of the potential which lies buried in them. We have also laid stress on the various analytical methods now available for drawing out patterns from them, 'deciphering' epidemics as we title the book. But we are aware that, despite some years of work, we have only begun to scratch the surface. We have limited ourselves to just six diseases and to just 100 cities. Many more diseases and many more cities remain to be analysed. We have not used morbidity figures, since they were available only for the United States, but crude (but robust) measures of mortality. In interpreting the data, we have had neither the data nor the skills to enter into current debates on the causes of mortality decline over both our 25-year and longer time spans, and which provide such an active arena of debate for economic historians, demographers, and historians of medicine. The battles between the nutritional hypotheses of McKeown and the public health hypotheses of his critics are left largely to one side. We fear that we shall be equally criticised by several camps for failing to confirm or deny their hypotheses. But the data we have used are, thanks to a massive exercise in data abstraction and checking, now available for others to use and we would welcome requests to have copies of our data archives.

All this work would not have been possible without the unswerving support of a large number of individuals and institutions. Our first and greatest debt is to the Wellcome Trust. They gave a grant to finance the writing of this book as part of a programme grant in the historical geography of epidemics. A second volume on *Island Epidemics* is under preparation. We owe a special debt of gratitude to Dr David Allen, secretary to the History of Medicine

Committee, and to its members for their continuing interest and support. The additional financial help given to fund hand-encoding of data when computer scanning of records failed to cope with the variable and unclear materials being used was especially appreciated.

In the USA, we paid a number of visits to the Centers for Disease Control and Prevention in Atlanta through the courtesy of Dr S. B. Thacker, chief of the Division of Surveillance and Epidemiology Branch, Epidemiology Program Office. There we worked closely and productively with Dr Donna F. Stroup. Elizabeth Cheney and Jill Ann Kirn from Georgia State University worked, under Dr Stroup's guidance, as CDC interns on aspects of the project, and they contributed both research help and computer mapping expertise. The librarians at both CDC and Emory University were helpful in digging out early epidemiological material and guiding us through the intricacies of the epidemiological records.

At Geneva, assistance was provided by two main sections of the World Health Organization. The Global Epidemiological Surveillance section gave us not only a working base but also access to a wealth of regular epidemiological reports. The splendid WHO library allowed us entry to much early epidemiological material from the League of Nations period not readily available elsewhere.

At Cambridge, the staff of the Drawing Office in the University's Department of Geography have long undertaken the major task of producing the bulk of the maps and diagrams over many volumes. But in this book there is a change, and it is a special pleasure for all the authors to thank Timothy Cliff who has drawn all the figures in this monograph. At both Cambridge and Bristol we thank Lesley Cliff, Margaret Reynolds, and Mary Southcott for undertaking the heavy task of entering up into massive data matrices the individual observations from the weekly public health records. They must have felt, as we often did, that there was no end in sight, and the final accuracy of the data owes much to their careful inputting and rechecking of material from tables that often changed their format in a whimsical way.

Finally, at Great Shelford, Chew Magna, and Nottingham, our families continued to give us their unfailing support. After a quarter-century researching together, the two senior authors feel that their excuses for jobs uncompleted and lawns uncut must by now be wearing even thinner than on the last volume. If this book throws even a little more light on the complex ways in which epidemics can be deciphered, then the credit will be more that of Brenda and Margaret than they would ever care to allow. They went well beyond the bounds of marital duty in spending hour after hour in the CDC archives in Atlanta painstakingly and painfully transcribing data from old bound volumes that were disintegrating unless handled with consummate care. We hope the occasional forays to Warm Springs or Civil War battlefields during our working trips to Atlanta will be some recompense.

1

Prologue: epidemics past

US Consulate,
Alexandria, Egypt,
— —, 1896

Sir:

The present epidemic of cholera in Egypt emphasizes the importance which attaches to international sanitation and the geography of disease.

Dr James F. Love

US Public Health Reports, vol. XI (1896), p. 861

1.1 Introduction

Throughout history, the fear of disease has been well founded. The Book of Revelation relates the story of the Four Horsemen of the Apocalypse. The picture revealed by the opening of the seals is grim indeed, but it was old even then. The first and second riders on their white and red horses represent wars

1

of conquest and civil war. The third horseman with his black horse represents famine. The fourth horse, ridden by Death, is 'sickly pale'. Death has an additional right – to kill by pestilence.[1] But, as the twentieth century has progressed, so the pace of the pale horse has slackened in many parts of the world under the onslaught of medical science and the global vaccination programmes of the World Health Organization, while war and famine have continued to surge ahead. Over the last 100 years, the spectacular falls in mortality from the classic infectious diseases, coupled with the apparent successes of global campaigns against smallpox and malaria, have brought a sense of security. Plagues and epidemics could be viewed as essentially historical phenomena, scourges which had devastated past human populations, but which had largely been eliminated by the advent of vaccines and antibiotics.

As late as 1970, W. H. Stewart, the then surgeon general, told the United States Congress that it was 'time to close the book on infectious diseases, declare the war against pestilence won, and shift national resources to such chronic problems as cancer and heart disease' (Garrett, 1993, p. 825). In a similar vein, the biologist John Cairns could write in 1975 that 'the western world has virtually eliminated death due to infectious diseases' (Cairns, 1978, p. 6). But the cheering was premature. Within the decade, a new pandemic disease, AIDS, was emerging that seems likely to kill in the next two decades as many victims as did smallpox in all previous years of the twentieth century. The re-emergence of malaria and tuberculosis as global killers and the recognition of a generation of apparently 'new' diseases such as Lyme and Ebola confirms that we need to be cautious in declaring plagues to be features of history.

The renewed interest in epidemic diseases has also given a fillip to studies of the behaviour of diseases in the past. Just as modern concerns about global warming have prompted an interest in the records of historical changes in climate, so there has grown in epidemiology the need to study the past to see if firm baselines can be established against which modern shifts in disease prevalence can be measured.

This book is a direct response to this challenge. It takes the mortality records for a critical period of disease change at the turn of the century, and shows how the data can be analysed to establish benchmarks against which both earlier and later trends in mortality from infectious diseases can be assessed. The benchmarks are set in the context of patterns of epidemics in previous centuries. They are eventually used to investigate the twentieth-century course for mortality in general as well as for a selection of infectious diseases. The factors which have lain behind the declines in mortality are also unravelled. Finally, the book looks forward by assessing the potential significance of infectious diseases in the coming century.

Our task not only has intrinsic value (this is the first time that the source we use has been studied at length), but it also has a wider interest as an example of the manner in which appropriate analyses can be undertaken and applied to other sources. In this chapter, we sketch how the volume evolved and what led it to take its present form.

1.2 The nature of epidemic diseases

Before we can consider the importance of epidemic diseases in the twentieth century, we must first define what we mean by an 'epidemic disease'. Accordingly, we address this issue in the next subsection. We then turn to an assessment of the significance of such diseases at the close of the present millennium in terms of their demographic impact and their variety. This assessment is carried out at two spatial levels: the global and the national.

1.2.1 Defining epidemics and epidemic diseases

(a) Origins of the term

The term *epidemic* comes from two Greek words: *demos* meaning 'people' and *epi* meaning 'upon' or 'close to'. It was used around 500 BC as a title for one major part of the Hippocratic corpus, but the section concerned was mainly a day-to-day account of certain patients and not an application of the word in its modern sense (Risse, 1993, p. 11). In addition to its wider usage in terms of public attitudes (for example, Burke's 'epidemick of despair'), the word has been used in the English language in a medical sense since at least 1603 to mean an unusually high incidence of a disease where 'unusually high' is fixed in time, in space, and in the persons afflicted as compared with previous experience. Thus the Oxford English Dictionary defines an epidemic as: 'a disease prevalent among a people or community at a special time, and produced by some special causes generally not present in the affected locality'. The parallel term, *epizootic*, is used to specify a disease present under similar conditions in a non-human animal community.

In the standard handbook of human communicable diseases, Benenson (1990, p. 499) defines an epidemic more fully as:

The occurrence in a community or region of cases of an illness (or an outbreak) clearly in excess of expectancy. The number of cases indicating presence of an epidemic will vary according to the infectious agent, size, and type of population exposed, previous experience or lack of exposure to the diseases, and time and place of occurrence; epidemicity is thus relative to usual frequency of disease in the same area, among the specified population, at the same season of the year.

Benenson's account goes on to stress that what constitutes an epidemic does not necessarily depend on large numbers of cases or deaths. A single case of a communicable disease long absent from a population, or the first invasion by a disease not previously recognised in that area, requires immediate reporting

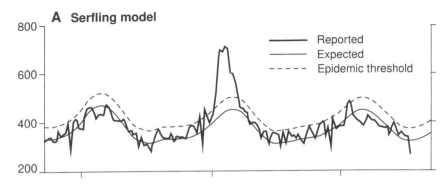

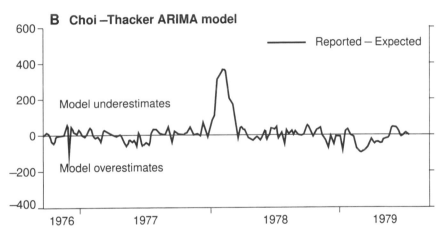

Figure 1.1. Definition of an epidemic in terms of reported and expected deaths. Reported and modelled weekly deaths from influenza and pneumonia for 121 cities in the United States, January 1976 to December 1979. The epidemic peak in the first few weeks of 1978 is defined in terms of the difference between the 'expected' number of deaths and those actually observed. Two different mathematical models developed by (A) Serfling and (B) Choi and Thacker are used to provide estimates from which the epidemic can be defined. For model details, see text and original source. Source: Cliff, Haggett, and Ord (1986), fig. 2.6, p. 22.

and epidemiological investigation. Two cases of such a disease associated in time and place are taken to be sufficient evidence of transmission for an epidemic to be declared.

The recognition of an epidemic implies that there is some benchmark against which an 'unusual' concentration of cases or deaths can be measured. In some instances, the benchmark will be zero reported cases but, in others, where the epidemic is a peak rising from a plinth of 'normal' incidence, complex methods of epidemic recognition may be called for (see fig. 1.1). Cliff,

Haggett, and Ord (1986, pp. 20–2) have reviewed the models used to separate epidemics of influenza from the background incidence of that disease, and we return to this topic in another context in section 4.4.2. The term *endemic* is used to describe the usual presence of a disease or infectious agent within a given geographical area. More rarely the term *hyperendemic* is used to describe a persistent intense transmission and *holoendemic* to describe a high level of infection which typically begins early in life and goes on to affect most of the resident population: many tropical areas with endemic malaria may be described as holoendemic (Benenson, 1990, p. 499).

(b) Types of epidemics

Epidemics of communicable disease are of two main types. A *propagated* epidemic is one that results from the chain transmission of some infectious agent. This may be directly from person to person as in a measles outbreak, or indirectly via some intermediate vector (malaria) or a microparasite. In some cases, indirect transmission may occur via humans (as in louse-borne epidemic typhus fever, or in a mosquito–man–mosquito chain with malaria). In others, the survival of the parasite is independent of man (thus *Pasturella pestis*, the cause of bubonic plague, is continually propagated through rodents, and the infection of man by an infected flea is in this respect a sideshow).

The second type of epidemic is a *common-vehicle epidemic* (Maxcy, 1973, p. 642) which results from the dissemination of a causative agent. In this case, the epidemic may result from a group of people being infected from a common medium (typically water, milk, or food) which has been contaminated by a disease-causing organism. Examples are provided by cholera and typhoid.

(c) Routes of transmission

The major routes of transmission for infectious diseases are listed in table 1.1. Many disease-causing organisms have several alternate routes, thus enhancing their chance of survival. The sequence of events in successful transmission involves release of the micro-organism from the cell, exit from the body, transport through the environment in a viable form, and appropriate entry into a susceptible host. This may be direct and essentially simple as in the case of the measles virus: the virus is shed from an infected cell and exits the body through exhalation, sneezing, and coughing as an aerosol. If a susceptible host is within range, the virus is inhaled and invades cells in the mucous membranes of the respiratory tract.

By contrast, other contagious diseases spread through a complex chain of contacts in which humans come only at the end. For example, the transmission of Lyme disease, a spirochetal disease attended by distinctive skin lesions and severe neurological abnormalities, depends on the life cycle of a tick (which may bite humans in summer), but also on mice, deer, and other zoonotic carriers.

Table 1.1. *Transmission of infections*

Route of exit	Route of transmission	Diseases	Route of entry
Respiratory	Aerosol	Chickenpox, diphtheria, influenza, Lassa fever, legionellosis, mumps, pertussis, pneumonia, poliomyelitis, rubella, smallpox, tuberculosis	? Mouth
	Salivary transfer	Hepatitis B, mononucleosis, mumps	Mouth
	Nasal discharges	Leprosy, smallpox	? Mouth
	Bite	Rabies	Skin
	Mouth: hand or object	Chickenpox, diphtheria, EBV in children, herpes simplex, pneumonia, smallpox	Oropharyngeal
Gastrointestinal tract	Stool: hand	Cholera, cryptosporidiosis enteroviruses, hepatitis A, poliomyelitis, salmonellosis, shigellosis, typhoid, paratyphoid	Mouth
	Stool: water, milk	Cholera, cryptosporidiosis, hepatitis A, tuberculosis	Mouth
	Stool: ground	Hookworm disease	Skin
	Thermometer	Hepatitis A	Rectal
Skin	Air	Poxviruses	Respiratory
	Skin: skin	*Molluscum cantagiosum,* yaws	Abraded skin
Blood	Mosquitoes	Arboviruses, dengue fever, malaria, yellow fever	Skin
	Ticks	Lyme disease, relapsing fever, Rocky Mountain spotted fever, togaviruses (group B)	Skin
	Blackflies	Onchocerciasis	Skin
	Lice	Typhus fever	Skin
	Fleas	Plague	Skin
	Blood transfusion	Hepatitis B, HIV	Skin
	Injection needles	Hepatitis B	Skin
Urine	Rarely transmitted	CMV, measles, mumps, rubella (congenital)	Unknown
Genital	Cervix	Chlamydial infections, gonorrhoeae, herpes simplex, CMV, HIV, syphilis	Genital
	Semen	CMV, HIV, syphilis	Genital
Placental	Vertical to embryo	CMV, HIV, leprosy, rubella smallpox, hepatitis B	Blood

Source and notes: Modified from A. S. Evans (1982), tab. 3, p. 10.
CMV=cytomegalovirus, EBV=Epstein–Barr virus.

1.2.2 The demographic impact of epidemic diseases

Infectious and parasitic diseases occupy the Tenth International Classification of Diseases (ICD) codes A00–B99, but at least 200 additional specific ICD codes reflect infection. Infectious diseases like measles represent a condition caused by a single virus attack, but some codes cover situations where infections may be secondary to other inciting events (for example, peritonitis). Despite decades of research and data collection, establishing the precise impact of infectious diseases at the world level remains difficult. Here we take our figures from the World Health Organization's (WHO) *World Health Report 1995* (1995c), although we recognise that the figures given there can be little more than rough estimates.

(a) International estimates

There are several ways in which an estimate may be made. One approach to measuring communicable diseases is through the deaths they cause – the mortality approach. Table 1.2 shows that infectious diseases occupy half of the top ten places as global killers.

Taken together infectious diseases and parasites take 16.4 million lives a year, ahead of heart disease which kills 9.7 million. Table 1.2 also shows that another way to measure disease is through disease incidence – the number of new cases of a disease each year. Again, the table illustrates the dominant position of infectious diseases (but note that the figures here are in 100,000s compared to 1,000s for deaths). Diarrhoea in children under five accounts for 1.8 billion episodes a year (and claims the lives of three million children). Acute lower respiratory conditions in children, sexually transmitted diseases, measles, and whooping cough remain major problems.

Yet other ways of measuring the disease burden are in terms of prevalence – the total number of people with a given condition – or the burden of disability that a disease causes. Global figures are hard to find and we know all too little about some major infectious diseases. Such fragments of information as we have at the world scale underscore the role of communicable diseases: for example, schistosomiasis has a prevalence of some 200 million cases on a worldwide scale, while 10 million people are permanently disabled by paralytic poliomyelitis.

A good example of the difficulty in estimating deaths from epidemic diseases is provided by measles. The number who now die from that disease each year is not known with precision. Aaby and Clements (1989) put the figure at well above 1 million:

Most global estimates indicate that more than 1 million children a year die from acute measles. The actual number of deaths may, however, be considerably higher than this. In addition, the impact of delayed mortality as a result of measles infection is only now being realized. Many months after they contract measles, children continue to

Table 1.2. *Communicable diseases as part of the global health situation (1993 estimates)*

Rank	Deaths Disease/condition	Deaths: number (000)	Incidence Disease/condition	Cases: number (00,000)
1	Ischaemic heart diseases	4,283	Diarrhoea under age five, including dysentery[b]	18,210
2	Acute lower respiratory infections under age five[a]	4,110	Acute lower respiratory infections under age five[b]	2,483
3	Cerebrovascular disease	3,854	Occupational injuries due to accidents	1,200
4	Diarrhoea under age five, including dysentery	3,010	Chlamydial infections (sexually transmitted)	970
5	Chronic obstructive pulmonary diseases	2,888	Trichomoniasis	940
6	Tuberculosis	2,709	Gonococcal infections	780
7	Malaria	2,000	Occupational diseases	690
8	Falls, fires, drowning, etc.	1,810	Measles	452
9	Measles	1,160	Whooping cough	431
10	Other heart diseases	1,133	Genital warts	320

Notes:
[a] Estimates for some diseases may contain cases that have also been included elsewhere; for example, estimates for acute lower respiratory infections and diarrhoea include those associated with measles, pertussis, malaria, and HIV.
[b] Estimates refer to number of episodes.
Source: WHO (1995c), tab. 1, p. 3.

experience higher levels of mortality and morbidity than those who do not. (Aaby and Clements, 1989, p. 443)

Berman (1991) estimates that acute respiratory infections cause four and a half million deaths among children every year, the overwhelming majority of which occur in developing countries. Of these, pneumonia associated with measles causes 15 per cent, or around 0.68 million deaths. But Markowitz and Nieburg (1991) put the proportion of deaths that are measles-related far higher, citing hospital- and community-based studies of acute respiratory infections which show that measles accounts for 6 to 21 per cent of the total morbidity, but 8 to 93 per cent of the total mortality.

Cliff, Haggett, and Smallman Raynor (1993) suggest that a figure for 1990 of two million deaths from measles is conservative but that it is probably of the right order of magnitude. While this yields a crude world death rate of only 1 per 2,500 population, the impact in terms of potential life lost (Cliff and

Haggett, 1988, p. 77) is much greater because most of these deaths are of young children.

(b) National estimates

An alternative approach to estimating the size of the disease burden is to use figures for a single country. For the United States, the Centers for Disease Control and Prevention (CDC) estimate that 83 per cent of all deaths from infections occur outside the 'classic' ICD disease codes 1–113: infections and infection-related deaths are important contributors to circulatory, respiratory, and gastrointestinal disease, to infant mortality and morbidity, and to arthritis. Infections complicate a wide range of injuries and have been found to cause malignancies in humans (Bennett, Holmberg, Rogers, and Solomon, 1987).

It is thus difficult to obtain a clear statistical picture of the real role of infectious diseases in causing mortality and morbidity. For this reason the Carter Center Health Policy Project reworked the available statistics for the United States and compared these with CDC Survey Data to provide a revised estimate of the effects of infectious diseases on morbidity and mortality. They concluded that 740 million symptomatic infections occur annually in the United States, causing 200,000 deaths per year. Such infections resulted in more than US$17 billion annually in direct costs, not including costs of deaths, lost wages, and productivity and other indirect costs. About 63,000 deaths are currently prevented annually and a further 80,000 deaths could be prevented by using current or soon-to-be available interventions.

Figure 1.2 summarises the Carter Center findings. This plots on logarithmic scales the number of deaths and number of cases for the main infectious diseases. Note that only diseases causing more than ten deaths or more than 1,000 cases per year are shown. The largest number of deaths (32,000) is caused by pneumococcal bacteria, followed by nosocomial deaths in acute (26,400) and chronic care (24,700). In terms of morbidity the largest number of cases is generated by the rhinovirus (125 million) that causes the common cold, followed by another group of viruses, influenza (20 million).

The figure illustrates only the leading 56 of the 117 specific infections considered in the Carter Center study. Although those not shown have fewer than ten deaths per year or fewer than 1,000 cases, they include many diseases which rank highly on the 'dread' factor. For example, amoebic meningo-encephalitis was recorded only four times in the United States in the year studied, but each resulted in death; rabies killed all ten of those infected, while half of the 100 cases infected with the cryptosporidiosis parasite died. The case-to-fatality ratio is marked by the diagonal lines in figure 1.2 for the more frequently occurring diseases. Those on or above the 1:10 diagonal include HIV, legionellosis, meningococcal invasions, and neonatal HSV.

Thus, although the last quarter-century has seen the global eradication of

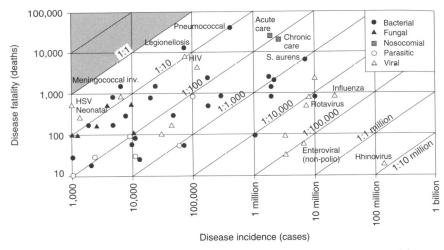

Figure 1.2. Annual mortality and morbidity from major infectious and parasitic diseases in the United States in the mid-1980s. Note that both disease fatality and disease incidence are plotted on logarithmic scales. The diagonal lines represent the case–fatality ratio. Source: drawn from data in Bennett, Holmberg, Rogers, and Solomon (1987), pp. 102 10; tab. 1, pp. 104–7.

one major human disease (smallpox) and major reduction in the incidence of others (notably measles and poliomyelitis), it has also witnessed the emergence of many new infections. In addition to AIDS, recognised more than a decade ago, we can add Legionnaires' disease, Lyme disease, and toxic shock syndrome. We also have outbreaks of African tropical diseases that occasionally erupt into middle-latitude consciousness, caused by the Lassa, Marburg, and Ebola viruses.

1.2.3 The increasing range of communicable diseases

In 1917, the American Public Health Association published the first edition of its pioneer handbook on *Control of Communicable Diseases in Man* (Benenson, 1990). It listed control measures for thirty-eight communicable diseases, all those then officially reported in the United States. Since 1917, the number listed has expanded steadily, so that the most recent edition of the handbook, the fifteenth, now details some 280 different diseases. Table 1.3 shows some examples of these emerging diseases, based on Morse's (1993, 1994) studies of viruses.

One of the disease groups that has shown the sharpest increase is that of the arboviruses (*ar*thropod-*bo*rne viruses). In 1930, only six viruses were known to be maintained in cycles between animal hosts and arthropod vectors like mosquitoes, gnats, and ticks. Only one of these, yellow fever, was known to

Table 1.3. *Examples of emerging virus diseases*

Virus family	Virus	Signs/symptoms	Natural host	Geographical range
Orthomyxoviridae	Influenza	Respiratory	Fowl, pigs	Worldwide
Bunyaviridae	Hantaan, Seoul, and other Hantaviruses	Haemorrhagic fever+renal syndrome+ respiratory stress	Rodent (e.g., *Apodemus*)	Asia, Europe, United States
	Rift Valley fever	Fever+haemorrhage	Mosquito; ungulates	Africa
Flaviviridae	Yellow fever	Fever, jaundice	Mosquito; monkey	Africa, South America
	Dengue	Fever+haemorrhage	Mosquito; human/monkey	Asia, Africa, Caribbean
Arenaviridae	Junin (Argentine haemorrhagic fever)	Fever, haemorrhage	Rodent (*Calomys musculinus*)	South America
	Machupo (Bolivian haemorrhagic fever)	Fever, haemorrhage	Rodent (*Calomys callosus*)	South America
	Lassa fever	Fever, haemorrhage	Rodent (*Mastomys natalensis*)	Africa
Filoviridae	Marburg, Ebola	Fever, haemorrhage	Unknown; ? primate	Africa
Retroviridae	HIV	AIDS	? Primate	Worldwide
	HTLV	Adult T-cell leukaemia, neurological disease	Human virus (? originally primate virus)	Worldwide with endemic foci

Note:
HIV=human immunodeficiency virus; HTLV=human T-cell leukaemia/lymphoma virus.
Source: Haggett (1994), tab. 1, p. 93; based partly on Morse (1994), tab. 1, p. 326.

cause disease in humans, although the other five caused epizootics and major economic loss in domestic animals (for example, African swine fever). Over the last sixty years, the number of arboviruses recognised has leapt from 6 to 504 worldwide (Lederberg, Shope, and Oaks, 1992). One-quarter of these are associated with viral diseases. North America alone now has around ninety different arboviruses and these include a few consistently associated with human disease: Colorado tick fever, California encephalitis, and dengue fever.

Most of the 'new' viruses discovered have probably existed for centuries, escaping detection because they existed in remote or medically little-studied populations or because they produced disease symptoms not previously recognised as being due to infectious agents. As with Marburg disease, they are recognised when they impinge on middle-latitude rather than tropical populations. Improvements in viral detection technology and in particular the invention of the polymerase chain reaction (PMR) method have opened up new frontiers in biology and medicine. It seems likely that the disease list will expand as links between previously unnoticed slow viral infections and chronic conditions (these include neurological problems and cancers) are unravelled.

The discovery of apparently new diseases raises afresh the question of where and when diseases originate, whether they will spread around the world, and whether new diseases will continue to be added to our existing list. Such questions have been given increased significance by the emergence, over the last decade, of AIDS as a major human disease. This has been accompanied by an unprecedented torrent of literature, some of it of geographical interest (Smallman-Raynor, Cliff, and Haggett, 1992). Notwithstanding this literature growth, one still unsolved question is when and where the epidemic of AIDS began. Conventional wisdom, based upon a variety of circumstantial evidence, is that the causative agent, the human immunodeficiency virus (HIV), jumped the species barrier from monkeys in Africa – possibly from the chimpanzee in Central Africa for HIV-1 and from the sooty mangabey in West Africa for HIV-2. Further, while we know that the epidemic spread of the disease in the United States began in 1981, there is increasing evidence that AIDS has been internationally present in a non-epidemic form for many years before the first epidemic cases, perhaps for some 150 years. Other scholars have argued for a much older origin (Ablin, Gonder, and Immerman, 1985).

(c)   Characteristics of new infectious diseases
We discuss the emergence of new infectious diseases in chapter 7, but such 'new' infectious diseases share a number of common features both with each other and with earlier historical manifestations: (a) the onset of the new diseases appears to be both sudden and unprecedented; (b) once the disease is recognised, isolated cases that occurred well before the outbreak are retro-

spectively identified; and (c) previously unknown pathogens or toxins account for many of the new infections.

Ampel (1991) suggests four factors which may explain these observations:

(1) The infection was present all along, but was previously unrecognised and unrecorded in the International Classification of Diseases (ICD). While this explanation may be true for progenitors of HIV, it is unlikely that toxic shock syndrome, Lyme disease, or AIDS existed in their present forms in a large number of patients for long before their recognition. We need to look further than a simple 'unrecorded' hypothesis.

(2) Pathogens responsible for these new diseases existed in the past but in a less virulent form. Some event, such as genetic mutation, then converted the organism to its virulent form. Rosqvist, Bolin, and Wolf-Watz (1988) have demonstrated that double-point mutations in the bacterium *Yersinia pseudotuberculosis* resulted in a marked increase in the virulence of this organism *in vitro*. Carmichael and Silverstein (1987) postulated that the marked increase in mortality associated with smallpox in sixteenth-century Europe could have been due to mutations in the causative virus, *variola*. Such events could also have occurred with regard to HIV-1. Finally, we note that the classic case of change to an already existing virus was the emergence of the Spanish influenza virus in 1918 (Cliff, Haggett, and Ord, 1986, p. 147).

(3) Environmental and behavioural changes provide a new environment in which the disease-causing organisms may flourish. Legionnaires' disease is related to the increased use of cooling towers and evaporative condensers from the 1960s; Lyme disease to the growth of deer population in woodlots that grew up on the abandoned fields of New England. Toxic shock disease is related to behavioural change, namely the increasing use of certain brands of tampons by menstruating women. Further back in time, the kinds of changes which accompanied agriculture may well have brought shifts in disease patterns. One hypothesis needing study is that malaria began to attack humans 10,000 years ago when Africans shifted from hunting on the savannah to farming in the forests.

(4) A new epidemic arises from the introduction of a virulent organism into a non-immune population (a so-called *virgin soil* epidemic) or to the arrival of new settlers in a previously unsettled area. This is a theme with rich historical parallels: one historically important example is the epidemic of smallpox that arrived in Mexico in 1520 with the Spanish conquistadores, decimating the native Aztec population; Cliff and Haggett (1985) have described the first introduction of measles into Fiji in 1875 in which around 25 to 30 per cent of the islands' population died within a two-month period. More recently, the spread of HIV provides a striking example of tropical to middle-latitude disease transmission.

Thus a historical review suggests that the emergence and persistence of new infectious diseases need very special conditions: there are many cases where diseases probably failed to emerge from population contact with a disease-bearing organism. For virus diseases, McKeown (1988, pp. 4–5) has noted that, when an infection comes into contact with a strong human host, three things may occur: the virus may fail to multiply and the encounter passes unnoticed; the virus multiplies rapidly and kills the host without being transmitted to another host; or virus and host populations (after a period of adaptation) settle down into a prolonged relationship which we associate with sustainable diseases. The relative probabilities we can attach to the three outcomes are unknown, but the fragmentary history of puzzling and unsustained disease outbreaks suggests that the third option is the rarest.

1.3 Evidence of past epidemics

From the present position of epidemic diseases, we now look back at a selection of the evidence for major epidemics in the past. We also consider the question of how we can know about the past and try to establish the protocols under which past epidemic events can be studied by analytical methods.

1.3.1 The pattern of past epidemics

In terms of its grip on the public imagination, the Black Death probably remains the most visible symbol of the power and influence of epidemic disease. In the year 1346 Europe, Northern Africa, and the Levant (the westward parts of the Middle East) had a population of the order of magnitude of 100 million (McEvedy, 1988). Within a decade, nearly a quarter of them had died and the population rise that had marked the evolution of medieval society had come to an abrupt end. The cause of what was known as the Great Dying or the Great Pestilence (it was only later that the term 'Black Death' emerged) was a bacterial disease carried by fleas that feed on rats, finally identified in 1894 by the French bacteriologist, Alexandre Yersin, as *Yersinia pestis*. The disease is thought to have emerged among marmots, large rodents native in Central Asia, and to have been introduced by fur traders moving along the Silk Road from Astrakhan and Saray. The subsequent spread to Kaffa, Constantinople, Egypt, Sicily, and Genoa (all infected by 1347) is shown in figure 1.3. As the time-contours on the map show, most of Europe was affected before the epidemic finally subsided in 1352.

Although the effects of the Black Death were catastrophic, they were not unique. Europe had seen a similar devastating outbreak of the disease in the reign of the Emperor Justinian in the sixth century. In 1356 a second outbreak of the plague occurred in Germany, and thereafter the plague returned to the continent with mournful regularity, although usually with decreased mortal-

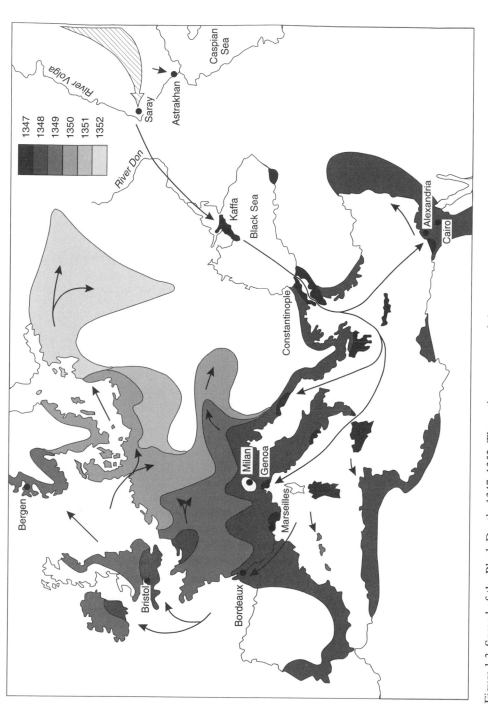

Figure 1.3. Spread of the Black Death, 1347–1352. The main routeways of the spread of bubonic plague from Central Asia through the Mediterranean to Southern and Northern Europe. Source: Brock (1990), fig. 1.1, p. 5.

ity. The reasons for the decline of the plague in advance of the advent of antibiotics remains a lively area of epidemiological controversy.

The Black Death of 1347 to 1352 is one of many tens of thousands of historically recorded disease outbreaks to which the term *epidemic* could properly be applied. Creighton's *History of Epidemics* (1894) and Kiple's *Cambridge World History of Human Disease* (1993) are major sources of information. Examples of some major epidemics over the past 2,500 years are summarised in table 1.4. The table does not pretend to be other than illustrative. The dates range from the Plague of Athens (430 BC) through to the current HIV and AIDS pandemic that is still in progress today. Note that, in terms of duration, some are for periods of a few days (the 28-day Legionnaires' outbreak in Philadelphia), while others persisted for years (the Black Death in medieval Europe). In spatial terms, the geographical extent varies from a single city (the Cartagena yellow fever outbreak of 1741), through to the worldwide AIDS epidemic.

To give a rough idea of the magnitudes of the epidemics, table 1.4 records the estimated crude mortality and the ratio of deaths to population. But, of course, these estimates are usually matters of considerable speculation. For example, the deaths attributed to measles in the 1875 Fiji epidemic vary from 28,000 to 40,000, with the bulk of scholarly opinion suggesting a figure of around 30,000. The rate of 1:4 deaths is an islands-wide average. Some parts of the Fijian archipelago were almost unaffected, while, in some islands, it was as high as 40 per cent (Cliff and Haggett, 1985). Still wider ranges apply to the totals and ratios given to the classical and medieval periods when the tally of total population, let alone mortality, was usually very poorly recorded.

1.3.2 Requirements for studying past epidemics

Before a past epidemic can be studied in a scientific as opposed to an anecdotal sense, several building blocks need to be in place. The aetiology and the epidemiology of the disease need to have been worked out, an agreed clinical definition must be struck, and an adequate recording system is required. We look at each in turn.

(a) Understanding the aetiology of infectious diseases

Understanding how epidemics are caused and how they operate demanded advances on several fronts. Lancaster (1990) has tabulated the dates on which the 'modern' causes of fifty major diseases were established (see table 1.5). The earliest date given by Lancaster is 1835 when Paget and Owen recognised the cause of trichinosis as due to an intestinal worm, *Trichinella spiralis*. The time pattern of discoveries over the next century is interesting: the rate of causal detection increased decade by decade from the 1830s until the 1880s when, in the golden age of bacteriology, the causes of nearly half the diseases listed were determined in a single decade.

This pattern reflects the tools available for clinical examination and laboratory analysis. The compound microscope was not developed commercially until 1840; versions of the electron microscope to allow virus recognition did not appear until 1932, and entered general scientific use only from c. 1940. Examination of human tissues through the freezing, supporting, and paraffin imbedding of samples was developed in 1843, 1853, and 1869 respectively. Stains for the study of cell structures began to be used from 1847.

Theory also played a critical role. Rokitansky's great text on systematic pathology was published between 1842 and 1846, while Virchow announced the cell theory in 1855. By the middle of the century, a small number of diseases had been shown to be caused by living organisms (see table 1.5) and Henle had given his closely reasoned account of the hypothesis that infectious diseases were not the result of unspecified 'miasmas' but transmitted by living organisms. The second half of the nineteenth century saw the heyday of bacteriological theory and practice with Louis Pasteur (1822–95), Ferdinand Cohn (1828–98), and Robert Koch (1843–1910) using the new laboratory tools to establish hypotheses of infection and contagion, often against entrenched opposition.

Since 1879 the abstracting journal, *Index Medicus*, has allowed the growth of medical knowledge to be tracked on an almost uninterrupted basis. Figure 1.4 plots the annual tally of publications over the last 110 years for one of the major infectious diseases studied in chapters 3–7 (measles) as an example of the way in which the build-up of knowledge can be portrayed in a quantitative form. This year-by-year bar chart should be compared with similar charts for six major diseases in chapter 7 (see figure 7.14).

(b) Understanding the epidemiology of infectious diseases
Alongside the advances that arose from improved clinical and laboratory examination stand breakthroughs in the field and in the analysis of the resulting data using mathematical models. One of the classic field investigations is Peter Panum's study of the Faeroe Islands measles outbreak of 1846 (Panum, 1847b) which laid the scientific foundation for understanding measles epidemiology (see plate 1.1). From an analysis of empirical data on measles cases in terms of their age, family position, location of residence, and pattern of contacts, Panum was able to state a series of seven epidemiological rules for the disease. The first related to the timing of the appearance of the rash:

The rule: That the contagium of measles may not cause disease phenomenon for some time after its introduction into the organism, and then only after an indefinite prodromal period, according to my observations always on the 13th or 14th day after exposure, was proved constant to me in a significant number of accurate observations. (Panum, 1847a; cited in Talbott, 1970, p. 748)

Table 1.4. *Examples of epidemic outbreaks in world history*

Timing	Location	Disease(s)	Estimated number of deaths	Estimated ratio deaths to population	Source
430 BC	Athens	Unknown (epidemic typhus or smallpox or ergotism)	?	1:4	Carmichael (1993c)
165–180	Old World	'Plague of Antoines': smallpox	>10,000 (Rome)	?	Zinsser (1935); Major (1943)
541–544	Eastern Mediterranean	'Plague of Justinian': bubonic plague	?	1:4	Carmichael (1993c)
1098–1099	Holy Land (First Crusade)	Epidemic diseases +famine	240,000	1:1.25	Zinsser (1935)
1241	Iceland	Smallpox	20,000	?	Hopkins (1983)
1271	Franconia, Germany	Rabies	30	?	Patterson (1993)
1346–1352	Western Europe	'Black Death': bubonic plague	20 million	1:4	Ziegler (1969)
c. 1430	Greenland	Smallpox	?	Near extinction	Hopkins (1983)
c. 1438	Paris, France	Smallpox	50,000	1:4	Hopkins (1983)

Date	Location	Disease	Deaths	Ratio	Source
1518–1519	Hispaniola	Smallpox	?	1:3 (natives)	Hopkins (1983)
1519–1520	Mexico	Smallpox	2–15 million	1:15–1:2	Hopkins (1983)
1524–1527	Peru	Smallpox	200,000	1:30	Hopkins (1983)
1563	Bahia, Brazil	Smallpox	?	>1:2	Hopkins (1983)
1587	Madrid	Smallpox	5,000	?	Hopkins (1983)
Late sixteenth century	Mexican Highlands	Epidemic typhus	>2 million	?	Harden (1993)
Early seventeenth century	Jamestown, Virginia	Typhoid	7,000	?	Le Baron and Taylor (1993)
1630	Nuremberg	Typhus+scurvy	8,000 (soldiers)	?	Zinsser (1935)
1637	Leipzig	Undefined pestilences	4,229	1:3.5	Prinzing (1916)
1699	Charleston, South Carolina	Yellow fever	179	1:17	Duffy (1953)
1702	New York City	Yellow fever	570	1:14	Duffy (1953)
1713–1714	Boston	Measles	150	1:80	Duffy (1953)
1741	Ireland	Famine, typhus, and dysentery	c. 300,000	1:6	Creighton (1965)
1741	Cartagena, Caribbean	Yellow fever	9,000	1:2	Cooper and Kiple (1993)
1781–1782	Pandemic	Influenza	>100,000 (Europe)	?	Patterson (1896)
1793	Philadelphia	Yellow fever	4,044	1:14	US Marine Hospital Service (1896)

Table 1.4. (*cont.*)

Timing	Location	Disease(s)	Estimated number of deaths	Estimated ratio deaths to population	Source
1795	New York [City?]	Yellow fever	700	1:57	US Marine Hospital Service (1896)
1801–1803	Haiti	Yellow fever	22,000 (French troops)	1:1.13	Zinsser (1935)
1808	St Mary's, Georgia	Yellow fever	c. 300	1:1.7	US Marine Hospital Service (1896)
1817	Calcutta, India	Cholera	4,000	1:60	Speck (1993)
1840–1855	Worldwide	Cholera	8,348 (Berlin)	1:50 (Berlin)	Speck (1993)
1857	Havana, Cuba	Yellow fever	2,058	1:102	Low (1920)
1870–1871	Paris (siege of)	Smallpox	75,167	1:29	Prinzing (1916)
1870	England and Wales	Whooping cough	c. 36,000	1:650	Hardy (1993c)
1874	England and Wales	Scarlet fever	24,922	1:943	Creighton (1965)
1875 (January–June)	Fiji, southwest Pacific	Measles+ sequelae	30,000	1:4	Cliff and Haggett (1985)
1889–1891	Pandemic	Influenza	60,000 (France)	1:625 (France)	Patterson (1986)

1899–1900	Alaska	'Great Sickness': measles + influenza	?	1:4 (Yukon–Kuskokwim Region)	Wolfe (1982)
1902–1904	Philippine Islands	Cholera	c. 200,000	1:40	de Bevoise (1995)
1903	Bombay City	Plague	20,788	1:47	Low (1920)
1909	Bahia, Brazil	Yellow fever	237	1:1,207	Low (1920)
1912	Bombay City	Cholera	1,790	1:547	Low (1920)
1918–1919	Worldwide	Influenza A	20 million	1:25 (India)	Jordan (1927)
1976 (July 20–August 16)	Philadelphia (Bellevue Stratford Hotel)	Legionnaires' disease	35 (veterans)	1:7 (veterans)	Fraser (1993)
1979 to present	Worldwide	AIDS	4,537 (Australia, to 30 September 1995)	1:3,527 (Australia, to 30 September 1995)	Australia, National Centre in HIV Epidemiology and Clinical Research (1996)

Table 1.5. *Discoveries of the causes of fifty major human diseases, 1835–1935*

Year	Disease	Modern name of organism	Discoverer
1835	Trichinosis	*Trichinella spiralis*	Paget, Owen
1843	Hookworm disease	*Ancylostoma duodenale*	Dubini
1849, 1876	Anthrax	*Bacillus anthracis*	Pollender, Koch
1853	Schistosomiasis	*Schistosoma mansoni*	Bilharz
1860, 1875	Amoebic dysentery	*Entamoeba histolytica*	Lambl, Loesch
1868	Leprosy	*Mycobacterium leprae*	Hansen
1868	Filiariasis	*Wuchereria bancrofti*	Wucherer
1873	Relapsing fever	*Treponema recurrentis*	Obermeier
1877–1878	Actinomycosis	*Actinomyces israeli*	Bollinger, Israel
1878–1879, 1881	Suppuration	*Staphylococcus aureus*	Koch, Pasteur, Ogston
1879	Childbed fever	*Streptococcus pyogenes*	Pasteur
1879, 1885	Gonorrhoea	*Neisseria gonorrhoeae*	Neisser, Bumm
1880	Malaria	*Plasmodium falciparum*	Laveran
1880, 1884	**Typhoid fever**	*Salmonella typhi*	Eberth, Gaffky, Klebs, Koch
1881	Suppuration	*Streptococcus pyogenes*	Ogston
1881	Rabies	*Rhabdovirus*	Pasteur
1882	Glanders	*Pseudomonas mallei*	Loeffler and Schutz
1882	**Tuberculosis**	*Mycobacterium tuberculosis*	Koch
1882	Pneumonia	*Klebsiella aerogenes*	Friedlander
1883	Erysipelas	*Streptococcus pyogenes*	Fehleisen
1883	Cholera	*Vibrio cholerae*	Koch
1883–1884	**Diphtheria**	*Corynebacterium diphtheriae*	Klebs, Löffler
1884–1889	Tetanus	*Clostridium tetani*	Nicolaeir, Kitasato
1886	Pneumonia	*Streptococcus pneumoniae*	Fraenkel
1886	Poliomyelitis	*Poliovirus hominis*	Medin
1886, 1892	Smallpox	*Poxvirus*	Buist, Guarnieri
1887	Cerebrospinal meningitis	*Neisseria meningitidis*	Weichselbaum
1887	**Scarlet fever**	*Streptococcus pyogenes*	Klein
1887	Undulant fever	*Brucella melitensis*	Bruce
1888	Food poisoning	*Salmonella enteritidis*	Gaertner
1889	Soft chancre	*Haemophilus ducreyi*	Ducrey
1892	Gas gangrene	*Clostridium welchii*	Welch
1894	Bubonic plague	*Yersinia pestis*	Kitasato, Yersin
1896	Botulism	*Clostridium botulinum*	Ermengem
1896	Bacillary dysentery	*Shigella shigae*	Shiga
1900	**Paratyphoid fever**	*Salmonella paratyphi*	Schottmuller
1901, 1903	Sleeping sickness	*Trypanosoma gambiense*	Forde, Bruce, Castellani
1903	Kala azar	*Leishmania donovani*	Leishman, Donovan
1905	Tick-borne relapsing fever	*Borrelia duttoni*	Dutton and Todd
1905	Syphilis	*Treponema pallidum*	Schaudinn and Hoffman
1906	**Whooping cough**	*Bordetella pertussis*	Bordet and Gengou

Table 1.5. (*cont.*)

Year	Disease	Modern name of organism	Discoverer
1909	American trypanosomiasis	*Trypanosoma cruzi*	Chagas
1909	Bartonellosis	*Bartonella bacilliformis*	Barton
1911, 1938	**Measles**	*Measles virus*	Anderson and Goldberger, Plotz
1912	Tularemia	*Francisella tularensis*	McCoy and Chapin
1915	Leptospirosis	*Leptospira icterohaemorrhagiae*	Inada
1916	Typhus	*Rickettsia prowazeki*	Rocha Lima
1916	Rocky Mountain spotted fever	*Rickettsia rickettsi*	Ricketts
1917	Chickenpox	*Herpesvirus*	Paschen
1933	Influenza	*Orthomyxovirus influenza A*	Smith, Andrewes, and Laidlaw

Source and note: Modified from Lancaster (1990), tab. 2.3.1, p. 16; tab. 2.3.2, p. 17.
The six diseases selected for study in chapters 3–7 are in bold type.

The other six were: (i) clinical symptoms do not develop until several days after exposure to the contagion; (ii) it is contagious only during eruption and efflorescence; (iii) there is no relationship between cowpox and measles; (iv) the disease does not occur twice in the same person; (v) it is not miasmic-borne but purely contagious; and (vi) isolation is the most certain means of arresting progress of its epidemic nature (Talbott, 1970, p. 748). Snow's observations on cholera, Ross's on malaria, and Gregg's on rubella are similarly part of this strong field tradition that has contributed to our understanding of the epidemiology of diseases.

The second advance in epidemiology that occurred outside the laboratory was in mathematical modelling. The critical discoveries using this approach are summarised in Bailey (1975, pp. 9–19), Fine (1979), and Dietz (1988). The first mathematical contribution to epidemiology is attributed to Daniel Bernoulli. In April 1760, Bernoulli, who was both a physician and a mathematician, gave a talk at the Royal Academy of Sciences in Paris in which he demonstrated the advantages of the heavily debated practice of inoculation against smallpox. Bernoulli used a logistic model to show that increased life expectancy resulted from inoculation.

Spatial spread: A fundamental step forward occurred in 1916 when Ross (Ross, 1916), already noted above as an outstanding field scientist, developed a general version of the Bernoulli model that incorporated population changes such as increase by birth and immigration, and decrease by death and

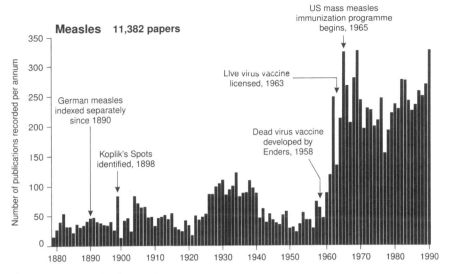

Figure 1.4. Growth of the scientific literature on infectious diseases. Number of publications each year on the virus disease, measles (rubeola) as recorded in *Index Medicus* (1879–1990). Source: Cliff, Haggett, and Smallman-Raynor (1993), fig. 1.7, p. 10.

emigration. The inclusion of components for immigration and emigration was a major development because it explicitly recognised the fact that communicable diseases may spread from one geographical area to another.

Population density: The Bernoulli–Ross models were designed for endemic rather than the epidemic situations discussed in this chapter: like that proposed by William Farr in 1866 to study cattle plague epidemics, they lacked the crucial aspect of epidemic models which relates the risk of acquiring the disease to the number of cases in the population. It was Ransome (1868; cited in Hilts, 1980) who first recognised the role of the density of susceptibles for the geographical spread of an epidemic:

At each successive period, therefore, of the duration of the disease, it advances at a constantly diminishing speed, until it reaches its highest point, when it suddenly falls at a rate, according to calculation, rather greater than it rose; but, according to our tables, probably owing to the lack of susceptible persons, it descends at about the same or a slower rate than it spread. (Ransome, 1868, p. 387)

Transmission mechanisms: Over the course of this century, two main types of epidemic model have been developed to account for the diffusion of disease in a population. The most extensively used is the general epidemic model which

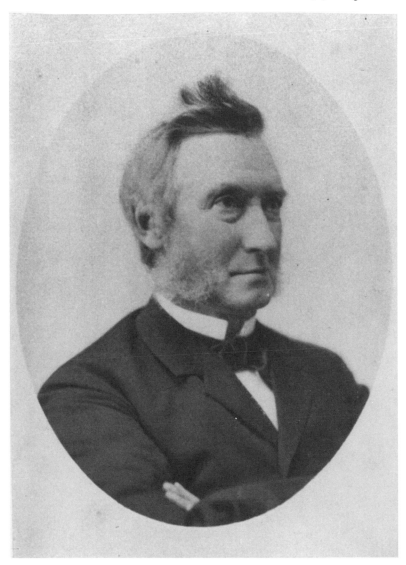

Plate 1.1. Peter Ludwig Panum (1820–1885). Panum's study of the measles outbreak of 1846 in the Faeroe Islands laid the scientific foundations for understanding the epidemiology of that disease. Source: Panum (1940), frontispiece.

depends upon the *mass action law* pioneered by Brownlee (1907) and Ross (1911). In mass action models, the total population is divided into two main subgroups, those with the disease (infectives) and those at risk (susceptibles). The mass action approach then allows the two groups to mix and studies the properties of the resulting epidemic. To the pioneers of the mass action approach, two names should be added: those of A. G. McKendrick (1912) who already at that time had formulated, apparently independently, the mass action assumption for epidemics which he applied to the transmission of venereal diseases and to malaria, and W. O. Kermack. Kermack and McKendrick collaborated from 1927 to 1939 and, in 1927, developed the celebrated threshold theorem which enables the interval between epidemics and their size to be studied (Kermack and McKendrick, 1927). According to this, the introduction of infectious cases into a community of susceptibles would not give rise to an epidemic if the density of susceptibles was below a certain critical value. Once the critical value was exceeded, then there would be an epidemic of magnitude sufficient to reduce the density of susceptibles as far below the threshold as it originally was above.

In contrast to the mass action approach, the second group of models, *chain binomials*, looked at person-to-person spread at the individual level. They were developed from a discrete time model for the spread of an infection in a susceptible population described in two lectures that Frost gave at Harvard in 1928. The first lecture was published only in 1976 (Frost, 1976). However, Dietz (1988) notes that, although Reed and Frost are credited with the major development of these models, the first chain binomial model was actually specified some forty years earlier by P. D. En'ko (1889; reprinted in English, 1989).

A definitive account of contemporary adaptations of these modelling strands is provided by Anderson and May (1991).

(c) Standardising disease recognition

The second requirement is an agreed clinical definition for each disease. Disease records for the past are often hard to match up with the specific diseases of today. Nonetheless, the precise classification of disease has been developing for over three centuries. Its roots lie in the statistical study of disease begun in the seventeenth century with John Graunt's analyses of the London Bills of Mortality. It continued in the eighteenth century with works by Francis de Lacroix, William Cullen, and the father of biological classification systems, Linneaus. Measles is one of the causes of death recorded by the parish clerks of London in the year 1766, along with other currently familiar names such as asthma, cancer, and smallpox, as well as some much less obvious today: 'Evil', 'St Anthony's Fire', and 'Rising of the Lights'. Figure 1.5 shows the record of deaths for measles in London from 1600 to 1850.

With the start of the General Register Office of England and Wales in 1837,

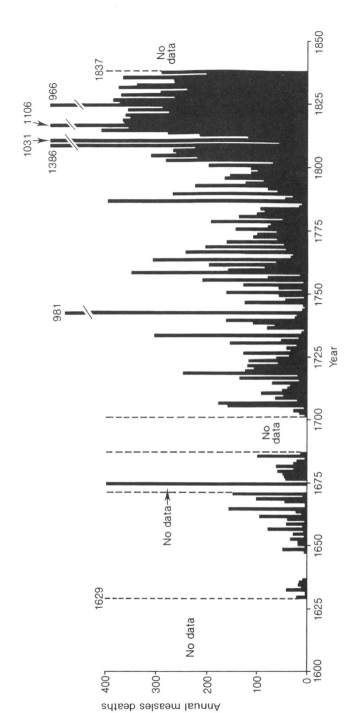

Figure 1.5. Annual mortality figures for an infectious disease, London, 1600–1850. Annual measles deaths taken from several tables in Creighton (1965), pp. 634–60. Source: Cliff, Haggett, and Smallman-Raynor (1993), fig. 3.4, p. 57.

attention was focused on improvement of disease classifications and on the promotion of international uniformity in their use. Israel (1990) has traced the history of the international classification of diseases from that point. The international importance of a statistical classification of diseases was so strongly recognised at the first International Statistical Congress held in Brussels in 1853 that the participants assigned to William Farr and Marc d'Espine of Geneva the task of preparing a 'uniform nomenclature of causes of death applicable to all countries' (Israel, 1990, p. 43). A compromise list of 138 rubrics was agreed at the next Paris congress in 1855.

Much revised at subsequent meetings, the Farr–d'Espine list formed a basis for the present International Classification of Diseases which began formally in Chicago in 1893 with the adoption by the International Statistical Institute of the Bertillon Classification of Causes of Death. In 1898, the American Public Health Association recommended the adoption of the Bertillon classification by the civil registrars of Canada, Mexico, and the United States, adding that the classification should be revised every ten years. The subsequent history of the classification in this century, now in its tenth revision, and its adoption by the Health Organisation of the League of Nations and subsequently by the World Health Organization is described at length by Israel (1990). Figure 1.6 illustrates the main chapters of the various revisions of the classification this century.

(d) Collection of mortality and morbidity statistics
The third requirement was that the records of deaths from a disease and its morbidity be collected on a sustained and systematic basis.

Mortality: In England and Wales, registration of deaths dates back to 1538 in the reign of Henry VIII when the clergy in every parish were required to keep a record of these events (see Benjamin, 1968, p. 43). An example of the London Bills of Mortality in the plague epidemic of 1665 appears in plate 1.2. Except for a brief period from 1653 to the Restoration, Henry VIII's requirement did not become statutory until the passage of the Births and Deaths Registration Act, 1836. While a few countries (for example, Sweden) predated England and Wales, the majority lagged by several decades.

Thus, although we have already seen in figure 1.5 that, for a disease like measles, we have some remarkable time series for deaths going back to the seventeenth century in London and some east coast North American cities, for most diseases there are little data of comparative value internationally before the middle of the nineteenth century. After this date, the public health movements that became established in many industrialising countries as a response to the perennial epidemics of diseases like cholera, typhoid, and scrofula that accompanied urbanisation produced a fundamental change in attitudes to disease recording.

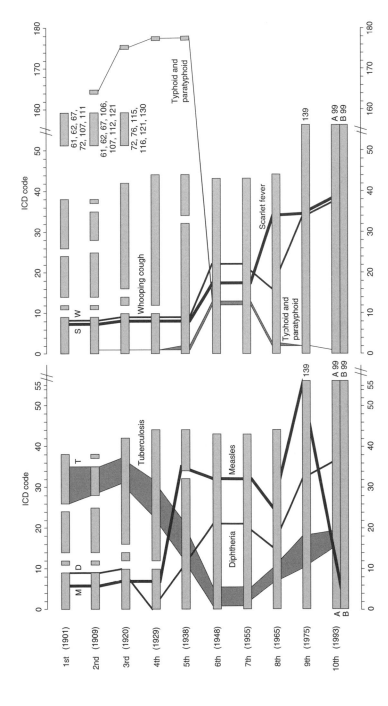

Figure 1.6. The International Classification of Diseases. Alignment of the main chapters for the first to the tenth revisions. The diseases studied are labelled.

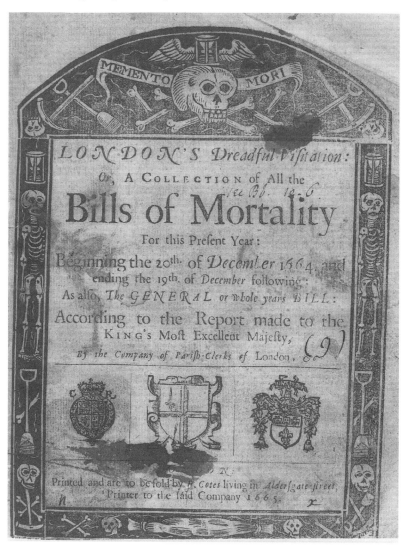

Plate 1.2. London Bills of Mortality, 1665. (Above) Cover bill for the year of the London plague epidemic of 1665 when 68,596 deaths were attributed to this disease. (Right and overleaf) Bill for the week ending 8 August 1665, showing deaths by parish and cause with 2,817 deaths from plague. Source: Cambridge University Library, rare books collection.

The Diseases and Casualties this Week.

Abortive	5	Infants		13
Aged	36	Kingsevil		2
Apoplexie	1	Leprosie		1
Childbed	25	Meagrome		1
Chrisomes	22	Mother		1
Consumption	130	Plague		2817
Convulsion	58	Plurisie		1
Cough	2	Purples		2
Distracted	1	Quinsie		3
Dropsie	32	Rickets		14
Drown'd in a Ditch at Saviours Southwark	1	Rising of the Lights		32
Feaver	314	Rupture		3
Flox and Small-pox	11	Scowring		3
Flux	1	Scurvy		3
Grief	3	Spotted Feaver		174
Griping in the Guts	70	Stilborn		11
Jaundies	2	Stone		3
Imposthume	16	Stopping of the stomach		10
		Suddenly		2
		Surfeit		85
		Teeth		90
		Thrush		4
		Tissick		3
		Ulcer		3
		Vomiting		1
		Wormes		18

Christned	Males	90	Buried	Males	2022	Plague 2817
	Females	88		Females	2008	
	In all	178		In all	4030	

Increased in the Burials this Week ——— 1016
Parishes clear of the Plague ——— 44 Parishes Infected ——— 86

The Assize of Bread set forth by Order of the Lord Maior and Court of Aldermen,
A penny Wheaten Loaf to contain Nine Ounces and a half; and three
half-penny White Loaves the like weight.

Plate 1.2. (*cont.*)

Morbidity statistics: A disease such as measles has been a notifiable disease in a few countries since the 1880s and, in some places (Denmark, for example), good historical records exist. Compulsory notification of infectious diseases in England and Wales dates from an Act of 1889, although records for a few urban areas are available for some decades earlier. Legislation requiring such notification exists in many countries while a number of others have voluntary reporting systems.

London 33	From the 1 of August to the 8.				1665	
	Bur.	Plag.		Bur.	Plag.	

London 33. From the 1 of August to the 8. 1665

Parish	Bur.	Plag.	Parish	Bur.	Plag.	Parish	Bur.	Plag.
St Alban Woodstreet	9	8	St George Botolphlane			St Martin Ludgate	2	2
Alhallows Barking	8	3	St Gregory by St Pauls			St Martin Orgars	2	1
Alhallows Breadstreet	3	1	St Hellen	3	2	St Martin Outwitch	2	2
Alhallows Grese	2		St James Dukes place	7	6	St Martin Vintrey	7	4
Alhallows Honylane			St James Garlickhithe			St Matthew Fridaystreet	1	
Alhallows Lesse		1	St John Baptist	2	1	St Maudlin Milkstreet	1	1
Alhallows Lumbardstreet	4	3	St John Evangelist			St Maudlin Oldfishstreet	2	2
Alhallows Staining	3	1	St John Zachary	1	1	St Michael Bassishaw	11	7
Alhallows the Wall	15	13	St Katharine Coleman			St Michael Cornhil	2	
St Alphage	14	5	St Katharine Creechurch	2	1	St Michael Crookedlane	1	
St Andrew Hubbard	1		St Lawrence Jewry	3	1	St Michael Queenhithe	2	1
St Andrew Undershaft	9	9	St Lawrence Pountney	1		St Michael Quern		
St Andrew Wardrobe	11	8	St Leonard Eastcheap			St Michael Royal	1	1
St Ann Aldersgate	5	1	St Leonard Fosterlane	11	11	St Michael Woodstreet	3	1
St Ann Blackfryers	21	15	St Magnus Parish	3	2	St Mildred Breadstreet	1	
St Antholins Parish			St Margaret Lothbury	9	6	St Mildred Poultrey	3	2
St Austins Parish			St Margaret Moses			St Nicholas Acons		
St Bartholomew Exchange	2		St Margaret Newfishstreet			St Nicholas Coleabby	1	1
St Bennet Fynck	1		St Margaret Pattons	1		St Nicholas Olaves	2	1
St Bennet Gracechurch			St Mary Abchurch	2		St Olave Hartstreet	4	2
St Bennet Paulswharf	9	2	St Mary Aldermanbury	5	1	St Olave Jewry		
St Bennet Sherehog			St Mary Aldermary	5	3	St Olave Silverstreet	17	8
St Botolph Billingsgate			St Mary le Bow	3	1	St Pancras Soperlane		
Christs Church	22	15	St Mary Bothaw	1	1	St Peter Cheap		
St Christophers			St Mary Colechurch			St Peter Cornhil	3	3
St Clement Eastcheap	1		St Mary Hill			St Peter Paulswharf	1	1
St Dionis Backchurch	2	1	St Mary Mounthaw			St Peter Poor	1	1
St Dunstan East			St Mary Sommerset	4	4	St Steven Colemanstreet	15	10
St Edmund Lumbardstr.			St Mary Stayning	1		St Steven Walbrook		
St Ethelborough	10	9	St Mary Woolchurch	2		St Swithin	3	1
St Faith	2	1	St Mary Woolnoth			St Thomas Apostle	10	8
St Foster	7	4	St Martin Iremongerlane			Trinity Parish	2	1
St Gabriel Fenchurch								

Christned in the 97 Parishes within the Walls —— 36   Buried —— 341   Plague —— 208

Parish	Bur.	Plag.	Parish	Bur.	Plag.	Parish	Bur.	Plag.
St Andrew Holborn	198	183	St Botolph Aldgate	103	81	Saviours Southwark	61	41
St Bartholomew Great	30	17	St Botolph Bishopsgate	180	133	S. Sepulchres Parish	325	205
St Bartholomew Lesse	12	6	St Dunstan West	26	20	S. Thomas Southwark	9	8
St Bridget	81	66	St George Southwark	60	39	Trinity Minories		
Bridewel Precinct	7	5	St Giles Cripplegate	691	356	At the Pesthouse	10	10
St Botolph Aldersgate	57	46	St Olave Southwark	143	64			

Christned in the 16 Parishes without the Walls—67   Buried, and at the Pesthouse—1993   Plague—1290

Parish	Bur.	Plag.	Parish	Bur.	Plag.	Parish	Bur.	Plag.
St Giles in the fields	290	259	Lambeth Parish	9	1	St Mary Islington	18	24
Hackney Parish	10	6	St Leonard Shoreditch	138	121	St Mary Whitechappel	177	158
St James Clerkenwel	148	136	St Magdalen Bermondsey	14	7	Rotherith Parish	3	2
St Kath. near the Tower	16	12	St Mary Newington	43	16	Stepney Parish	204	136

Christned in the 12 out Parishes in Middlesex and Surry—53   Buried—1105   Plague—879

Parish	Bur.	Plag.	Parish	Bur.	Plag.	Parish	Bur.	Plag.
St Clement Danes	61	42	St Martin in the fields	304	143	St Margaret Westminster	199	178
St Paul Covent Garden	29	16	St Mary Savoy			whereof at the Pesthouse		39

Christned in the 5 Parishes in the City and Liberties of Westminster—22   Buried—   Plague—450

K

Plate 1.2. (*cont.*)

Where collected, statistics are generally published on a weekly or monthly basis for each responding public health authority area within a country. For England and Wales, the relevant document is the registrar general's *Weekly Return*, published for each of the local authority areas into which the country is divided. The return is based on the data supplied by individual physicians to the medical officer of health for a given area for each week (ending on a Friday). Variations in the relative ease of clinical identification and attack

Table 1.6. *England and Wales: estimates of notification completeness*

Disease	Completeness
Acute poliomyelitis	Notification fairly complete
Cerebrospinal fever	Notification fairly complete
Diphtheria	Notification fairly complete
Scarlet fever	Notification fairly complete
Respiratory tuberculosis	Probably nine-tenths notified
Typhoid and paratyphoid	Probably four-fifths notified
Measles	About two-thirds notified
Pneumonia	From a third to a quarter notified
Whooping cough	From a quarter to a fifth notified
Erysipelas	Defective to an indeterminate degree
Non-respiratory tuberculosis	Defective to an indeterminate degree
Dysentery	Notification only fractional

Source: Benjamin (1968), p. 171.

rates mean that the statistical reporting differs considerably from disease to disease (see table 1.6).

In the case of measles, for example, detailed clinical studies suggest that this disease was generally underrecorded in the United Kingdom in the pre-vaccination period prior to 1965, so that reported cases would need to be multiplied by a correction factor of between 1.5 and 2.0 to give a more realistic estimate of the number of cases.

1.4 The search for a global data source

In this section, we describe the steps which led us to select the particular source of epidemic disease data whose analysis forms the substance of this book. Our overall concern was to find a source which was, at least in some measure, international in nature rather than one that reflected the epidemic history of just one particular country. We look first at the general time period in which the search was concentrated, then at the general characteristics we required of the data, and finally explain how far the selected source stands up to these requirements. Figure 1.7 summarises in chart form the main datasets we considered and the time periods for which they are available.

1.4.1 Windows of opportunity

(a) Time constraints
After a lengthy review of mortality statistics in his classic *Expectations of Life*, Lancaster (1990, p. xiv) concludes that:

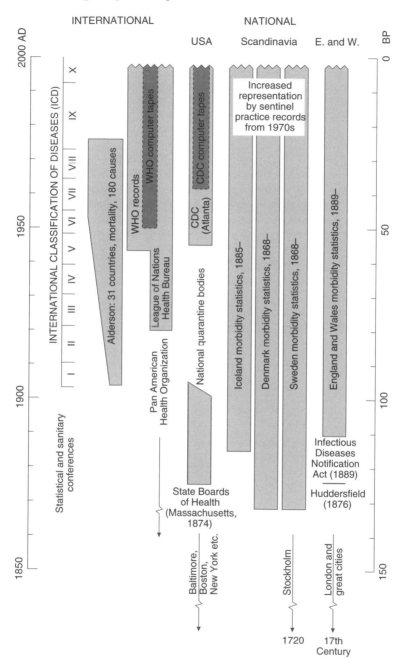

Figure 1.7. Disease data. Time span of archival records, 1850–2000.

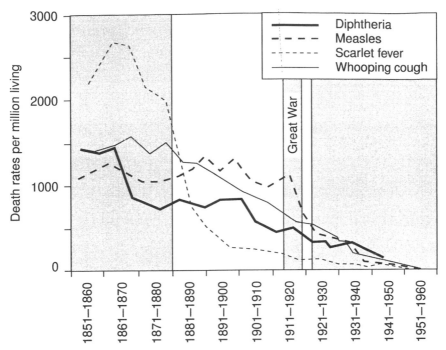

Figure 1.8. Historical trends for infectious disease mortality, England and Wales, 1851–1960. Historical record of disease mortality for a 110-year period to show the 'window of opportunity' between 1880 and 1920. Areas outside that time zone are stippled as are the Great War years. Source: Ramsay and Emond (1978), fig. 83, p. 181.

For those hoping to follow the course of individual diseases over a long period of time, the most optimistic statement can be that, notwithstanding the various revisions of international classifications, some diseases can be traced back to 1880 (and others earlier still) with some confidence.

We followed Lancaster's advice and drew an imaginary cut-off line at 1880 and concentrated our search after that point.

At the other end of the calendar, the creation of the World Health Organization in 1948 and its predecessor, the Health Committee of the League of Nations, in 1921 established a basis for at least a partial international recording system (see the appendices of this book for details). We have used the publications of both heavily in our earlier study of the changing epidemiology of measles (see Cliff, Haggett, and Smallman-Raynor, 1993, especially chapters 8–11). But, from the viewpoint of the present task, they suffered from the singular disadvantage highlighted in figure 1.8: they began to record changes in mortality at too late a stage in epidemiological history to pick out the dramatic falls for some of the most common infectious diseases. By 1923, at least six major diseases (diphtheria, measles, scarlet fever, tuberculosis, typhoid, and whooping cough) had halved their death rates from the turn of the century.

This consideration gave an upper cut-off point to our search and, in broad terms, we now concentrated upon the time window from 1880 to the early 1920s. In practice, the window had to be closed still further since the Great War of 1914–18 interrupted normal recording of mortality in some countries. Inclusion of the war years and the immediate aftermath was rejected on a second ground. The Great War caused the wholesale dislocation of civilian populations in many areas and led to the breakdown of normal medical care. This created disease patterns which might be expected to make the detection of longer-term trends more difficult. Our search period was accordingly narrowed still further to the 1880–1914 time band.

(b) Space constraints
The second dimension used to determine a possible source was that of geographical space. Given the pattern of political and economic development which obtained in the 35-year window between 1880 and 1914, the only countries likely to have assembled and retained international data on infectious diseases were those which already had a well-established state medical and health service. Using criteria such as the proportion of death registrations and the number of qualified physicians per 100,000 population, Alderson (1981) was able to find only thirty-one countries which he regarded as providing adequate mortality data for the period 1901–75.

But a number of the countries in Alderson's list did not begin to report until well into the twentieth century (for example, Hungary from 1916). So, if we leave in Alderson's list just those countries that were reporting in 1901 (roughly halfway through our search period), then we are left with only sixteen. Of these, most were European (Austria, Belgium, Denmark, England and Wales, Finland, France, Italy, Netherlands, Norway, Portugal, Scotland, Spain, and Switzerland), two were North American (Canada, United States of America), and one Asian (Japan). The valuable Japanese historical epidemiological sources have been reviewed by Jannetta (1987) but, since any relevant material would be in Japanese, this country was dropped on language and accessibility grounds. Our search was concentrated in the epidemiological publications and archives on both sides of the North Atlantic, using principally the libraries of the Centers for Disease Control and Prevention, Atlanta, the World Health Organization, Geneva, and the School of Hygiene and Tropical Medicine, London. A list of the sources considered is given in the appendices to this book.

1.4.2 Requirements for an international source

To choose a single usable source from which to trace past epidemics from the remaining possibles, we followed Alderson's lead and set up a series of ideal 'experimental conditions' which we hoped our source might meet.

These ideal conditions embodied four basic requirements:

(a) *Global coverage*: We were looking for a source which would cover not just a single country but provide a global cross-section. As with the later League of Nations and WHO data, we were aware that any such source would have to report (albeit in a selective or edited form) the raw material provided by a given country. Even in the 1990s, no international epidemiological agency has the resources to collect data independently (except occasionally by special surveys), and the figures used represent the end-result of a long process of reporting (or non-reporting) with many opportunities for error (see the review in Cliff and Haggett, 1988, pp. 65–92).

(b) *Geographical precision*: To allow spatial analysis, it was important that any data should be as geographically precise as possible. Ideally, readings should be for a small spatial unit rather than countrywide in extent. Given that medical services and death registration rates were higher in urban than in rural areas, it was likely that such a precision requirement would lead to a restriction to city-by-city data rather than data collected on a small area basis.

(c) *Temporal precision*: In order to allow time series analysis, it was necessary to identify a source which reported on a fine time scale. Many epidemic diseases have sharp peaks of morbidity and mortality which persist for a period of a few weeks or months. Annual data would not be good enough to capture these extreme events or to allow their spatial transmission to be traced; a data source which reported on at least a monthly basis would be necessary to give this temporal precision.

(d) *Range of infectious diseases*: To allow contrasts in epidemic behaviour to be observed it was necessary to select a source which reported mortality for a range of epidemic diseases. As figure 1.8 shows, the behaviour of infectious diseases has been very varied over the period since the middle of the nineteenth century, and we wished to be able to analyse that variability. In addition to our basic requirements for a study of disease change, we wanted to include examples of diseases for which the analytical results would have practical ramifications for control. Measles and whooping cough are merely two which fit this requirement. We explore this link further in chapter 7.

1.4.3 The United States Weekly Reports as a global source

After sifting through a large number of possible sources, we eventually selected the United States *Weekly Abstract of Sanitary Reports* (latterly the *Public Health Reports*) as our data source. The nature of this source is considered in detail in chapters 2 and 3. Here, we outline in a summary form the extent to which the *Weekly Abstract* meets our four 'experimental conditions' described in section 1.4.2.

(a) *Global coverage*: From the outset, the *Weekly Abstract* was established to provide an international record of infectious disease activity. As described in chapter 2, the origin of the *Weekly Abstract* rests with the US National Quarantine Act of 1878. This Act legislated for the collection and publication of sanitary reports from those overseas locations with which the United States had commercial interests. These interests had extended to every continent by the 1870s, and this global coverage is reflected in the pages of the *Weekly Abstract*. The parallel development of this source as the domestic disease surveillance report for the United States serves to augment its global coverage. It survives today as an epidemiological data source for the United States as the Centers for Disease Control and Prevention's *Morbidity and Mortality Weekly Report*.

(b) *Geographical precision*: In accordance with this requirement, the basic spatial unit for which information is available in the *Weekly Abstract* is the city. Here, the term 'city' is used to refer to a settlement with defined administrative boundaries. As described in chapter 3, reporting cities ranged in size from large metropolises of several millions (for example, London and New York) to small settlements of just a few hundred inhabitants. Although the *Weekly Abstract* does not define the areal extent of the reporting cities, such information is readily obtained from census material and other historical documents.

(c) *Temporal precision*: An important characteristic of the *Weekly Abstract* is the temporal precision of the epidemiological data. The 1878 Quarantine Act stipulated that sanitary reports should be submitted on a weekly basis. Although a small number of reporting cities were unable to meet this demand, and there were delays in submission, as its name implies, the calendar week forms the basic reporting interval in the *Weekly Abstract*.

(d) *Range of infectious diseases*: Up to eleven infectious diseases were recorded in the *Weekly Abstract* during the period examined in this book, 1888–1912. These included the four great quarantine diseases – cholera, plague, smallpox, and yellow fever – and seven other conditions perceived as a threat to the health of the United States – diphtheria, enteric fever (typhoid and paratyphoid fevers), measles, scarlet fever, tuberculosis, typhus fever, and whooping cough. These eleven include three major

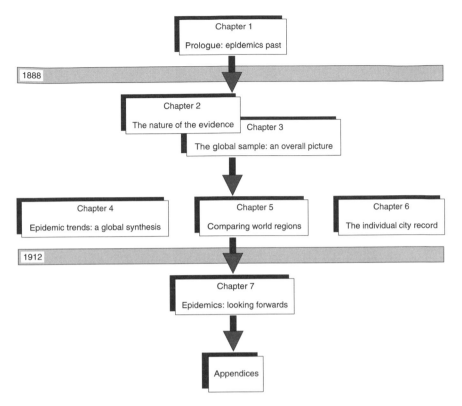

Figure 1.9. Organisation of the book. Schematic diagram of the sequence of topics covered in this volume. The year lines, 1888 and 1912, delimit the main time period covered in the book.

groups of causative agent (viruses, bacteria, and *Rickettsiae*) and span a range of epidemiological experiences in the late nineteenth and early twentieth centuries. Moreover, while some of the diseases no longer pose a threat to the human race (smallpox), others, such as cholera, measles, and tuberculosis, remain at the forefront of disease control concerns as the twentieth century draws to a close.

1.5 Organisation of the book

The structure of the book is laid out in figure 1.9. The opening chapter is essentially a prologue to the main part of the volume. Chapter 2 introduces the archival source that is the basis of our analysis, the *Weekly Abstract*, which was prepared weekly from 1878 by the United States Marine Hospital Service under this and other titles. The chapter outlines the ways in which the data were collected around the world, and the environment which led both to their publication and to the eventual demise of non-US records. Chapter 3 provides a preliminary analysis of the material, indicating how six infectious diseases (diphtheria, enteric fever, measles, scarlet fever, tuberculosis, and whooping cough) were eventually chosen from the eleven listed above, and why 100 cities were selected for special study.

The next three chapters are essentially analytical, subjecting the data matrix (6 diseases and all causes×100 cities×1,304 weeks) to a range of statistical examinations. Chapter 4 conducts the analysis at the global level, concentrating on the worldwide picture as shown by the average values calculated from the 100 cities and the broad conclusions that can be drawn from them. Chapter 5 changes the focus and breaks the world down into ten separate regions. This allows comparisons to be drawn between regions and throws light on the different epidemiological stages reached in different parts of the globe. Finally chapter 6 brings the focus down still further, studying the evidence that is yielded by the disease traces of individual cities. Special attention is paid to the cities of North America and then to those of the British Isles.

The last part of the book, chapter 7, looks at what has happened to mortality from different diseases since the picture drawn in the three previous chapters was completed in 1912. It portrays the twentieth-century course both for mortality in general and for the six marker diseases, and tries to probe the factors which lay behind the declines of mortality. In recent years, there has been a revolution of interest in infectious diseases, and so chapter 7 also looks forward and assesses the potential significance of infectious diseases in the coming century.

An important addendum to the book is provided by the appendices. Bearing in mind space limitations, these give a comprehensive review of epidemiological and associated demographic sources.

2

The nature of the evidence

Health of Rio de Janeiro. – This appears to me a very serious matter, and foreign nations are so deeply interested in it, and their interests and lives so seriously implicated, that it, perhaps, arises to the importance of an international question.

R. Cleary, Sanitary Inspector, US Marine Hospital Service
Weekly Abstract of Sanitary Reports, vol. IX (1894), p. 311

2.1 Introduction

Chapter 1 outlined the rationale for our selection of the US *Weekly Abstract of Sanitary Reports* as a data source for a global study of epidemic history between 1887 and 1912. This chapter sets the scene for the remainder of the book by describing the development, structure, and scope of that archive. We begin, in section 2.2, by placing the *Weekly Abstract* within the broad context of the nineteenth-century US public health movement and, more especially, the operation of the US Marine Hospital Service. The multifarious duties of the Marine Hospital Service included the preparation of the *Weekly Abstract* and the nature and extent of this publication is considered in sections 2.3 and 2.4. Finally, sections 2.5 and 2.6 address the crucial issue of the reliability of the numerical information included in the *Weekly Abstract*.

2.2 Origins of the *Weekly Abstract*

The *Weekly Abstract* was the brainchild of the US Marine Hospital Service, the forerunner of the US Public Health Service. In this section we briefly describe the history of the Marine Hospital Service and the factors that prompted US concerns with international sanitary conditions. The sequence of events that led to the formal establishment of international disease surveillance by the United States is then traced, and the nature and extent of the consular system through which the surveillance system operated is outlined.

2.2.1 Background: the US Marine Hospital Service (USMHS)

The history of the US Marine Hospital Service (USMHS) dates back to July 1798 and the passage of the Act for the Relief of Sick and Disabled Seamen. The Act provided for a federal tax of 20¢ to be levied each month on merchant sailors. The revenue was to provide health care for ailing sailors, with surplus monies used for the finance of marine hospitals (R. C. Williams, 1951; Furman, 1973; Bordley and Harvey, 1976; Greene, 1977; Bienia, Stein, and Bienia, 1983). During the next sixty years the USMHS expanded to include twenty-seven hospitals. But the Civil War was to decimate this system; only five hospitals remained operative in the immediate post-war period with medical care essentially restricted to acute conditions (Bienia, Stein, and Bienia, 1983). One remedial response, in 1871, was to create the post of supervising surgeon of the Marine Hospital Service. The first person to occupy this position was John M. Woodworth (plate 2.1). As described in section 2.2.3, Woodworth was to play a pivotal role in the subsequent development of international disease surveillance and the establishment of the *Weekly Abstract*.

2.2.2 Risk of disease importation

For much of the early history of the North American colonies, the populations were too sparse to hold many infectious diseases in endemic form. Diseases such as smallpox and yellow fever would, occasionally, be introduced

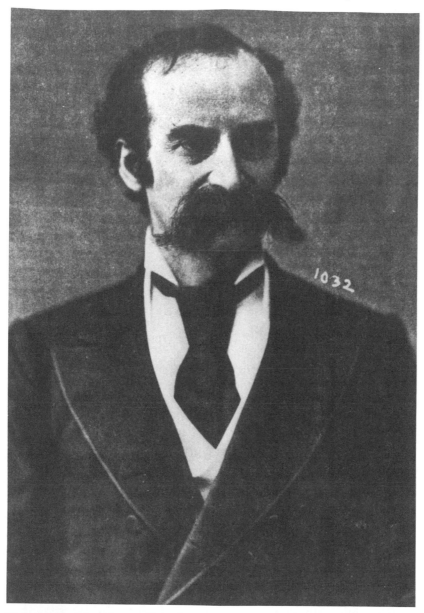

Plate 2.1. Dr John Maynard Woodworth (1837–1879). Supervising surgeon and supervising surgeon general, US Marine Hospital Service, 1871–9. Source: Furman (1973), p. 122.

into southern ports by ships sailing from Latin America and the Caribbean, but the epidemics would rarely be sustained.[1] The epidemiological isolation of the colonies in these early years was bolstered by long sea journeys in small sailing ships, shipboard epidemics usually having run their course well before the colonies were reached. But this situation was to change dramatically in the nineteenth century. The expanding international interests of the fledgling United States, coupled with advances in transport technology and high-level immigration, effectively eroded its epidemiological isolation.

Growth in international shipping: One important factor for the increased risk of disease importation was the rapid growth in ships destined for the United States from foreign ports. This growth is charted in figure 2.1 for the half-century period from 1850. The line trace plots the number of vessels embarking annually for the United States from foreign ports, while the tonnage of shipping is plotted as the bar chart. Figure 2.1 shows that the volume of shipping spiralled from about 10,000–12,000 vessels each year in the 1850s to a peak of almost 26,000 in the late 1870s, falling thereafter to 20,000–22,000 vessels a year in the 1890s as the size of individual vessels increased. During the same interval, tonnage grew by an order of magnitude, from less than 2 million tons in 1850 to around 22 million tons in 1900.

The proportion of these ships which were carrying infectious diseases, contracted at the port(s) of embarkation, will never be known with any certainty. However, figure 2.2 is based on information collated by the USMHS and shows the monthly series of deaths on vessels sailing to the United States from foreign ports for a sample period from July 1883 to June 1894.[2] The upper graph, which plots deaths by all causes ($n=859$), shows an oscillatory motion with summer highs associated with the immigration season. The remaining two graphs plot deaths attributable to tuberculosis (centre graph) and a selection of other major infectious diseases (lower graph). Together, infectious diseases accounted for some 13 per cent of all shipboard deaths. Tuberculosis was the most prevalent killer, maintaining a low but constant level throughout the observation period. Reports of deaths from other infectious diseases were a sporadic phenomenon.

Developments in transport technology: The threat of the introduction of infectious diseases was made doubly secure by the increase in the size and speed of ocean-going vessels. Here, the succession of steam over sail from the middle of the nineteenth century was to prove critical. Figure 2.3A traces the nineteenth-century growth in steam-powered vessels by plotting the number of steamships built annually in the United States between 1800 and 1889. The first US-manufactured steamships were launched in 1812 and, by the 1860s, the United States was manufacturing 250–450 steamships each year.

An indication of the increase in speed associated with steamships may be

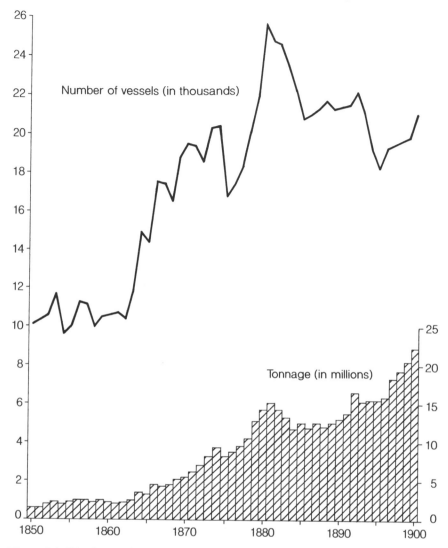

Figure 2.1. Number and tonnage of foreign vessels entering the United States, 1850–1900. Source: data from US Department of the Treasury, Bureau of Statistics (1850–1900).

gained from figures 2.3B and 2.3C. Figure 2.3B plots, by year of construction, the maximum speed of large steamships in global operation in 1901.[3] Maximum speeds of 12–14 knots in the 1850s were superseded by vessels capable of 15–17 knots in the 1870s and 18–20 knots in the 1880s. Some idea of the resulting breakdown in the epidemiological isolation of the United

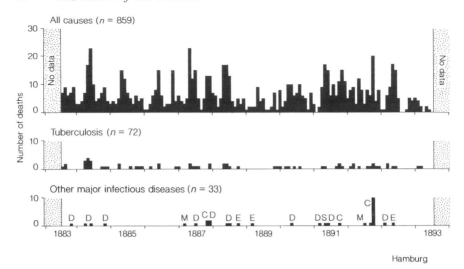

Figure 2.2. Deaths on voyages from foreign ports to the United States, July 1883–June 1894. *Upper*: all causes. *Centre*: tuberculosis. *Lower*: other major infectious diseases (C denotes cholera; D, diphtheria; E, enteric fever/typhoid fever; M, measles; S, scarlet fever). Source: data from US Marine Hospital Service (1884–94).

States can be gained from 2.3C which plots changes in the length of transatlantic voyages for a 370-year period from 1620. From a sailing time of over three weeks in 1830, the length of the voyage had more than halved to ten days by the mid-1840s, only to halve again by the first decade of the twentieth century.

Many of the voyage times plotted in figure 2.3C were record times associated with Blue Riband crossings. Scheduled journey times were, of course, rather longer. To illustrate this, figure 2.3D plots a sample of scheduled journey times for regular voyages between the US city of San Francisco and selected foreign ports (identified by numerical code) in 1890. The distance of the journey is plotted on the horizontal axis, against journey time on the left-hand vertical axis. An alternative way of measuring journey time is in transmission generations[4] and so, for comparison, the average number of generations required to sustain one sample infectious disease (measles, studied later in this book) throughout the voyage is plotted on the right-hand vertical axis. The names of the ships undertaking the voyages are given in italics. The chart shows that, in 1890, Sydney and Hong Kong lay more than sixty days (some four measles virus generations) from San Francisco. The Central American city of Panama lay some three generations away, whilst the Mexican port of Guaymas lay just one generation away.

Figure 2.4 extends the analysis of figure 2.3D by plotting the estimated

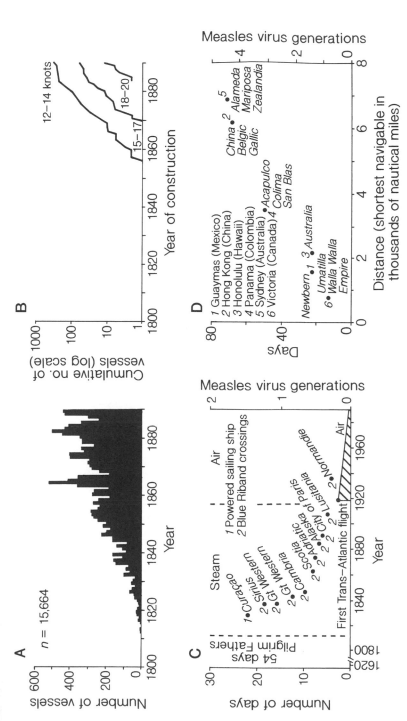

Figure 2.3. International connectivity of the United States. (A) Number of steamships built in the United States, 1800–89. (B) Speed of large steamships (2,000 tons or greater) in global operation in 1901, by year of construction. (C) Atlantic voyage times, 1620–1990. (D) Voyage times for scheduled sailings between the United States and international Pacific ports, July 1890; names of vessels are shown in italics while foreign origin/destination ports are indicated by the numerical key. Sources: US Department of the Treasury, Bureau of Statistics (1890), tab. 83, pp. 1000–1; US Department of the Treasury, Bureau of Navigation (1901), appendix O, pp. 382–3; US Department of the Treasury, Bureau of Statistics (1891), tab. 63, opposite p. 1174; Cobh Heritage Museum, Cobh, Ireland.

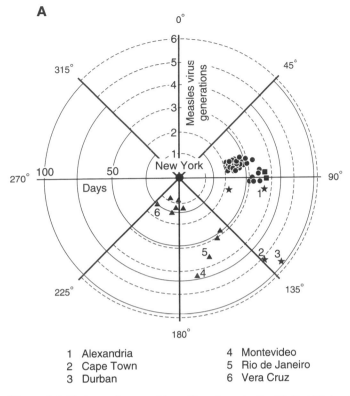

A

1 Alexandria   4 Montevideo
2 Cape Town   5 Rio de Janeiro
3 Durban   6 Vera Cruz

Figure 2.4. Estimated steamship sailing times to the United States from fifty-six foreign ports. (A) To New York. (B) To San Francisco. Destination ports in the United States are placed at the centre of the charts, while foreign ports are located according to their bearing on Bartholomew's *The Times* pseudo-conical world projection. Cartesian distance between origin and destination ports is scaled to estimated sailing times (in days) by the shortest navigable route in 1890 (solid circles). For reference, the average number of transmission generations required to sustain one viral disease (measles) throughout the voyage is indicated (pecked circles). Sources: data from US Department of the Treasury, Bureau of Navigation (1901), appendix N, pp. 361–81; US Department of the Treasury, Bureau of Statistics (1891), tab. 63, opposite p. 1174.

steamship sailing times from sample foreign ports to New York (A) and San Francisco (B) during the 1890s.[5] New York and San Francisco, which were principal reception points for international shipping destined for the east and west coasts respectively, have been placed at the centre of the charts. Foreign ports have been oriented according to their bearing from the two cities.[6] The cartesian distance from the centre of the charts to each foreign port is scaled to estimated sailing times (in days), and is to be read against the horizontal

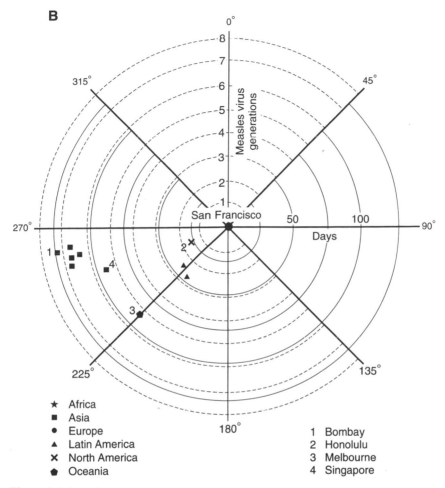

Figure 2.4. (*cont.*)

axes and marked in 25-day intervals by full circles. For reference, the average number of transmission generations required to sustain our sample infectious disease (measles) throughout the voyage is indicated by the broken circles, to be read against the vertical axes. The ports have been categorised according to their continental location (Africa, Asia, Europe and Latin America, North America, and Oceania) with sample ports named.

Figure 2.4A indicates that New York was within easy epidemiological reach of many African, Asian, European, and Latin American ports. In most instances, voyage times were well below seventy-five days or approximately four measles virus generations. San Francisco was rather more distant from many major international ports of Asia and Oceania. However, it is apparent

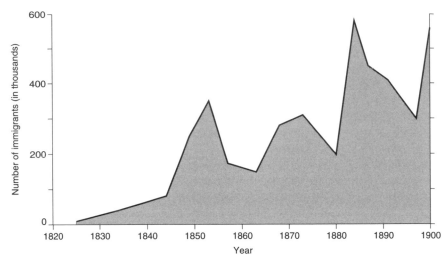

Figure 2.5. Levels of foreign immigration, United States, 1820–1900. Source: adapted from Keely (1979), fig. 1, p. 13.

for both New York and San Francisco that a single incubating case of measles on departure from some Latin American ports would still be active on arrival in the United States, with the potential to spark an epidemic.

Immigration: Not only did the volume and speed of shipping destined for the United States increase dramatically; so, too, did the number of immigrants arriving from foreign locations where infectious diseases were rife. To illustrate this, figure 2.5 plots the number of immigrants entering the United States between 1820 and 1900. Although the number of immigrants fluctuated from time period to time period, there is an underlying growth from just a few thousand towards the start of the observation period to several hundred thousand at the close of the nineteenth century (Keely, 1979).

2.2.3 *Establishment of the* Weekly Abstract

The risk of importation of infectious diseases into the United States was to serve as the stimulus for the establishment of the *Weekly Abstract*; the evolution of international disease surveillance and the *Weekly Abstract* is traced in figure 2.6.

One critical factor was the appointment in 1870 of John Maynard Woodworth as the first supervising surgeon (later supervising surgeon general) of the Marine Hospital Service (plate 2.1). Woodworth contended that the most effective way to halt the spread of epidemic disease in the United States was to prevent it from entering the country. His first move was to revive the

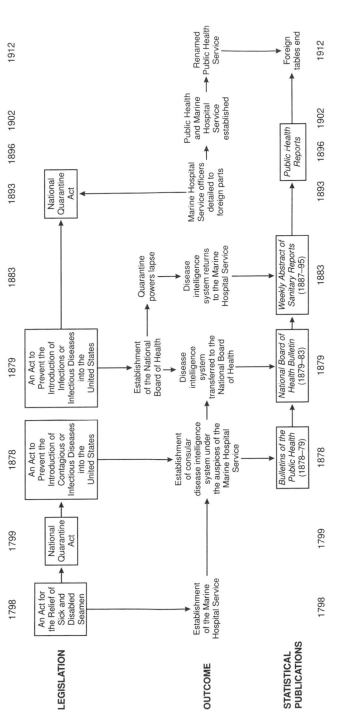

Figure 2.6. Critical dates in the development of disease surveillance in US public health records, 1798–1912.

Quarantine Law of 1799 by ordering USMHS personnel to familiarise themselves with local quarantine regulations (see figure 2.6). Probably more significant, however, was his contribution to the report on the *Cholera Epidemic of
1873 in the United States* commissioned by Congress in 1874.[7] His 25-page
preface, 'The Introduction of Epidemic Cholera Through the Agency of the
Mercantile Marine: Suggestions of Measures of Prevention', argued that
infectious diseases were permitted to break out in the United States because
insufficient information was to be had of disease activity in foreign locations.
In the context of the 1873 epidemic of cholera in the United States, he suggested that:

If the health-officer at the port of New York, for instance, had been aware of the facts
which were subsequently ascertained concerning . . . Sweden, Holland, and Russia,
there is no reason to doubt but that such measures would have been resorted to . . . as
would have effectually prevented the transportation of the cholera-poison.[8]

To address the problem, Woodworth urged the president of the United States
to instruct consular officials to inform the State Department of infectious diseases prevailing in their jurisdictions:

A circular letter from his Excellency the President, through the Department of State,
instructing consular officers to place themselves in communication with the health
authorities of their respective localities; to advise promptly, by cable[9] if necessary, of
the outbreak of cholera (or other epidemic disease) at the ports or in any section in
communication therewith; to inspect all vessels clearing for United States ports with
reference to the original and intermediate as well as the final port of departure of emi-
grants thereon; and to report, always by cable, the sailing and destination of any such
vessel carrying infected or suspected passengers or goods – this would be the first step.[10]

Woodworth proposed that the resulting information should be collated and
circulated to port health officers and other concerned parties. He concluded
that:

International sanitary action is too remote, and the steps toward it have been too vac-
illating in the past to admit of much hope from it in the near future. But the acquisi-
tion and diffusion of general sanitary knowledge is a matter in which each nation for
itself may engage . . . Let the General Government do its share in collection and publishing the information – a work which it alone can do.[11]

The 1878 Quarantine Act: Woodworth's call for an international disease surveillance system materialised on 29 April 1878 with the passage of the
National Quarantine Act. The title of the Act was explicit: 'An Act to Prevent
the Introduction of Contagious or Infectious Diseases into the United States'
(figure 2.6). Not only did the Act grant the USMHS powers of detention over
vessels originating from areas infected with epidemic disease, it also directed
consular officers in foreign ports to forward weekly reports of sanitary conditions prevailing in their jurisdictions to the USMHS. This information was to

be collated by the supervising surgeon general, and circulated in the form of a weekly abstract to USMHS officers and other interested parties. As described more fully in section 2.3.1, the first number was issued on 13 July 1878 under the title *Bulletins of the Public Health*.

The 1893 Quarantine Act: The National Quarantine Act of 1893 was to extend further the international powers of the USMHS. This Act authorised the detailing of USMHS medical officers to US consulates in order to assist in preventing the importation of contagious or infectious diseases into the United States. Because of outbreaks of cholera in Europe, a number of medical officers were immediately assigned to consulates there.

2.2.4 The US consular system and international disease surveillance

The idea of an international disease surveillance system which operated through consular officials was by no means new. Indeed, similar systems had been implemented in the city states of the Mediterranean as early as the fourteenth century (see, for example, Carmichael, 1993b; Cipolla, 1981, 1992). What was new, however, was the global scale of the operation mandated under the 1878 Quarantine Act.

Consulates were, first and foremost, commercial interests; consuls were appointed by the United States to promote and protect overseas trade, to direct shipping and navigation, and to assist US nationals. We briefly comment on the origins, growth, and geographical extent of the US consular system. We then examine the means by which the consular sanitary information, required under the 1878 Quarantine Law, was forwarded to the USMHS.

Origins and growth: The evolution of the US consular system has been outlined by a number of workers (see, for example, Johnson, 1898; Stuart, 1952; Barnes and Heath Morgan, 1961; Plischke, 1967; Kennedy, 1990), and we draw on their accounts here. The roots of the system are usually traced back to 1775 and the American War of Independence, when the Continental Congress dispatched agents to sound out public opinion in Europe regarding the relationship of the colonies with Great Britain.[12] The first fully fledged US consuls were appointed under Article XXXI of the 1778 Treaty of Amity and Commerce. This treaty permitted France and the United States to maintain consuls in each other's ports (Kennedy, 1990). Subsequent treaties paved the way for consulates in Morocco in 1787 and the Netherlands in 1792 (Plischke, 1967).

The subsequent growth of the consular system is graphed in figure 2.7. The lower line trace plots the number of consulates worldwide between 1790 and 1930, while the upper line trace plots the number of officers engaged in the consular service. The eighty years to 1870 were a period of major expansion

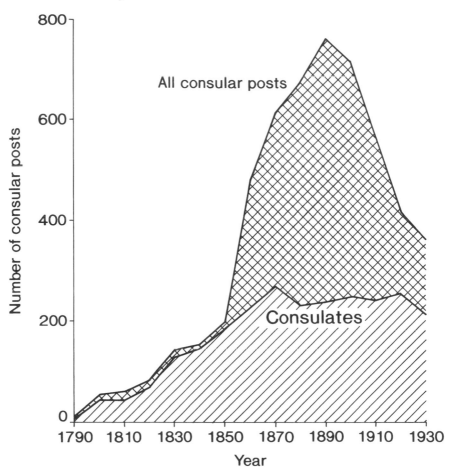

Figure 2.7. Growth of the US consular service, 1790–1930. The total number of consular posts (including commercial agencies) and consulates is shown. Source: data from Barnes and Heath Morgan (1961), appendix 4, tab. B, p. 350.

in the consular service; the number of consulates grew from just a handful in 1800 to over 200 in 1870. Meanwhile, the large increase in the number of consular officials from the middle of the nineteenth century largely reflected the financially lucrative practice of consular agents attached to consulates (Barnes and Heath Morgan, 1961).

Geographical extent: The numerical increase in the number of consulates during the nineteenth century was accompanied by geographical expansion, itself a reflection of the expanding commercial interests of the United States.

From its initial foci in Europe and the Caribbean Basin in 1800, by the late 1880s the consular system had assumed a global pattern. The pattern is described in detail in section 2.4.1, but it included much of the Caribbean Basin and Latin America, Northern, Central, and Southern Europe, the St Lawrence Seaway, and parts of Africa and Asia.[13]

Many consulates were located in the major urban centres of the most powerful trading nations, in cities such as London, Paris, and Rome. But other consulates were situated in small settlements, rarely heard of then as now. The rationale was that, even in these small ports with populations of only a few hundred, the goods on US ships had to be certified (Mattox, 1989). In other instances, consulates represented once major trading centres which had diminished in importance with swings in trade and the associated routes of shipping traffic (Mattox, 1989).

Sanitary dispatches: As described in section 2.2.3, the 1878 Quarantine Act required consuls to submit weekly reports of the sanitary conditions prevailing in their jurisdictions. The information was usually drawn from local disease surveillance reports although, as we describe in section 2.5, other sources were not unknown.

Most of the sanitary reports reached the USMHS, via the State Department, in the form of consular dispatches. Examples of consular dispatches are reproduced in plate 2.2.

Sanitary dispatches rarely exceeded more than a few lines when favourable health conditions prevailed. But severe epidemics and poor sanitary conditions usually warranted much more information. Under these circumstances, dispatches frequently stretched to several handwritten pages and provided detailed qualitative and quantitative information pertinent to the health of the consular city. Under other conditions, dispatches simply served to refute popular rumours, to report the medical research of local luminaries, or as a call for action on the part of the USMHS. Newspaper clippings, journal articles, commissional reports, and sundry other enclosures added further substance to the dispatches.

2.3 Nature of the *Weekly Abstract*

2.3.1 Background

The provision of sanitary reports fell within the jurisdiction of a well-developed commercial intelligence system as evidenced by consular reports in the form of *Reports on the Commercial Relations of the United States*[14] and *Reports from the Consuls*.[15] Notwithstanding this, sanitary reports from the consuls were, at first, apparently irregular and unreliable.[16] Two years after the initiation of the reporting system, in the summer of 1880, a Joint Resolution

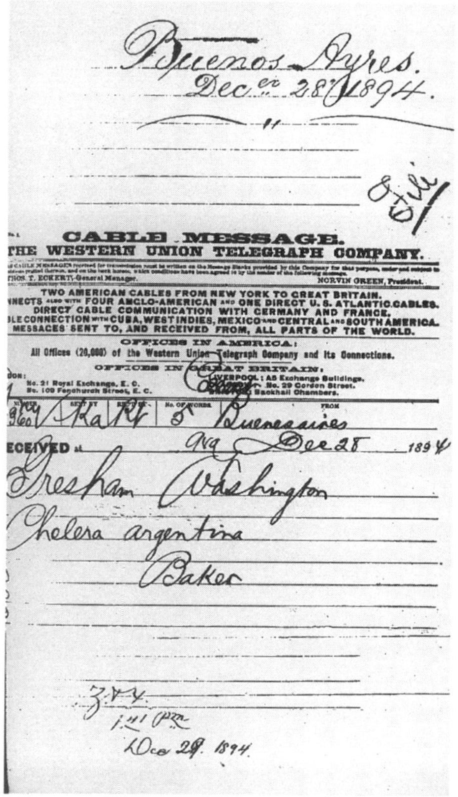

Buenos Ayres.
Dec. 28 1894.

CABLE MESSAGE.
THE WESTERN UNION TELEGRAPH COMPANY.

THOS. T. ECKERT, General Manager. NORVIN GREEN, President.

TWO AMERICAN CABLES FROM NEW YORK TO GREAT BRITAIN.
CONNECTS ALSO WITH FOUR ANGLO-AMERICAN AND ONE DIRECT U. S. ATLANTIC CABLES.
DIRECT CABLE COMMUNICATION WITH GERMANY AND FRANCE.
CABLE CONNECTION WITH CUBA, WEST INDIES, MEXICO AND CENTRAL AND SOUTH AMERICA.
MESSAGES SENT TO, AND RECEIVED FROM, ALL PARTS OF THE WORLD.

OFFICES IN AMERICA:
All Offices (20,000) of the Western Union Telegraph Company and its Connections.

OFFICES IN GREAT BRITAIN:
LONDON: No. 21 Royal Exchange, E. C. No. 109 Fenchurch Street, E. C.
LIVERPOOL: 45 Exchange Buildings.
GLASGOW: No. 29 Gordon Street.
BRADFORD: Backhall Chambers.

960 | Ka | Rf | 5 | Buenosaires

RECEIVED at 9 A Dec 28 1894

Gresham Washington
Cholera argentina
Baker

1.41 PM
Dec 29. 1894.

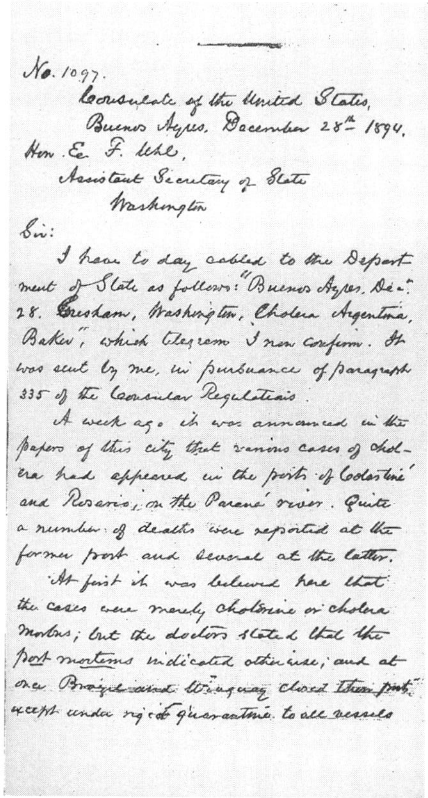

No. 1097.

Consulate of the United States,
Buenos Ayres, December 28th 1894.

Hon. E. F. Uhl,
Assistant Secretary of State
Washington

Sir:

I have to day cabled to the Department of State as follows: "Buenos Ayres, Dec. 28. Gresham, Washington, Cholera Argentina, Baker", which telegram I now confirm. It was sent by me, in pursuance of paragraph 335 of the Consular Regulations.

A week ago it was announced in the papers of this city that various cases of cholera had appeared in the ports of Colastine and Rosario, on the Paraná river. Quite a number of deaths were reported at the former port and several at the latter.

At first it was believed here that the cases were merely cholerine or cholera morbus; but the doctors stated that the post mortems indicated otherwise; and at once ~~Brazil and Uruguay closed their ports~~ except under rigid quarantine to all vessels

ARGENTINA.

Cholera in Argentina.

BUENOS AYRES, *December 28, 1894.*

SIR: I have to-day cabled to the Department of State as follows—"Buenos Ayres, December 28. Gresham, Washington. Cholera, Argentina. Baker"—which telegram I now confirm. It was sent by me, in pursuance of paragraph 335 of the Consular Regulations.

A week ago it was announced in the papers of this city that various cases of cholera had appeared at the ports of Colastine and Rosario, on the Parana River. Quite a number of deaths were reported at the former port and several at the latter.

At first it was believed here that the cases were merely cholerine or cholera morbus; but the doctors stated that the post mortems indicated otherwise; and at once Brazil and Uruguay closed their ports except under rigid quarantine to all vessels arriving from the Argentine Republic.

A few days after cases of what was also pronounced to be cholera appeared here in Buenos Ayres; and to-day the Argentine national authorities have so far recognized the existence of the disease as to issue a decree closing all the up river ports and requiring all vessels to enter here.

No deaths have yet occurred here from cholera, though a number of cases have been sent to the lazaretto or "Casa de Aistamiento;" but it is my opinion that no Asiatic cholera has appeared in this city, or, indeed, this country, and that the cases reported were the usual cholera morbus, which to some extent appears here every year during the hot weather, the result of improper diet or other excesses.

In view, however, of the decree of the Government I have deemed it my duty to cable, as I have done, to the Department.

I have the honor to be, sir, very respectfully, your obedient servant,

E. L. BAKER,
United States Consul.

Plate 2.2. Examples of consular sanitary dispatches. *Left*: a telegram dated 28 December 1894 from Eugene Baker, consul to Buenos Aires, Argentina, informing the State Department of the presence of cholera. *Centre*: a letter to confirm the telegram. *Right*: reproduction of the letter in the *Weekly Abstract*.

of the Senate and House of Representatives called for an international sanitary conference to discuss the 'untrustworthy evidence obtainable in some cases as to the sanitary conditions of suspected foreign ports' and the means by which 'a uniform and satisfactory system of Bills of Health, the statements in which shall be trustworthy as to the sanitary condition of the port' could be established.[17]

As mentioned in section 2.2.3, the 1878 Quarantine Act required publication of the consular sanitary reports as a weekly abstract and this was begun as *Bulletins of the Public Health* on 13 July of that year (plate 2.3, left). Issue no. 1 consisted of just twenty-three lines of text and detailed the sanitary conditions prevailing in Cuban ports, and the occurrence of yellow fever in Florida and cholera on British troop ships in the Mediterranean.[18] However, the *Bulletins* soon expanded to include reports of disease activity in major cities around the world; by December 1878, the *Bulletins* contained summaries of morbidity and mortality in places as far-flung as Brazil, China, Singapore, and Ireland.[19]

Publication of the *Bulletins* was suspended on 24 May 1879, after just forty-six issues, when powers under the 1878 Quarantine Act were temporarily transferred from the USMHS to the newly created National Board of Health (see figure 2.6).[20] The National Board of Health continued to publish the consular reports in the weekly *National Board of Health Bulletin*. The quarantine powers of the National Board of Health were to lapse in 1883 and charge of the 1878 Quarantine Law again returned to the USMHS (R. C. Williams, 1951). But it was to be a further four years before the surgeon general of the USMHS, John B. Hamilton (plate 2.4), was to regain the initiative; publication of the consular sanitary reports recommenced in January 1887 as the *Weekly Abstract of Sanitary Reports* (plate 2.3, centre). With new legislation under the 1893 National Quarantine Act,[21] the *Weekly Abstracts* were further extended and volume XI, published in January 1896, appeared under the new title *Public Health Reports* (plate 2.3, right). For convenience, throughout this book we refer to this series of publications as the *Weekly Abstract*; full details of the individual volumes, 1878–1912, are given in section 1 of appendix A to this book.

2.3.2 *Domestic disease surveillance*

Although the *Weekly Abstract* was a vehicle for the dissemination of international sanitary information, it also assumed the role of the domestic disease surveillance report of the United States. The early editions restricted domestic information to brief statements, largely for port cities and quarantine stations. But, in June 1888, the *Weekly Abstract* began to tabulate disease reports for major US cities. This initiative continues today in the form of the US Centers for Disease Control and Prevention's *Morbidity and Mortality Weekly Report*.

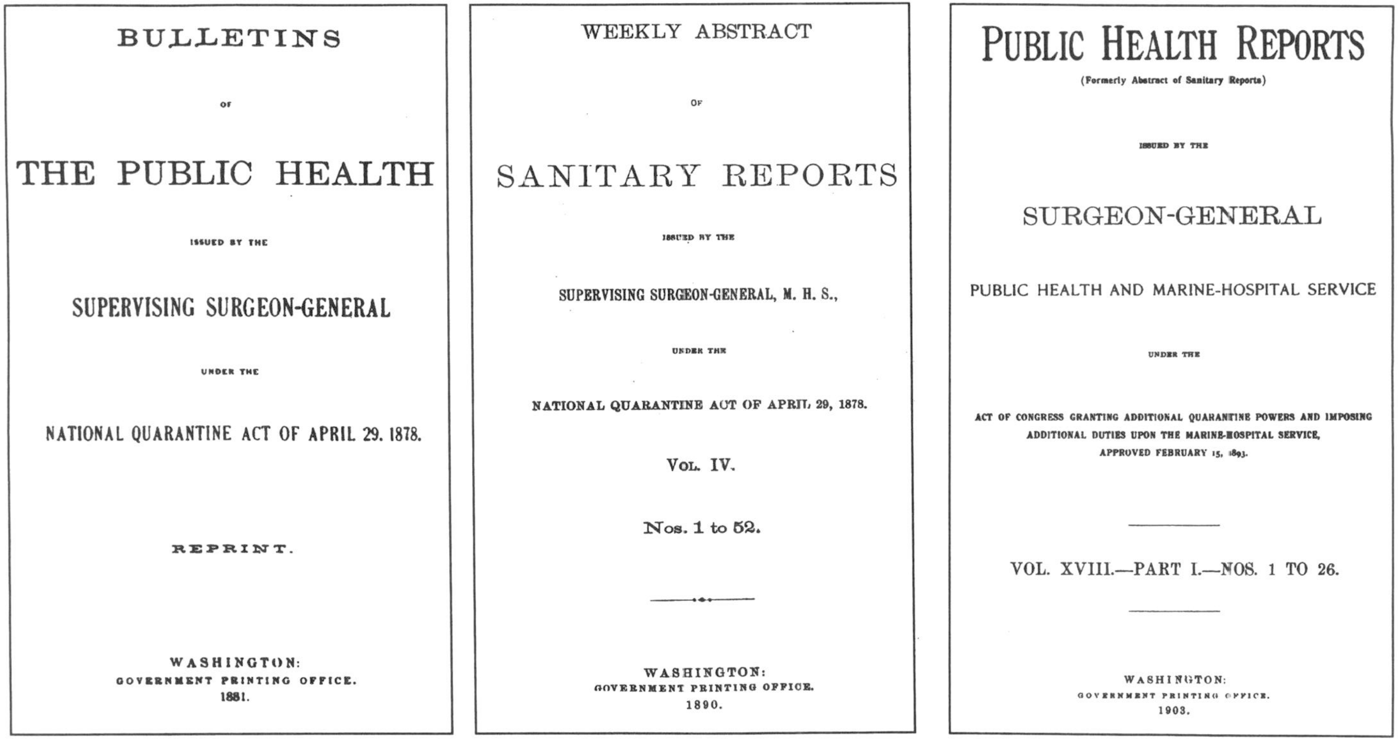
BULLETINS

OF

THE PUBLIC HEALTH

ISSUED BY THE

SUPERVISING SURGEON-GENERAL

UNDER THE

NATIONAL QUARANTINE ACT OF APRIL 29. 1878.

REPRINT.

WASHINGTON:
GOVERNMENT PRINTING OFFICE.
1881.

WEEKLY ABSTRACT

OF

SANITARY REPORTS

ISSUED BY THE

SUPERVISING SURGEON-GENERAL, M. H. S.,

UNDER THE

NATIONAL QUARANTINE ACT OF APRIL 29, 1878.

VOL. IV.

Nos. 1 to 52.

WASHINGTON:
GOVERNMENT PRINTING OFFICE.
1890.

PUBLIC HEALTH REPORTS

(Formerly Abstract of Sanitary Reports)

ISSUED BY THE

SURGEON-GENERAL

PUBLIC HEALTH AND MARINE-HOSPITAL SERVICE

UNDER THE

ACT OF CONGRESS GRANTING ADDITIONAL QUARANTINE POWERS AND IMPOSING ADDITIONAL DUTIES UPON THE MARINE-HOSPITAL SERVICE, APPROVED FEBRUARY 15, 1893.

VOL. XVIII.—PART I.—NOS. 1 TO 26.

WASHINGTON:
GOVERNMENT PRINTING OFFICE.
1903.

Plate 2.3. Front covers of the *Weekly Abstract* under its various aliases. *Left*: volume I appeared in 1878 as the *Bulletins of the Public Health*. *Centre*: after a gap of nine years, volume II emerged in 1887 as the *Weekly Abstract of Sanitary Reports*. *Right*: the *Weekly Abstract* was renamed *Public Health Reports* in 1896.

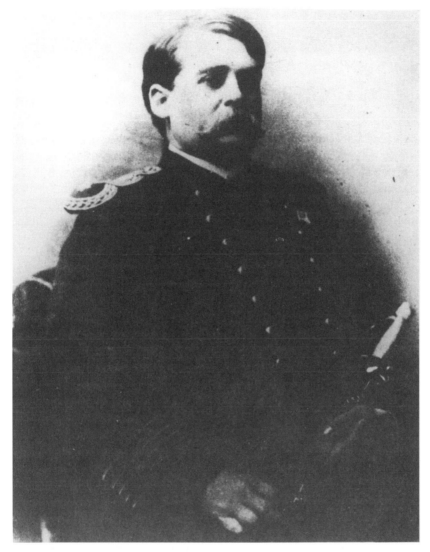

Plate 2.4. Dr John B. Hamilton (1847–1898). Surgeon general, US Marine Hospital Service, 1879–91. Source: Furman (1973), p. 15.

2.3.3 Circulation, size, and structure of the Weekly Abstract

The first issue of the *Weekly Abstract* was less than a page long and circulated to 1,000 'subscribers' (Hunter, 1978). By 1899, some 2,400 copies were distributed each week to public health officers, consuls, and sanitarians, the average length having increased to well over forty pages. The circulation and size of the publication remained close to these levels throughout the first decade of the twentieth century.[22]

Figure 2.8 outlines the structure and content of a typical edition of the *Weekly Abstract* from the turn of the century. Each weekly edition was divided into two main sections: United States (upper path in figure 2.8); and Foreign and Insular Cities (lower path). We comment on each in turn.

United States (upper path in figure 2.8). Here, written and tabular statements of quarantine activities, immigration, disease occurrence, and meteorological conditions in the United States were reproduced. The contributions included reports from surgeons of the USMHS, immigration and quarantine officers, and local and state health officials. In addition, four standard tables appeared on a weekly basis:

(i)   immigration tables, stating the name of immigrant vessels arriving in the week, the number of immigrants aboard, the date and port of arrival, and the port of departure;

(ii)   meteorological tables, summarising the weather conditions prevailing at various US stations during the week;

(iii) quarantine tables which listed, for national, state, and municipal quarantine stations, all quarantine activities during the previous week;

(iv)   mortality from all causes, and major infectious diseases, in US cities during the week.

Foreign and Insular (lower path in figure 2.8). Here, epidemiological information received from consuls, chargés d'affaires, officers of the USMHS, and various other officials located in cities around the world was reproduced. The section was divided into three main parts:

(i)   tables of morbidity from major quarantinable diseases (cholera, plague, smallpox, and yellow fever) worldwide;

(ii)   reports of consular officials and, later, sanitary inspectors regarding the health conditions prevailing in major cities around the world;

(iii) mortality tables, listing deaths from all causes, and major infectious diseases, in foreign cities during each week. These tables formed the overseas equivalent to the domestic mortality tables listed for the United States under (iv), above.

The substantive analyses in chapters 4–6 of this book are based on the statistical information contained in the weekly mortality tables for United States and foreign cities; these tables are charted on the far right of figure 2.8. It is to the nature of these weekly mortality tables that we now turn.

2.4 The weekly mortality tables

Weekly tabular information on deaths from all causes and from major infectious diseases for some overseas cities first appeared in the *Weekly Abstract* in

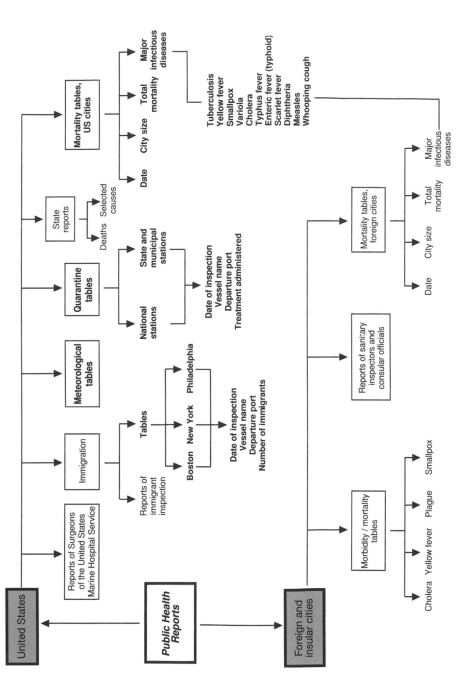

Figure 2.8. Typical structure of an issue of the *Weekly Abstract*, circa 1900.

volume II, number 55, 1887. The earliest of these tables is reproduced in plate 2.5. The table consisted of a matrix with twenty-two cities by seven diseases, together with the population of each city and the total number of deaths from all causes. From July 1888, the mortality tables for foreign cities were supplemented by a parallel table of mortality in selected US cities.

These mortality tables were published every week for a quarter of a century until Rupert Blue's appointment as surgeon general in 1912 (plate 2.6). He reviewed the publications of the US Public Health Service and decided to continue the reporting only for the United States and its territories. The last foreign tables to be published appeared in the issue of 12 December 1912, although separate entries for cholera, yellow fever, plague, and smallpox (the 'plague' diseases) continued.[23]

2.4.1 Extent of the mortality tables

The weekly tables of mortality published the numbers of reported deaths from selected diseases in a given week. The surgeon general's office printed what had come to hand that week, rather than by, for example, week of occurrence on a regular basis. Reports might refer to records from some previous week, depending upon the lag in reporting; reporting delays of up to six weeks were not uncommon. Sometimes, late reports from a distant city, or a tardy respondent, were simply aggregated for periods longer than a week. Under these circumstances, the information was published outside the main tables. Even the term, 'week', is not without ambiguity: most respondents related their figures to a week ending on a Friday or a Saturday, but other closing days are not unknown.

Number of cities reporting: Usually two to three pages of each report were devoted to the table of deaths from infectious diseases in overseas cities. The table of deaths in US cities was of a similar length. As figure 2.9 indicates, however, the number of cities for which reports of mortality were available varied over time. For foreign cities, the number reporting began at less than thirty but, by 1894, had risen to over 100. It remained at that level until 1908 when the coverage began to contract until the series was discontinued in 1912. For United States cities, the pattern is more complex with an isolated reporting peak in 1894, followed by a trough, and then a steady rise up to 1912.

Location of foreign reporting cities: Not all cities were reported continuously, particularly those in foreign locations. So, although the number of cities included in the foreign mortality tables rarely exceeded 140 in a given week, these were drawn from an overall sample of more than 200 cities that, at some time or another, found their way into the table.

As described in section 2.2.4, the geographical distribution of overseas

MORTALITY TABLE, FOREIGN CITIES.

Cities.	Week ended.	Estimated population.	Total deaths from all causes.	Deaths from—						
				Cholera.	Yellow fever.	Small-pox.	Typhus fever.	Enteric fever.	Scarlet fever.	Diphtheria.
Calcutta	January 22	433,219	237	18	22	5		15		
Guayaquil	February 10	35,000	70		24	15		19		
Guayaquil	February 17	35,000	92							
Paris	February 26	2,260,045	1,211			4		42	6	55
Rheims	February 26	98,083	56			1		2		2
Genoa	February 26	179,403	130			3		2		
Leghorn	February 27	101,172	82							
Rome	January 15	364,511	163			2		3	1	6
Bristol	February 26	223,695	100						5	
Warsaw	February 19	431,572	220			6				
Glasgow	February 25	545,678	250				1		3	2
Edinburgh	February 26	258,629	104						11	
Leith	February 26	72,297	27							
Palermo	February 26	250,000	115					2		1
Leipsic	February 26	170,000	71							5
Toronto	March 5	120,000	40					2	1	7
Rotterdam	February 19	190,521	93							
Kingston, Canada	March 11	15,109	15							
Havre	February 26	112,074	65							
Rotterdam	February 12	190,521	88							
Cadiz	February 26	65,028	54							
Gibraltar	February 20	23,631	11							
Matamoras	March 5	12,000	5							

Plate 2.5. The first weekly table of mortality in foreign cities to appear in the *Weekly Abstract* (vol. II, no. 55, dated 17 March 1887). The table was published on a weekly basis until December 1912.

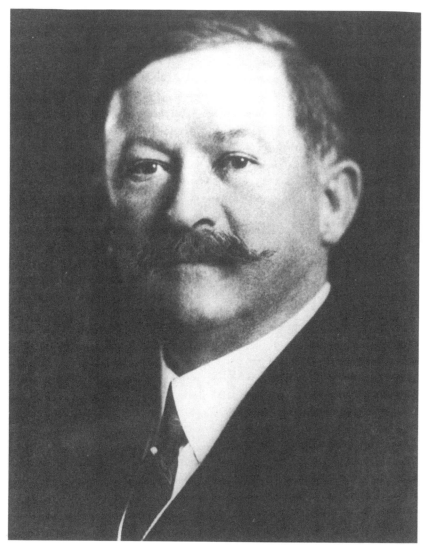

Plate 2.6. Rupert Blue (1867–1948). Surgeon general, US Marine Hospital Service, and surgeon general, US Public Health Service, 1912–20. Source: Furman (1973), p. 282.

reporting cities was determined by the international trading interests of the United States. On 1 December 1888, towards the beginning of the publication of the foreign disease tables, the United States operated 277 consulates worldwide. An additional thirty-nine commercial agencies were also registered.[24] The locations of these 316 institutions are indicated by the circles in figure

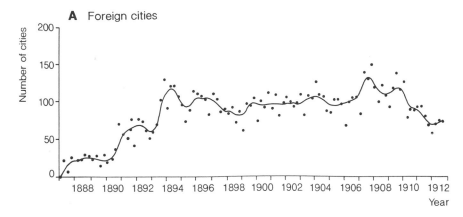

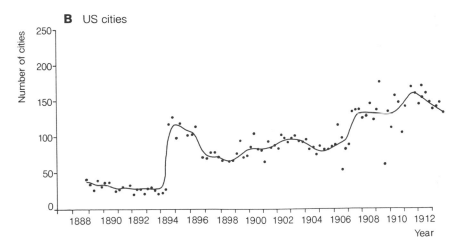

Figure 2.9. Number of cities for which mortality reports were published in the *Weekly Abstract*, 1887–1912. Points are based on a sample count of the first week in each quarter with moving means shown by the continuous line. (A) Foreign cities. (B) United States cities.

2.10. Major concentrations of consular offices occur in Central America and the Caribbean Basin, along the St Lawrence waterway and the Canadian Great Lakes, Northern and Central Europe, and in the Mediterranean Basin. Small clusters are also to be seen in the southern cone of South America and along the coast of China. Elsewhere, in Africa and Asia, consulates and commercial agencies were restricted to the ports of a few major cities.

The 316 cities plotted in figure 2.10 depict the maximum extent of the disease surveillance system if all institutions had submitted reports in 1888. In fact, only fifty or so institutions submitted reports in that year; reporting cities

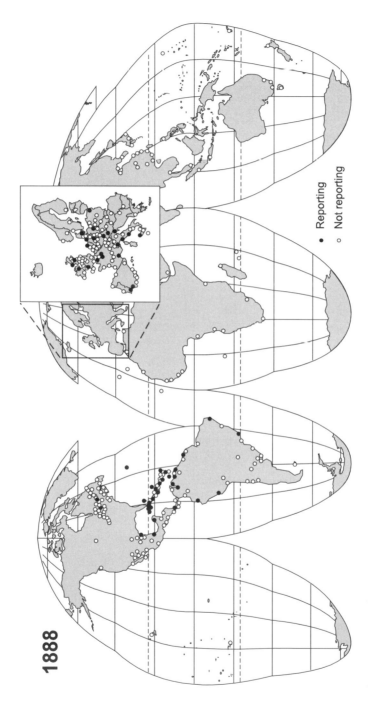

1888

Figure 2.10. Location of US consulates and commercial agencies in operation in 1888. Offices submitting mortality reports in this year are indicated by black circles. Source: US Department of State (1889).

Reporting
Not reporting

are identified by the black circles. At this time, the disease reporting network was biased to parts of the Caribbean Basin, the northern shores of the Mediterranean, and Northern Europe. Five years later, in 1893, the global distribution of consulates and commercial agencies had changed only little.[25] But the number of consular offices that submitted sanitary reports had expanded dramatically to include two-thirds of consular institutions; cities from which sanitary reports were received in 1893 are plotted in figure 2.11.

Disease coverage: In addition to deaths from all causes, deaths from eleven different diseases were recorded in the mortality tables at some time or another during the 26-year period, 1887–1912: cholera, diphtheria, enteric fever (typhoid and paratyphoid), measles, plague, scarlet fever, smallpox, tuberculosis, typhus fever, whooping cough, and yellow fever. But, as we describe more fully in chapter 3, records for five of these diseases (cholera, plague, smallpox, typhus, and yellow fever) are so incomplete that we doubt if their analysis would prove worthwhile. Figure 2.12 shows the trends in city reporting for six diseases for which records are much more continuous. All show some evidence of cyclicity. But the most striking trend for both foreign and United States cities is the rapid increase in the number reporting tuberculosis since it was first recorded in the lists in 1899.

2.5 Data quality, I: evidence from the consuls

In this section and the following one, we attempt to provide an insight into the quality and reliability of the statistical data included in the mortality tables of the *Weekly Abstract*. This analysis serves as a precursor to the systematic consideration of data quality in section 3.3. Here, we begin our assessment with a review of the statements and views of the consuls and others actively engaged in the procurement and submission of diseases statistics from overseas locations. Then, in section 2.6, we cross-check the data from the weekly mortality tables with the domestic surveillance reports of sample countries and cities.

2.5.1 Qualitative statements

The *Weekly Abstract* makes numerous references to factors that impinged on the quality of the sanitary information from overseas cities. We review these factors under five headings: disease surveillance and vital registration; unofficial data sources; communications difficulties; political expediency; and consular practice.

Disease surveillance and vital registration: For some locations, the quality of reported mortality statistics was undoubtedly good. In the summer of 1892, for example, the consul to Kingston, Jamaica, could boast that

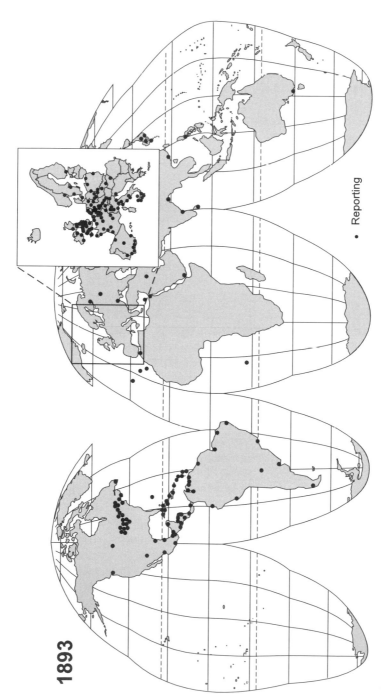

Figure 2.11. Location of US consulates and commercial agencies submitting mortality reports in 1893. The worldwide distribution of consulates and commercial agencies had changed little from the pattern of 1888 (see figure 2.10). Source: US Department of State (1893).

• Reporting

1893

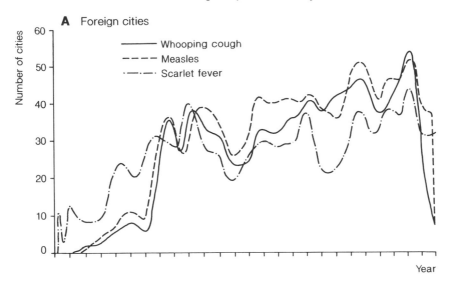

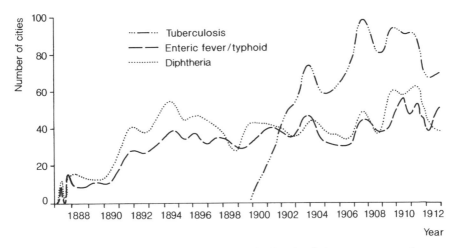

Figure 2.12. Number of cities recording mortality for six of the most commonly reported infectious diseases. (A) Foreign cities. (B, overleaf) United States cities. Note that counts are formed from non-zero reports published in the first week of each quarter, 1887–1912.

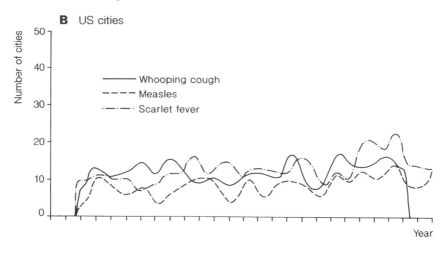

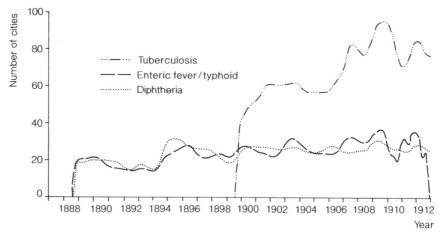

Figure 2.12. (*cont.*)

[T]he small area, density of population, vigorously enforced compulsory laws providing for the prompt registration of all births and deaths, and the fact that each neighbourhood is provided with a local office for registration, render these [sanitary] reports
accurate.[26]

Such favourable conditions, however, tended to be the exception rather than
the rule. The problems were particularly acute in those consular jurisdictions
of sub-Saharan Africa and Asia where local authorities paid scant regard to
the collection of mortality statistics.[27] Even in those places with reasonably
well-established disease surveillance systems, consular officials encountered
numerous difficulties in meeting the remit of the Quarantine Laws.[28] The

sudden onset of an epidemic was often accompanied by an exodus of the local populace and, with them, the physicians from whom mortality statistics could be obtained.[29] Many cities simply did not have the resources for all fatalities to be attended by a diagnosing physician,[30] and the local surveillance systems could be severely limited in geographical extent and population coverage,[31] while conflicting diagnoses merely complicated the situation.[32]

Unofficial data sources: Under these circumstances, some consuls turned to unofficial sources for their sanitary reports; private contracts with physicians, the accounts of coffin manufacturers, body counts in public wash houses, and financial rewards for the diagnosis of a disease were variously cited in official communications.[33] In 1899, the US consul to Beirut reported the inadequacies of his own novel approach:

I made a contract with the grave diggers of each cemetery . . . to furnish me, for a certain pecuniary consideration, the number of burials and the cause of death in each case during a given week . . . [B]ut I regret to say that in many cases my representatives failed to obtain the desired information . . . The method is expensive and not altogether satisfactory in its results.[34]

Communications difficulties: Poor lines of communication could prove formidable obstacles to the timely submission of the sanitary reports. In April 1893, for example, W. Stanley Hollis, consul to Mozambique, informed the State Department that it would be impossible to submit sanitary reports on a weekly basis since mail steamers visited the port only once a month.[35] Such obstacles to communication were not restricted to remote African jurisdictions; Thomas E. Heenan presented the State Department with a graphic account of communications difficulties experienced in some Russian locations:

The mails . . . are very irregular and are usually several days late, if, indeed, they arrive at all. The rivers and streams are swollen to such an extent as to render crossing extremely dangerous. It is only a few weeks ago that I received a mass of pulp, all that was left of a very large mail . . . the mail wagon or cart having been overturned in the Syr Daria River.[36]

Political expediency: Sanitary reports frequently alluded to the role of political expediency in the withholding of information during the course of an epidemic.[37] Certainly, it was not always in the best economic interests of a city for the authorities to give details of the occurrence of a disease, and information was to be had at a price. In the summer of 1892, for example, the consul to Odessa reported in guarded tones that

a death . . . occurred from Asiatic cholera at Raakha . . . on the line of the Transcaspian Railway . . . I requested permission to cable the information [to the State Department], but the governor-general [of Tashkent] was not willing that I should do so . . . As this is a military government, the governor-general's wishes are equivalent to a command.[38]

In a subsequent dispatch he reported that

There is a sort of feeling that the authorities are holding back something, and that cholera is more prevalent than the official reports show . . . I am not in a position to express an opinion.[39]

It was not unknown for local authorities to turn to internment to avoid dissemination of information regarding the progress of an epidemic.[40] The consul to St Petersburg acknowledged that foreign sources often knew more about occurrences in Russia than the Russians themselves,[41] whilst outbreaks of quarantinable diseases were often greeted with strenuous official denials.[42]

Consular practice: Political reprisals and internment were not the only risks faced by consuls in meeting the remit of the quarantine laws. All too often, the surveillance record was interrupted by the death of consuls from the epidemic diseases they were supposed to be monitoring (plate 2.7).[43]

Question marks also surrounded the reliability and commitment of some consular officials in meeting their remit. For some, submission of a weekly sanitary report simply proved too much effort,[44] while evidence for poor consular practice in disease reporting can be found in the pages of the *Weekly Abstract*. In 1892, for example, the consul-general to Berlin described the consul to Stettin as 'not animated with the deepest devotion to the public interests of the United States' in his failure to execute the Quarantine Laws.[45] The ineptness of other consular officials is manifested in the highly conflicting reports occasionally received from the same location.[46] But such observations appear to have been the exception rather than the rule, and evidence for a conscientious approach to consular duties abounds.[47]

2.5.2   Quantitative assessments

Only rarely did consular officials attempt to provide quantitative assessments of the completeness of disease reporting. Consul Comfort, consul to the Indian city of Bombay during a severe outbreak of human plague in 1897, for example, used vital registration records to estimate the reporting completeness of plague mortality at somewhat less than 25 per cent.[48] In a similar vein, Acting Assistant Surgeon Wilson analysed independent sets of mortality records to estimate the completeness of disease surveillance in the Cuban city of Santiago in 1904; he estimated a 6 per cent overreporting of deaths from all causes, and attributed the figure to disinterments and reburials consequent to the war.[49]

2.6   Data quality, II: cross-checks

The statements from the consuls provide only brief glimpses into the integrity of the sanitary information included in the mortality tables of the *Weekly*

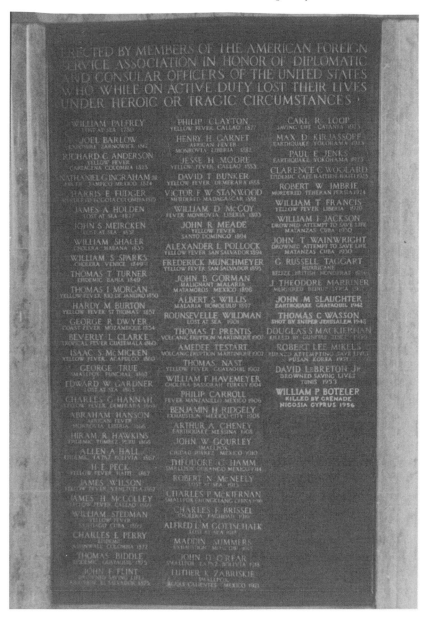

Plate 2.7. Memorial (US Department of State, Washington, DC), to honour US Foreign Service officers who lost their lives under heroic or tragic circumstances. Causes of death are clearly visible on the plaque; no fewer than forty officers lost their lives to disease. Source: Barnes and Heath Morgan (1961), opposite p. 227.

Table 2.1. *Twenty-eight sample cities common to the* Weekly Abstract *and the* Registrar General's Weekly Return

For each city, weekly data relating to deaths from all causes and four infectious diseases (diphtheria, measles, scarlet fever, and whooping cough), 1887–1912, have been abstracted from both surveillance reports.

Asia	Continental Europe	United Kingdom
Bombay	Amsterdam	Birmingham
Calcutta	Berlin	Cardiff
Madras	Brussels	Edinburgh
	Budapest	Glasgow
	Christiania	Leeds
	Copenhagen	Liverpool
	Hamburg	Manchester
	Moscow	Newcastle upon Tyne
	Paris	Sheffield
	Prague	Sunderland
	St Petersburg	
	Stockholm	
	Trieste	
	Venice	
	Vienna	

Abstract, and then only for overseas (non-US) cities. A critical question remains as to the reliability of the mortality statistics published in the *Weekly Abstract* relative to the domestic surveillance statistics of the cities involved. That is, through processes of misreporting and underreporting, did the consular surveillance system serve to distort the basic mortality data collected by individual cities? To address this question, in this section we cross-check data from the mortality tables of the *Weekly Abstract* with other contemporary disease surveillance reports.

2.6.1 Cross-checks with national sources: England and Wales

For the period of unbroken disease reporting in the *Weekly Abstract*, 1887–1912, the contemporary *Registrar General's Weekly Return for England and Wales* published weekly mortality statistics for cities of England and Wales.[50] As described in section 2 of appendix A to this book, these domestic records were further supplemented by weekly mortality tables for a selection of twenty to thirty 'Colonial and Foreign' cities. Table 2.1 lists twenty-eight sample cities which were covered by both the *Weekly Abstract* and the *Registrar General's Weekly Return*. Geographically, the sample includes ten UK cities, three Asian cities, and fifteen cities of continental Europe. These twenty-eight cities form a subset of the 120 cities initially selected for detailed statistical analysis in chapters 4–6; see section 3.3 for full details.

Although the mortality tables of the *Weekly Abstract* record deaths for up to twelve categories (all causes and eleven infectious diseases), only five categories (all causes, diphtheria, measles, scarlet fever, and whooping cough) are common to both the *Weekly Abstract* and the *Registrar General's Weekly Return*. For each of these five categories, the weekly series of mortality in the twenty-eight sample cities were abstracted from both surveillance reports for the period 1887–1912. The resulting 140 pairs of city- and mortality-specific time series (5 diseases×28 cities) permit an assessment of the statistical concordance of the data contained in the two surveillance reports.

Patterns in space: Table 2.2, which groups the twenty-eight sample cities by major geographical division (see table 2.1), compares the number of deaths recorded in the two reports for the entire period, 1887–1912. The upper part of the table shows the total number of deaths recorded from all causes in the *Weekly Abstract* (column 1) and the *Registrar General's Weekly Return* (column 2). The percentage completeness of the *Weekly Abstract* relative to the *Registrar General's Weekly Return* [=(column 1 / column 2)×100)] is given in column 3. The equivalent information for total deaths due to the four infectious diseases appears in the lower part of the table.

Table 2.2 shows that the number of deaths recorded in the *Weekly Abstract* falls short of the *Registrar General's Weekly Return* in all geographical areas and mortality categories. For deaths from all causes, the relative completeness of the *Weekly Abstract* ranges between 73 per cent (continental Europe) and 89 per cent (Asia) with an aggregate of 77 per cent. The aggregate for infectious diseases is marginally lower at 73 per cent, but again with marked geographical variations.

It should be noted that the statistics in columns 1–3 of table 2.2 make no distinction between underreporting attributable to (i) missing weekly data units and (ii) discrepancies in levels of mortality reported by correspondents. The question of missing data units is considered in detail in sections 3.2.1 and 3.3 but, to examine the issue briefly here, column 4 of table 2.2 lists the number of deaths recorded in the *Weekly Abstract* and which occurred in thirteen-week (that is, quarterly) periods for which no weekly data units were missing. Column 5 lists deaths published in the *Registrar General's Weekly Return* for the equivalent periods.[51] Comparison of columns 4 and 5 reveals that the estimated percentage completeness of the *Weekly Abstract* (column 6) ranges close to 100 per cent. It is concluded that data differences in the *Weekly*

Table 2.2. *Completeness of mortality statistics in the* Weekly Abstract *relative to the* Registrar General's Weekly Return, *1887–1912*

	Deaths (n=1,357 weeks)[a]			Deaths (complete quarters only)[b]		
	Weekly Abstract[c]	*Weekly Return*[d]	Completeness (percentage)[e]	*Weekly Abstract*[c]	*Weekly Return*[d]	Completeness (percentage)[e]
All causes						
Asia	1.70	1.91	89	0.99	0.88	113
United Kingdom	1.64	2.09	78	1.10	1.12	98
Continental Europe[f]	4.57	6.29	73	2.12	2.12	100
Total	7.92	10.29	77	4.21	4.12	102
Four infectious diseases[g]						
Asia	0.01	0.02	50	0.00	0.00	100
United Kingdom	0.11	0.16	69	0.05	0.05	100
Continental Europe[f]	0.25	0.34	74	0.09	0.09	100
Total	0.38	0.52	73	0.14	0.14	100

Notes:
[a] Deaths in millions documented in 1,357 calendar weeks, 1887–1912.
[b] Deaths in millions documented in quarterly periods for which complete weekly records are available, 1887–1912.
[c] *Weekly Abstract of Sanitary Reports.*
[d] *Registrar General's Weekly Return.*
[e] Deaths documented in the *Weekly Abstract* as a percentage of deaths documented in the *Registrar General's Weekly Return.*
[f] Excluding the United Kingdom.
[g] Diphtheria, measles, scarlet fever, and whooping cough.

Abstract and the *Registrar General's Weekly Return* arise from missing data units rather than variations in levels of reported mortality.

Patterns in time: Figure 2.13 charts, on a quarterly basis, the completeness of the *Weekly Abstract* relative to the *Registrar General's Weekly Return* for deaths from all causes (graph 2.13A) and four infectious diseases (graph 2.13B). For each graph, the bar chart measures the absolute difference in the number of deaths recorded in the two sources [(*Weekly Abstract*)–(*Weekly Return*)], and is to be read against the left-hand vertical axis. This axis is intersected by the horizontal axis at $y=0$; points below the horizontal mark periods when the *Weekly Abstract* was in deficit, while points above the horizontal mark periods of excess. The line trace plots the percentage completeness of the *Weekly Abstract* relative to the *Weekly Return* and is to be read against the right-hand vertical axis. This axis is intersected by the horizontal at $y=100$; points below the horizontal mark periods of underreporting in the *Weekly Abstract*, while points above the horizontal mark periods of overreporting.

Figure 2.13 shows that the statistical completeness of the *Weekly Abstract* improved during the nineteenth century as sample cities were increasingly drawn into the US surveillance system. The completeness of deaths from all causes (graph 2.13A) grew steadily at an average rate of 8 per cent per annum, from a low of 2 per cent in 1887 to over 90 per cent in 1899. Thereafter it fluctuated about a roughly constant mean before plummeting in the final year of the series. Deaths from infectious diseases (graph 2.13B) followed a broadly similar pattern, but with a steep rise in completeness in the 1890s.

Statistical comparisons of serial behaviour: From an analytical viewpoint, it may be argued that the absolute completeness of a disease dataset is less important than its ability to accurately describe the serial form of epidemic events. In this context, it is useful to cross-check the serial patterns of mortality documented in the *Weekly Abstract* with those recorded in the *Weekly Return*.

Correlation analysis provides a simple check on the coherence, or statistical similarity, of two data series (see Cliff, Haggett, Stroup, and Cheney, 1992). In the present instance, Pearson's product-moment correlation coefficient, r, was computed for corresponding pairs of mortality series from the *Weekly Abstract* and the *Registrar General's Weekly Return* for each of the twenty-eight sample cities. The average correlation coefficients for the twenty-eight cities, by geographical division and disease, are given in table 2.3; statistically significant and positive coefficients ($p=0.05$ level, two-tailed test) are marked with an asterisk. The table indicates that, on average, statistical similarities exist between the series for the United Kingdom and continental Europe. In contrast, three of the five mortality categories for Asian cities are non-coherent or dissimilar in serial form.

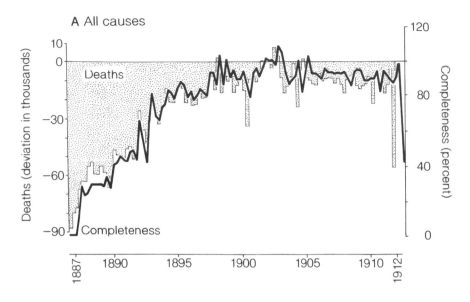

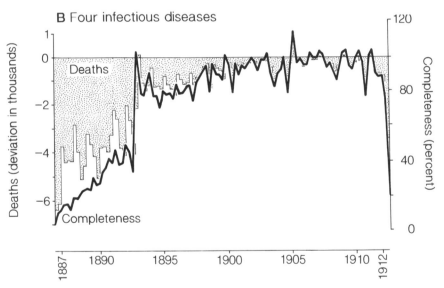

Figure 2.13. Estimated completeness of mortality reporting for twenty-eight cities recorded in the *Weekly Abstract*, by quarter, 1887–1912. (A) Deaths from all causes. (B) Aggregate deaths from four diseases (diphtheria, measles, scarlet fever, and whooping cough). *Returns of the Registrar General of London* represent the standard against which estimates are formed. Bar graphs show absolute levels of reporting completeness; negative values identify periods of deficit in the *Weekly Abstract*. Line traces show the estimated percentage completeness of the *Weekly Abstract*.

Table 2.3. *Coherence of mortality series from the* Weekly Abstract *and the* Registrar General's Weekly Return

For each of three geographical regions, the table shows the average correlation coefficients between corresponding pairs of mortality series in twenty-eight cities, 1887–1912.

Region	All causes	Diphtheria	Measles	Scarlet fever	Whooping cough
Asia	0.757*	−0.064	0.647*	−0.006	−0.034
Continental Europe[a]	0.360*	0.623*	0.650*	0.704*	0.490*
United Kingdom	0.415*	0.769*	0.651*	0.460*	0.655*

Notes:
* Significant at $p=0.05$ level (two-tailed test).
[a] Excluding United Kingdom.

2.6.2 Cross-checks with local sources: Baltimore

In this section, the mortality tables of the *Weekly Abstract* are cross-checked with local records of the US city of Baltimore. Local mortality statistics for this city are provided in the appendices to Howard's (1924) classic book *Public Health Administration and the Natural History of Disease in Baltimore, Maryland, 1797–1920*, and we use those data here. We restrict our analysis to deaths from all causes and six infectious diseases (diphtheria, enteric fever, measles, scarlet fever, tuberculosis, and whooping cough).

For the period 1887–1912, table 2.4 shows the number of deaths by mortality category according to the local disease records of Baltimore (column 1) and the *Weekly Abstract* (column 2). The percentage completeness of the *Weekly Abstract* relative to the local records [(column 2/column 1)×100] appears in column 3.

Table 2.4 shows that a total of 224,869 deaths were registered for Baltimore in the *Weekly Abstract*. This represents a shortfall of 38,559 on the 263,428 deaths recorded by the Baltimore Department of Health, yielding a relative reporting completeness for the *Weekly Abstract* of 85 per cent. Notably, the *Weekly Abstract* includes only half the deaths from tuberculosis recorded in the local health department statistics, reflecting the late introduction of tuberculosis as a separate disease in the *Weekly Abstract* in 1899. For other diseases, reporting completeness varies between 73 per cent (diphtheria) and 91 per cent (scarlet fever).

The serial completeness of the *Weekly Abstract* relative to the local statistics is examined on an annual basis in figure 2.14. For deaths from all causes, graph 2.14A plots the total mortality registered in the *Weekly Abstract* (bar chart) and the local health department records (line trace). The percentage

Table 2.4. *Deaths in Baltimore from selected causes, 1887–1912*

Completeness of statistics in the *Weekly Abstract* relative to local disease statistics.

	Number of deaths		Completeness (percentage)[b]
	Baltimore[a]	*Weekly Abstract*	
Diphtheria	5,496	4,007	72.9
Enteric fever	4,800	4,103	85.5
Measles	1,343	1,022	76.1
Scarlet fever	1,514	1,371	90.6
Tuberculosis	34,611	17,591	50.8
Whooping cough	1,787	1,426	79.8
All causes	263,428	224,869	85.4

Notes:
[a] Local disease reports from Howard (1924).
[b] Percentage completeness of the *Weekly Abstract* relative to local health department reports.

difference between the two series is plotted in 2.14B. Here, values below the horizontal axis mark years when the *Weekly Abstract* was in deficit, while values above the horizontal mark years of excess. Graphs 2.14A and B display wide annual fluctuations in the relative completeness of the *Weekly Abstract* during the nineteenth century, although the two series approach parity after 1900.

Graphs 2.14C and D repeat the analysis of 2.14A and B for the six infectious diseases (diphtheria, enteric fever, measles, scarlet fever, tuberculosis, and whooping cough). Because tuberculosis was not included as a separate cause of death in the *Weekly Abstract* until 1899, the broken line in 2.14C shows health department records with tuberculosis excluded; deaths including tuberculosis are indicated by the solid line. Similarly, graph 2.14D shows the percentage difference between the *Weekly Abstract* and local health department records with tuberculosis excluded (bar chart to 1899) and included (line trace).

If tuberculosis is excluded for the period to 1899, graphs 2.14C and D indicate that the relative completeness of the *Weekly Abstract* mimics the pattern for all causes in A and B; the period to 1900 is characterised by wide annual fluctuations but, from 1900, the two sources approximate parity. However, the inclusion of tuberculosis for the period to 1899 results in a relative deficit of 60 per cent or more in the *Weekly Abstract*.

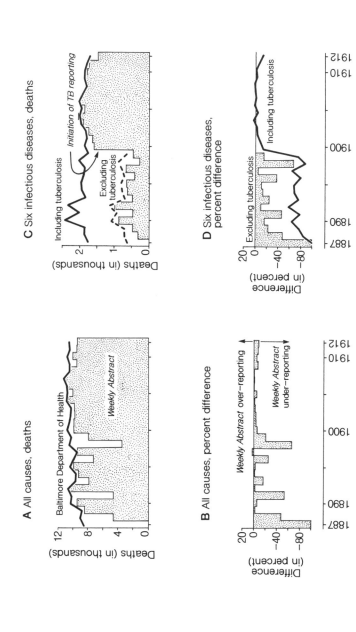

Figure 2.14. Completeness of mortality reporting in Baltimore, 1887–1912. Assessment of the completeness of mortality records abstracted from *Weekly Abstract* against those of the Baltimore Department of Health. (A) Annual series of deaths from all causes based on *Weekly Abstract* (bars) and Baltimore Department of Public Health (line trace). (B) Percentage difference in the two series of graph A; negative values mark underreporting of *Weekly Abstract* relative to the records of the Department of Health while positive values mark overreporting. (C) Annual series of deaths from six diseases (diphtheria, enteric/typhoid fever, measles, scarlet fever, tuberculosis, and whooping cough) based on *Weekly Abstract* (bars) and Baltimore Department of Public Health (line traces). (D) Percentage difference in the series of graph C; again, negative values mark underreporting of *Weekly Abstract* relative to the records of the Department of Health while positive values mark overreporting.

2.7 Conclusions

In this chapter, we have outlined the rationale for the establishment of an international disease surveillance system by the United States in the late nineteenth century. The initiative was prompted by the increased volume, speed, and capacity of commercial shipping destined for the United States from foreign ports. The steam age had bought many parts of the world within just a few days' or weeks' sailing time from the United States, and with this came the increased threat of imported epidemics. In response, the 1878 Quarantine Law provided the mechanism by which US health officials could monitor epidemics around the globe. After a faltering start, by 1888 the USMHS had established a regular system for the circulation of this information in the form of the *Weekly Abstract of Sanitary Reports*.

For the 25-year period to 1912, each edition of the *Weekly Abstract* included tables of mortality in US and overseas cities. These tables provide the raw data for the substantive analyses in chapters 4–6 of this book. As described in section 2.3, the tables record deaths from all causes and up to eleven infectious diseases in some 350 cities worldwide. The quality of the data undoubtedly varies from city to city. But cross-checks with other national and local disease surveillance reports suggest that, with careful selection, the data for some cities and diseases are of sufficient integrity to provide useful insights into global epidemic history. It is to the selection of these cities and diseases that we now turn.

3

The global sample: an overall picture

US Marine Hospital Service,
Rio de Janeiro, Brazil,
— —, 1896.

Enteric fever. – There were 272 fatal cases of this disease during the year . . .

Tuberculosis still continues to make its usual ravages . . .

Measles, scarlatina, diphtheria, influenza, and whooping cough. These diseases
only appear sporadically, and, with the exception of the last two, are very
fatal.

R. Cleary, Sanitary Inspector, US Marine Hospital Service
Public Health Reports, vol. XII (1897), p. 162

3.1 Introduction

In the previous chapter, we discussed the origins and subsequent development of the *Weekly Abstract of Sanitary Reports,* and we outlined the scope of the information that the serial contains for both diseases and cities. Numerical information on eleven diseases and deaths from all causes was reported at one time or another during the published life of the *Weekly Abstract,* and some 350 cities (150 in the United States, 200 elsewhere) appeared for varying spans of time. From this collection, we ultimately selected six diseases and 100 cities for analysis. In this chapter, we examine the rationale for our selections. In the first half of the chapter, we focus upon our six target diseases of diphtheria, enteric fever, measles, scarlet fever, tuberculosis, and whooping cough. We discuss the reasons for our choice, and then outline the causes and aetiology of each. Our consideration of the six diseases is concluded with a brief history of their epidemiologies from their presumed origins up to the start of our study period at the end of the nineteenth century.

In the second half of the chapter, we turn our attention to the 100 cities. The process by which we arrived at this 100 from the c. 350 potentially available is outlined. We then go on to examine the geographical and population size distributions of those selected before turning our attention to the city–disease matrix for each disease. Here, issues of data reliability and completeness of reporting on a city-by-city basis are paramount. The chapter is concluded with a classification of the cities on the basis of their time series of reported crude mortality from each of the six diseases.

3.2 The infectious diseases

Since we shall be frequently referring to specific infectious diseases in the following five chapters, it is useful at this early point to set out the nature of the six diseases (as seen from a late twentieth-century perspective) eventually chosen for analysis. We set out here the reasons for their selection (section 3.2.1), the clinical nature of each disease (section 3.2.2), and their comparative epidemiology (section 3.2.3). Finally, we look backwards from our study period of 1888–1912 and comment on the origin and early history of the diseases up to the end of the nineteenth century (section 3.2.4).

3.2.1 Selecting the six diseases

As we noted in chapter 2, crude mortality from eleven different diseases was reported at one time or another during the 26-year life of the *Weekly Abstract.* The diseases are: cholera, diphtheria, enteric fever (typhoid and paratyphoid fevers), measles, plague, scarlet fever, smallpox, tuberculosis, typhus fever, whooping cough, and yellow fever. But records for five of these (cholera, plague, smallpox, typhus, and yellow fever) are either so incomplete or unreliable that we doubt if their analysis would prove worthwhile; see sections 2.5 and 2.6. The principal difficulty in working with the records for these five diseases arose from the fact that reports were almost always presented as part of a textual account, so that the data were not regularly tabulated in the conventional sense. The figures that appear in these accounts frequently reflected what the writer judged to be significant epidemiological events in a particular city in a given week. This does not mean that these accounts are without interest – indeed, they are an important way of adding flesh and colour to the numerical record, and of judging what was internationally important in a particular week. But they are not tractable for the kinds of numerical analyses employed in this book because of the overwhelming proportion of missing observations when the data are abstracted from the qualitative accounts. This is because a disease/city that experienced a sharp rise in mortality in one week might return to 'the norm' in another, and so disappear from the text account even though deaths were still occurring. Because of these difficulties, we were left with the regularly tabulated diseases of diphtheria, enteric fever, measles, scarlet fever, tuberculosis, and whooping cough, along with deaths from all causes.

But how accurate are mortality counts of these diseases likely to be? Some guidance is provided in an outstanding exemplar of historical–epidemiological research, *The Epidemic Streets: Infectious Disease and the Rise of Preventive Medicine, 1856–1900*, where Hardy (1993a) analyses at length the reliability of the data for infectious diseases in England and Wales in the second half of the nineteenth century. She concludes that, for the communicable diseases as a group, the registration data categories may, on the whole, be taken as fairly reliable. *Diphtheria* in England was, as Hardy emphasises, a 'new' disease when it appeared in 1856. By the 1880s, its reliability in registration had settled down but its mortality levels need to be considered alongside those of croup and quinsy. Overall, registration for diphtheria was less reliable than for the other three childhood diseases. Of the *enteric fevers* typhoid and typhus are very similar in symptoms and were not distinguished in the registrar general's reports after 1869. Given its distinctive rash, *measles* might be distinguished from other infection-induced rashes without too much difficulty but, since measles deaths were often due to subsequent respiratory complications, registered measles deaths may have underestimated mortality levels. Diagnoses of *scarlet fever* are likely to have been reliable although it had only been separated from diphtheria from 1859. But Hardy warns that it is the registration data for respiratory *tuberculosis* should be treated with greatest caution. Diagnosis became more precise during the course of the nineteenth century (with the advent of auscillation and the stethoscope), but many deaths were registered as bronchitis, pneumonia, or even typhoid, depending on the symptoms present in the final stages. *Whooping cough* was a widespread and very familiar disease of childhood. Further comments on the reliability of mortality statistics by diseases are given by W. Luckin (1980).

3.2.2 *The clinical nature of the six diseases*

We now take each of the six diseases in turn and describe their leading characteristics. Given that each is fully described in any standard textbook of infectious diseases, we rely wholly on the excellent brief accounts given in the small work which since its first publication in 1917 has been the *vade mecum* of epidemiologists worldwide: *Control of Communicable Diseases in Man* (15th edn, Benenson, 1990). Unless otherwise specified material in this section is based on this source.

(a) Diphtheria
Diphtheria (ICD-10-CM A36)[1] is an acute bacterial disease which mainly affects parts of the respiratory tract: the tonsils, pharynx, larynx, and nose (Benenson, 1990, p. 138). Occasionally it may affect other mucous membranes or skin (for example, the conjunctivae or genitalia) and wounded tissues. The characteristic lesion is caused by the liberation of a specific cytotoxin; it is marked by patches of an adherent greyish membrane with a surrounding inflammation. It gains its name from this membrane (Greek: *diphtheria*, for 'shield' or 'membrane') which forms in the respiratory tract in severe cases of infection.

(b) Enteric fevers
The term 'enteric fever' was used in the *Weekly Abstracts* as generalised term to cover typhoid (ICD-10-CM A01.0) and paratyphoid fevers (ICD-10-CM A01.1–A01.4): both are generalised infections of the bowel (Benenson, 1990, p. 469). Typhoid fever is a systematic bacterial disease characterised by the slow onset of a sustained fever and a variety of other symptoms which include headache, malaise, anorexia, slowness of the heart, 'rose spot' rash on the trunk, non-productive cough, constipation more commonly than diarrhoea (in adults), and involvement of the lymphoid tissues. Paratyphoid fever presents a similar clinical picture, but tends to be milder, and the case–fatality rate is much lower.

(c) Measles
Measles (ICD-10-CM B05) is a highly communicable virus disease (Benenson, 1990, pp. 269–70). It is characterised by a prodromal fever, conjunctivitis, coryza, cough, and Koplik's Spots on the buccal mucosa. A characteristic red blotchy rash appears on the third to seventh day, beginning on the face, becoming generalised, lasting four to seven days and sometimes ending in 'branny' desquamation. Complications may result from viral replication or

bacterial superinfection, and include otitis media, pneumonia, diarrhoea, and encephalitis. Evidence of measles pathology has been found in the ear, eye, thymus, lung, liver, intestine, spleen, kidney, bladder, and bone. Measles is presently a more severe disease in developing countries, especially among very young and malnourished children, in whom it may be associated with haemorrhagic rash, protein-losing enteropathy, mouth sores, dehydration, diarrhoea, blindness, and severe skin infections; the case–fatality rate may be 5–10 per cent or more.

(d) Scarlet fever

Scarlet fever (ICD-10-CM A38) is an acute infectious disease characterised by the sudden onset of soreness when swallowing, fever, and headache (Benenson, 1990, pp. 411–12). Clinical characteristics may include all those symptoms associated with a streptococcal sore throat (or it may be linked with a wound, skin, or puerperal infection), as well as enanthem, strawberry tongue, and exanthem. The rash is usually a fine erythema, commonly punctate, blanching on pressure, often felt (like sandpaper) better than seen and appearing most often on the neck, chest, in folds of the axilla, elbow, and groin, and on inner surfaces of the thighs. Typically, the rash does not involve the face, but there is flushing of the cheeks and circumoral pallor. High fever, nausea, and vomiting often accompany severe infections. A range of complications, principally affecting young children, add to the dangers of the disease. These include anaemia, otitis media, rheumatic fever, and meningitis. In rare cases, scarlet fever appears in severe septic or toxic forms.

(e) Tuberculosis

Tuberculosis (ICD-10-CM A15–A19) is a mycobacterial disease important as a cause of disability and death in many parts of the world (Benenson, 1990, p. 457). The initial infection usually goes unnoticed; tuberculin sensitivity appears within a few weeks. Lesions commonly heal, leaving no residual changes except occasional pulmonary or tracheobronchial lymph node calcifications. Approximately 95 per cent of those initially infected enter this latent phase from which there is lifelong risk of reactivation. In approximately 5 per cent of cases, the initial infection progresses directly to *pulmonary tuberculosis* or, by lymphohaematogenous dissemination of bacilli, to pulmonary, miliary, meningeal, or other extrapulmonary involvement. Serious outcome of the initial infection is more frequent in infants, adolescents, and young adults. *Extrapulmonary* tuberculosis is much less common than pulmonary. It may affect any organ or tissue and includes tuberculous meningitis, acute haematogenous (miliary) tuberculosis, and involvement of lymph nodes, pleura, pericardium, kidneys, bones and joints, larynx, skin, intestines, peritoneum, and eyes. *Progressive* pulmonary tuberculosis arises from exogenous reinfection or endogenous reactivation of a latent focus remaining from the initial infection. If untreated, about half the patients will die within a two-year period.

(f) Whooping cough

Whooping cough (ICD-10-CM A37) is an acute bacterial infection of the respiratory tract, which includes both pertussis (ICD-10-CM A37.9) and parapertussis (Benenson, 1990, p. 319). Parapertussis is clinically indistinguishable from pertussis but has a milder form. The disease has an insidious onset with an initial catarrhal stage combined with an irritating cough that gradually becomes paroxysmal, usually within one to two weeks. The condition lasts for one or two months, sometimes longer. The paroxysms are marked by repeated violent coughs and may be followed by a characteristic crowing or high-pitched inspiratory 'whoop'; it is this cough which gives the disease its popular name. The paroxysms often end with the vomiting of a clear, tenacious mucous substance. The symptoms are most acute in children: infants less than six months old and adults often do not have the typical whoop or cough paroxysm.

3.2.3 Comparative epidemiology of the six diseases

In this subsection we briefly compare and contrast those epidemiological features of the six diseases which bear on their historical interpretation. We consider in turn (a) their causes, (b) the reservoirs of infection, (c) the mode of transmission, (d) the incubation period, (e) communicability, and (f) the question of susceptibility and resistance. As in the previous section, we rely largely on the standard accounts given in Benenson (1990). Unless otherwise specified material in this section is based on this source.

(a) Causes of the diseases

Four of the diseases (enteric fever, scarlet fever, tuberculosis, and whooping cough) are now known to be caused by different bacteria. A fifth (measles) is a virus disease and a sixth (diphtheria) is caused by a bacterium which is subsequently infected by a bacteriophage. Table 3.1 summarises their main features.

Diphtheria (plate 3.1A). The cause of diphtheria is infection by a bacteria, *Corynebacterium diphtheriae* (so named for its clubbed shape, Greek: *koryne*, or 'club') which occurs in three different biotypes, *gravis*, *mitis*, or *intermedius* (Benenson, 1990, p. 138). Local lesions are produced by a toxin which results from infection of the bacteria by a corynebacteriophage containing the gene, *tox*. Non-toxigenic strains of the bacteria rarely produce local lesions.

Enteric fever (plate 3.1B). The infectious agent for typhoid fever is a member of one of the largest and most widespread families of bacteria on earth with nearly

Table 3.1. *The six marker diseases*

Principal features affecting their epidemic characteristics.

Disease	Agent	Reservoir	Transmission	Incubation period	Infectious period	Susceptibility
Diphtheria	*Corynebacterium diphtheriae* containing the gene *tox*	Man	Generally contact with patient or carrier	2–5 days	Usually 2 weeks or less; rarely more than 4 weeks	All; recovery not always followed by lasting immunity
Enteric fever	*Salmonella typhi; S. paratyphi*	Man for typhoid and paratyphoid; rarely domestic animals for paratyphoid	Food and water contaminated by faeces of infectives	1–3 weeks	Usually 1–2 weeks; 10% for 3 months; 2–5% permanent in absence of treatment	General, especially the young
Measles	Measles virus of the family *paramyxoviridae*	Man	Airborne droplets	8–12 days	7–9 days	Historically all: infection confers lifelong immunity; vaccination after 1963
Scarlet fever	*Streptococcus pyogenes* producing erythrogenic toxin	Man	Direct or intimate contact with patients or carriers	1–3 days	Untreated, 10–21 days; 2 days post-penicillin	All; second attacks rare
Tuberculosis	*Mycobacterium tuberculosis* and *M. africanum* primarily from humans; *M. bovis* primarily from cattle	Primarily man; historically diseased cattle	Airborne droplets; ingestion of untreated dairy products from infected cattle	4–12 weeks	Historically, as long as viable tubercule bacilli discharged in sputum; a few days to a few weeks with modern treatments	All; 6–12 months after infection
Whooping cough	*Bordetella pertussis; B. parapertussis*	Man	Airborne droplets	7–10 days	Up to 3 weeks without treatment; 5 days when treated with erythromycin	All; prolonged/lifelong immunity after attack

Note:
Figures in the literature for the lengths of the incubation and infectious periods vary considerably, and we have quoted middle values.

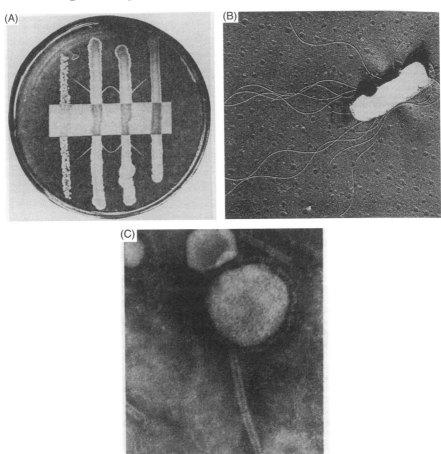

Plate 3.1. Causative microbiological agents of the six diseases. (A) Diphtheria: gel diffusion test for toxin-producing *Corynebacterium diphtheriae* (source: Myrvik and Weiser, 1988, fig. 15.2, p. 245). (B) Enteric fever: electron micrograph of *Salmonella typhi* (source: Ramsay and Emond, 1978, fig. 106, p. 262). (C) Measles: electron micrograph of measles virus (source: Ramsay and Emond, 1978, fig. 42, p. 80). (D) Scarlet fever: beta-hemolytic *streptococcus* on membrane of human mouth cell (source: Sherris, 1990, fig. 16.3, p. 297). (E) Tuberculosis: *Mycobacterium tuberculosis* in lung tissue (source: Myrvik and Weiser 1988, fig. 27.1, p. 379, left). (F) Whooping cough: tracheal cell infected with *Bordetella pertussis* (source: Sherris, 1990, fig. 23.3, p. 410).

two thousand serotypes recognised (Benenson, 1990, p. 469). But, almost unique amongst the salmonellae, *Salmonella typhi* (the typhoid bacillus) is adapted to human beings alone. The bacillus is very variable and presently 106 types can be distinguished by phage typing. For paratyphoid fever, the corresponding bacillus is *Salmonella paratyphi* for which three serotypes (A, B, and

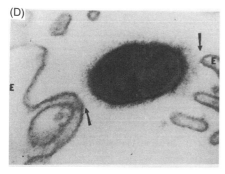

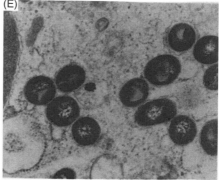

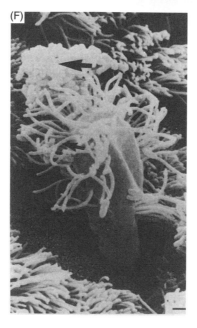

Plate 3.1. (*cont.*)

C) are presently recognised. Of the three, paratyphoid B is the most common, A is less frequent, and C is extremely rare. The two typhoid bacilli are members of a family of bacilli named after D. E. Salmon who, in the 1880s, discovered an organism (*Salmonella cholerasuis*) responsible for bacteremia in humans and diarrhoea in swine (LeBaron and Taylor, 1993, p. 107).

Measles (plate 3.1C). The infectious agent for measles is the measles virus, a member of the genus *Morbillivirus* of the family *paramyxoviridae* (Benenson, 1990, p. 270). Measles is the type species of this genus which lists distemper (dogs), rinderpest (cattle), and peste-des-petits ruminants (sheep and goats) among its members. There is a single serotype of the measles virus, and it is not currently distinguishable from other members of the paramyxovirus family by electron microscopy.

Scarlet fever (plate 3.1D). Scarlet fever is one of a variety of diseases caused by the streptococci group of bacteria: the other diseases include streptococcal sore throat, impetigo, erysipelas, and puerperal fever (Benenson, 1990, p. 413). The specific group, *Streptococcus pyogenes*, consists of approximately eighty serologically distinct types that vary greatly in time and geographical distributions. Group A streptococci producing skin infections are usually of different serological types from those associated with throat infections and, in scarlet fever, three immunologically different types of erythrogenic toxin (A, B, and C) have been demonstrated.

Tuberculosis (plate 3.1E). The infectious agents of tuberculosis spread primarily from humans are two types of bacteria, *Mycobacterium tuberculosis* and *M. africanum*. A third, *M. bovis*, is spread primarily from cattle (Benenson, 1990, pp. 457–8). Other mycobacteria may occasionally produce a disease which is clinically indistinguishable from tuberculosis and the specific aetiologic agents can be identified only by culture of the organisms.

Whooping cough (plate 3.1F). The infectious agent of whooping cough is the pertussis bacillus, *Bordetella pertussis*, while *B. parapertussis* causes parapertussis (Benenson, 1990, p. 319).

(b) Disease reservoirs
A disease reservoir is the place where an infectious agent normally lives and multiplies and on which it depends primarily for survival. For three of our six diseases (measles, scarlet fever, and whooping cough) the sole reservoir is the human population, *Homo sapiens*. For diphtheria the situation is slightly more complex, for *Corynebacteria* are widely distributed throughout the world, even though the only known reservoir of *C. diphtheriae* is man. The reservoir for both typhoid and paratyphoid is the human population plus, rarely, domestic animals for paratyphoid. A carrier state may follow from an acute illness or mild or even subclinical infections. Faecal carriers are more common than urinary carriers and the chronic carrier state is most common among persons infected during middle age, especially females. For tuberculosis the reservoir is primarily but not solely man. In some areas, diseased cattle may serve as a focus; this was an important reservoir during our study period. Other primates, badgers, or other mammals have been recorded as minor reservoirs.

(c) Modes of transmission
Respiratory transmission is the main mechanism of spread for three of the six diseases: measles, tuberculosis (pulmonary or laryngeal), and whooping

cough. For these sicknesses, expiration in all its forms, but especially coughing and sneezing, will produce airborne droplets infected with the causative agent. Direct contact with the nasal or throat secretions of infected persons will also cause propagation. But while the airborne route is the most important mechanism of transmission, for none of them is it exclusive. Measles can be spread, less commonly, by articles freshly soiled with nose and throat secretions. A second important pathway for tuberculosis during our study period was intestinal: the disease was frequently caused by drinking raw milk or eating unpasteurised dairy products prepared from the milk of tuberculous cattle. For tuberculosis, a third pathway may be the direct invasion of tissues through mucous membranes or through breaks in the skin, but this is extremely rare (Benenson, 1990, p. 459). Tuberculosis in forms other than pulmonary or laryngeal is generally not communicable.

For diphtheria and scarlet fever, the transmission pathways are more complex. Diphtheria is spread predominantly by contact with a patient or carrier. Very occasionally, transmission has been recorded after contact with articles soiled by discharges from lesions of infected persons and via unpasteurised milk (Benenson, 1990, p. 139). Christie (1974) observes that even dust around the bed of a diphtheria patient can remain infective for weeks. The mode of propagation for scarlet fever is by direct or intimate contact with patients or carriers. The infection is only rarely passed through indirect contact with objects or hands. Nasal carriers are particularly likely to transmit disease.

For enteric fever the mode of transmission of the bacteria is by food and water contaminated by the faeces and urine of patients and carriers: thus, where pure water and uncontaminated food can be assured, typhoid transmission is minimal. During our main study period, from 1888 to 1912, this disease was common if only because the proper separation of sanitation from fresh water supplies was still under development in many cities. Today, the most important transmission path varies widely from one part of the world to another: from shellfish contaminated by sewage discharge to vegetables fertilised by nightsoil.

(d) Comparative incubation periods

The incubation periods for five of the six diseases are short, ranging up to twenty-one days; see figure 3.1. The diseases are, in rank order from the shortest: scarlet fever (usually one to three days and only rarely longer), diphtheria (two to five days but occasionally longer), whooping cough (commonly a week to ten days, rarely exceeding fourteen days), measles (about ten days, varying from seven to eighteen days), and typhoid (one to three weeks; for paratyphoid, the period is one to ten days).

By comparison with these five diseases, the incubation period for tuberculosis is long. The time interval from initial infection through to a

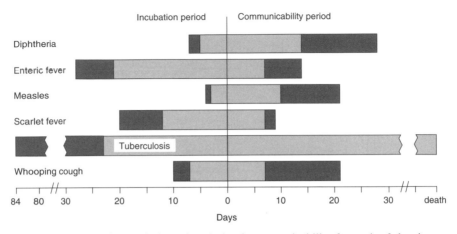

Figure 3.1. Incubation periods and periods of communicability for each of the six diseases. Bars are divided to show lower (light stipple) and upper (dark stipple) estimates of the duration of each period.

demonstrable primary lesion or to a significant tuberculin reaction is commonly four to twelve weeks. The risk that an initial infection will lead to progressive pulmonary or extrapulmonary tuberculosis is greatest within the first year or two from primary infection, and it is possible for tuberculosis to persist for a lifetime as a latent infection.

(e) Differing periods of communicability
The length of the period during which a disease can be passed from one person to another is clearly critical to its infectiousness. In the case of both tuberculosis and enteric fever, this period is a long one. For tuberculosis, the period of communicability for an infected person is in theory as long as viable tubercle bacilli are being discharged in the sputum (Benenson, 1990, p. 460). Untreated or inadequately treated patients may remain intermittently sputum-positive for years. The degree of communicability is a complex function of (a) the number of bacilli discharged, (b) the virulence of the bacilli, (c) the adequacy of ventilation, (d) exposure of the bacilli to sunlight or UV light, (e) the opportunities for bacilli to be converted into aerosols by coughing, sneezing, talking, or singing, and (f) the age of the patient (children with primary tuberculosis are generally not infectious). For enteric fever, the period of communicability is as long as the bacilli appear in the excreta (Benenson, 1990, p. 460). In the case of typhoid, it is usually from the first week throughout convalescence. With paratyphoid, it is commonly one to two weeks. About one in ten of untreated typhoid fever patients will discharge bacilli for three months after the onset of symptoms, and up to one in twenty become permanent

typhoid carriers. In the case of paratyphoid, some infected persons may become permanent carriers in their gall bladders.

At the other end of the time spectrum are measles and scarlet fever. For measles, the period of communicability is just a few days, extending from slightly before the beginning of the prodromal period to four days after the appearance of the rash; however, communicability is low after the second day of rash. Scarlet fever also has a brief period of communicability. In untreated and uncomplicated cases, it is ten to twenty-one days but, in untreated conditions with purulent discharges, this may be extended to weeks or months.

Whooping cough and diphtheria fall between these two groups of extremes. Pertussis is highly communicable from the early catarrhal stage up to the paroxysmal cough stage. Despite a persisting spasmodic cough with a whoop, communicability gradually decreases and becomes negligible for ordinary non-family contacts in about three weeks. For diphtheria, Benenson (1990, p. 139) records very variable periods of communicability, dependent on when virulent bacilli have disappeared from discharges and lesions. This is usually reported as two weeks or less and seldom more than four weeks. For the rare chronic diphtheria carrier, the period of communicability may be longer and clinical accounts suggest this may extend to six months or more.

(f) Susceptibility and resistance
Susceptibility and resistance to the six diseases is variable and still not fully understood. The simplest case is measles where susceptibility is general: all persons who have not had the disease (or who have not been successfully immunised) are susceptible. The immunity acquired after disease is permanent. Infants born to mothers who have had the disease or who have been vaccinated are immune for approximately the first six to nine months of life, depending on the amount of residual maternal antibody at the time of pregnancy and the rate of antibody degradation.

Like measles, susceptibility to whooping cough is universal, but there is no clear evidence of effective transplacental immunity in infants. It is predominantly a childhood disease; incidence rates of reported disease are highest under five years of age (Benenson, 1990, p. 319). As with measles, immunisation against the disease is now possible.

Susceptibility to scarlet fever is general. Many persons develop either antitoxic or type-specific antibacterial immunity, or both, through asymptomatic infection. Antibacterial immunity develops only against the specific M-type of group A streptococcus that induced the infection, and this may last for years. Second attacks of scarlet fever are rare, but may occur (Benenson, 1990, p. 415). Susceptibility to both typhoid and paratyphoid diseases is general, and this is increased in individuals with gastric achlorhydria (Benenson, 1990, p. 470). Relative specific immunity follows recovery from clinical disease and asymptomatic infection, but this is not sufficient to protect against a subsequent ingestion of large numbers of organisms. Thus immunity seems to be relative and can be overcome by administration of a sufficiently large dose of bacilli.

Prior to the development of immunisation, susceptibility to tuberculosis was universal. The most hazardous period for the development of clinical disease is the first six to twelve months after infection, and it is highest among four age groups: children under three years of age, adolescents, young adults, and the very old. In this last cohort, disease may generally be attributed to the reactivation of long-latent infections. Lifelong immunity is not conferred by infection.

3.2.4 The history of the six diseases prior to 1900

Succinct histories of each of the six diseases studied here are given at length in Kiple's monumental *Cambridge World History of Human Diseases* (1993) and we draw heavily on the scholarly account given there in this section. Our purpose is to highlight those points in the earlier history of the diseases that bear on the 1888–1912 study period. The consequent course of the diseases in the twentieth century is deferred until chapter 7.

(a) Diphtheria

With diphtheria, as with most infectious diseases, questions of the location and timing of their origin lie outside the span of recorded historical research and may extend back into palaeopathology. Thus Carmichael (1993a, p. 682) suggests that although diphtheria was described in the early modern period as a 'new' disease this should be regarded with caution. English (1985) notes that diseases resembling diphtheria were described in classical Greek medical literature (Risse, 1993) and in European medical writing from the sixteenth century. The aetiology of diphtheria was not was worked out until 1884 by Klebs and Löffler (only two years after Robert Koch's classic paper on the germ theory of disease), but Bretonneau, a French physician from Tours, had described the specific clinical features of the disease and given it its name in the 1820s. From his clinical and post-mortem findings he stressed the presence of a pseudomembrane as diagnostic of the disease.[2]

Unlike cholera and yellow fever, both seen as severe epidemic threats, diphtheria in the middle of the nineteenth century was widely regarded as a disease of poverty. Crowded conditions in cities were thought to favour spread of the disease and, before the germ theory of disease was elaborated, diphtheria was widely accepted to be a 'filth disease, largely favouring the poor' (Carmichael, 1993a, p. 681). The periodic peaks in diphtheria mortality received little attention from clinicians. Gale (1959, p. 93) suggests that the modern history of diphtheria in England began with the wave of prevalence which started about 1855. Simon's second report to the Privy Council for the year 1859 has a section of 160 pages about it. He says that the disease was almost unknown to British doctors until 1855 but that, in the four years since then, it had become widespread. As is usual when an epidemic disease which has been rare becomes common, importation from abroad was blamed and, at first, diphtheria was known as the 'Boulogne sore-throat'.

If it was imported, it seems to have spread quickly. At first, it was overshadowed by deaths from scarlet fever but, by the quinquennium 1886–90 (overlapping the start of our survey period), it took the lead. Although the bacillus appeared to lead to subclinical infection during endemic periods, more virulent strains appear to have dominated in the epidemic outbreaks. In epidemics, fatality rates for affected children ranged from one-third to one-half: Carmichael (1993a, p. 681) notes that occlusion of the airway and consequent sudden suffocation was an especially feared cause of death in young children.

(b) Enteric diseases
For the physicians of ancient Greece, the non-specific symptoms of the enteric diseases meant that they appeared to be very similar to many other gastrointestinal infections. As a result, they attracted little special comment. However, LeBaron and Taylor (1993, p. 1075) note that Hippocrates described a case of what appears to have been typhoid, and that Caesar Augustus was cured of a fever with typhoid-like characteristics by the use of cold baths. From the scant evidence it is likely that typhoid and paratyphoid fever are very old diseases of human populations, probably more than 2,000 years old.

The role of typhoid fevers in causing major epidemic outbreaks was noted by the early seventeenth century: typical was the outbreak at Jamestown, Virginia, when 6,500 out of 7,500 colonists died. Later in the same century, a British physician, Thomas Willis, catalogued the symptoms, signs, and course of a disease he called 'putrid malignant fever', which was clearly typhoid (LeBaron and Taylor, 1993, p. 1075). It was not until the 1830s that Pierre Louis in France and William Gerhard in the United States were able to separate out typhoid fever and typhus as separate entities. Typhus is now reserved for the two rickettsial diseases, epidemic-louse borne typhus fever (ICD-10-CM A75.0) and murine typhus fever (ICD-10-CM A75.2).

We can gain some idea of the relative importance of typhoid compared with a number of other epidemic diseases by examining data for London given in Gale (1959, p. 136) for 1849, the year immediately following the first Public Health Act (1848). The year 1849 is an especially interesting one in which to take another look at the prevailing epidemic diseases of London (see section 1.3.2) because it coincided with the major cholera epidemic investigated by John Snow in the first edition of his classic, *On the Mode of Communication of Cholera*. In comparing Gale's data with those given in section 1.3.2, it must be remembered that the Registration Area was much larger than that of the

Bills of Mortality and that the information collected, although still defective, was much more complete. In 1849, the Registration Area had a population of 2,360,000, and 68,755 deaths were recorded. Of these deaths, 26,243 were ascribed to the seven principal epidemic diseases: with typhus and typhoid (2,482 deaths), third after cholera (14,125) and diarrhoea (3,463).

Another indicator of the mortality from enteric fevers comes from military records. During the Spanish–American War of 1898, one-fifth of the American army fell ill from typhoid fever, with a mortality six times the number of those who died of wounds (LeBaron and Taylor, 1993, p. 1075). Two years later in the South African (Boer) War, this disastrous experience was virtually repeated among British troops.

It was not until 1882 that Carl Eberth and Edwin Klebs finally identified the typhoid bacillus in intestinal lymph nodes (LeBaron and Taylor, 1993, p. 1075). But as early as the 1830s there were clear clinical definitions of typhoid and in the next decade the English physician William Budd demonstrated that typhoid was spread from infected individuals to new hosts by means of water and food. But Budd's views were opposed by the 'spontaneous generation' school. It was not until the British Public Health Act (1875) was passed that sanitary practices were improved along the lines recommended by Budd. Within a decade, typhoid mortality in Britain was halved.

(c) Measles

Cliff, Haggett, and Smallman-Raynor (1993, pp. 45–67) have traced the early history of measles from its emergence as a crowd disease in the cities of the river valleys of the Middle East, probably some 5,000 years ago, to the brink of the modern period starting in the middle of the nineteenth century. If 5,000 years is correct, then measles and man have been in close association for some 130,000 virus generations and some 200 human generations. It is likely that the virus jumped the species barrier to man from its relative, distemper in dogs (see section 3.2.3).

The greatest geographical change in the distribution of the disease up to 1840 resulted from the increasing number of locations worldwide where human populations clustered, both in sufficient numbers and at sufficient density to provide a continuous reservoir of susceptible people for the virus to prosper. Until 1492, these reservoirs were confined to the Old World but, from the early sixteenth century, we have clear evidence of measles invading the New World and contributing to massive population loss as both it and other new infections were introduced into an Amerindian population that lacked any antibody protection.

We have enough fragments of data for the last few centuries to be able to plot the spread of the disease. Thus, by the Tudor period in England, we have records of measles as a major illness, showing the same cyclical behaviour which is so characteristic of measles today. By 1840, all the evidence points to measles as a highly aggressive and commonplace infectious disease of both the Old and New Worlds, as well as Africa and Asia.

From 1840, our scientific understanding of the disease enters the modern period. The diffusion of measles to global coverage continued as the virus spread through Australia and invaded the Pacific islands during the second half of the nineteenth century. As new areas were reached for the first time, catastrophic levels of mortality were often experienced. For example, the Fiji epidemic of 1875 resulted in a c. 25–30 per cent death rate (Cliff, Haggett, and Smallman-Raynor, 1993, pp. 133–4), while that in mainland Alaska in 1900 carried rates of mortality that reached 40 per cent among the isolated Indian populations (Wolfe, 1982).

Although the mode of transmission was understood in general terms from the nineteenth century, identification of the causative agent, a virus, had to await the development of the electron microscope (see section 1.3.2); the virus was eventually isolated in 1954 by J. F. Enders and T. C. Peebles.

(d) Scarlet fever
Scarlet fever and diphtheria have in common the symptom of a sore throat, and the early history of the two diseases is therefore confused. Sydenham described *febris scarlatina* in 1675. At the end of the eighteenth century, Willan identified three types of scarlet fever: (a) *scarlatina simplex* with a rash and no sore throat, (b) *scarlatina anginosa* with a rash and sore throat, and (c) *scarlatina maligna*, a very severe form with sloughing of the soft tissues of the throat and mouth and profound toxaemia (Gale, 1959, p. 90).

In the light of modern knowledge about streptococcal sore throat, Gale estimates that, while major epidemics of scarlet fever occurred during the eighteenth century in England and Wales, there were long intervals between them. He also suggests that, at the end of the century, the disease became milder. This mild phase of scarlet fever lasted until about 1830. From then on, the disease began to increase in severity again and, in the first two and a half years of civil registration (1836–9), the number of deaths attributed to this cause rose sharply. In 1840, deaths nearly doubled and, for a generation after, scarlet fever and associated streptococcal infections were the most formidable prevailing form of infectious disease among the infectious diseases of childhood (Ramsay and Emond, 1978, p. 181). The chart in figure 1.8 indicates that the disease completely outweighed diphtheria, measles, and whooping cough as causes of mortality among those under fifteen years of age. Different strains of streptococci produced different amounts of toxin and epidemics thus varied greatly in severity, with mortality rates ranging from zero to 30 per cent. Creighton (1894, p. 726) says of this period: 'The enormous number of deaths from scarlatina during some thirty or forty years in the middle of the nineteenth century will appear in history as one of the most remarkable things in our epidemiology.'

The year of highest mortality was 1863 when the death rate among children under fifteen was 3,966 per million living. The marked decline in mortality from scarlet fever began in the 1860s and continued steadily up to the start of our survey period. During the 1880s, the disease continued to be widely prevalent but it began to decline as a cause of death and, by the 1890s, its character was again relatively mild, although not as mild as it has become today. This decline in severity was first apparent in Britain and Western Europe, although a malignant form remained present in Russia and Eastern Europe for the first few decades of the twentieth century (Hardy, 1993b, p. 992). A full understanding of scarlet fever was not achieved until the twentieth century (sce chapter 7), although streptococci were first isolated from the blood of scarlet fever patients by Edward Klein in 1887.

(e)   Tuberculosis
Of the six diseases included in this study, the evidence for great antiquity is strongest for tuberculosis (Johnston, 1993, p. 1059). Skeletons carrying lesions apparently caused by spinal tuberculosis have been identified from Stone Age skeletons and from Egyptian mummies around 5,000 years old. Early evidence of tuberculosis scars on the lungs of a mummified body comes from the early Han dynasty (206 BC–AD 7).Tuberculosis appears to have been carried to the New World by the movement of peoples from Asia; there is skeletal evidence of the disease from 800 BC in North America and from AD 290 in South America.

The rich historical evidence in early Greek and Chinese literature about tuberculosis in its various forms is summarised by Rene Dubos and Jean Dubos in their classic study of tuberculosis, *The White Plague* (1953). Although the idea of a single cause for the different forms of tuberculosis was advanced by Laennec at the start of the century, it was not until the experimental work by Villemin in 1865 and Koch in 1882 that the present concept of tuberculosis as a single disease caused by the tubercle bacillus emerged. Until then, the various clinical manifestations were given separate names and they were thought of as different diseases. The terms *phthisis* or *pulmonary consumption* (often shortened to *consumption*) were used to label pulmonary tuberculosis. *Scrofula* described tubercular infections of the lymph glands surrounding the neck. *Lupus vulgaris* was the term used to describe tuberculosis of the skin.

Mortality from tuberculosis has been historically associated with population growth in cities. In sixteenth-century England, tuberculosis caused about one-fifth of all deaths at mid-century with the greatest concentrations of the disease in London. In Japan at the same time, phthisis had become widespread in the rapidly growing administrative capital of Edo. But it was during the eighteenth century, however, that the world's great epidemics of tuberculosis began. They were especially intense in those countries (England, the United

States, Italy, and France) that experienced the greatest urbanisation and industrialisation (Johnston, 1993, p. 1059). Tuberculosis was so rampant that autopsies showed that close to 100 per cent of some urban populations, such as those of London, Paris, and other major industrial cities, had at some point in their lives developed the disease (although they had died from some other cause). By the early nineteenth century, rates of mortality from tuberculosis in most major US cities ranged from 400 to 500 per 100,000 population.

Mortality in the nineteenth century behaved as a diffusion wave. Johnston (1993, p. 1059) notes that rates in the older industrial countries of Western Europe and the United States started to decline after 1860, whereas in the then developing industrial countries of the time (including Eastern European nations and Japan), major tuberculosis epidemics were not to start until the end of the nineteenth century.

The epidemiology of tuberculosis illustrates the principle of multifactorial causation. The tubercle bacillus is a necessary but not sufficient condition for the development of the disease. The necessary co-factors can be divided into (a) host-dependent factors and (b) environment-dependent factors. The former include age, gender, and genetic factors; the latter crowding, nutrition, and working conditions. A full discussion of the role of such factors is provided by Johnston (1993, pp. 1060–1).

Early treatment of tuberculosis involved a wide range of quackeries. But, by the middle of the nineteenth century, open air therapies had become increasingly popular. In the 1880s, luxury sanitoria for the wealthy proliferated and, about 1900, state-sponsored sanitoria began to be created in Western Europe, North America, and Japan. The effectiveness of this treatment and others is considered in section 7.2.5.

(f) Whooping cough
In an extensive review of the literature, Hardy (1993c, p. 1095) argues that the history of whooping cough prior the twentieth century is obscure, and she was unable to trace back the disease with certainty before the middle of the sixteenth century. August Hirsch (1886) suggests that the native habitat of the disease was originally Northern Europe. But the existence of a widespread folklore with regard to its treatment may indicate a more ancient existence in such places as southern India and Malabar (Hardy, 1993c, p. 1095). It was almost certainly unknown to the ancient world. Creighton (1894) also notes that there is little reference to whooping cough in early medical writings. He suggests a possible reason for this may be that it was generally left to the management of parents and nurses, and that it may also have been thought of as a complication of other diseases rather than as a disease in its own right. There is, however, a reference to 'the kink' in a medieval prescription book.

The first medical description of a severe epidemic of whooping cough is that given by Baillou of Paris in 1578. Although he wrote of the disease as a familiar affliction, for which there seemed to be several names already, the prevalence of the disease remained largely obscure until the middle of the eighteenth century. Sydenham mentions it under the name pertussis 'which we call hooping cough' but always in association with another disease – in one instance with measles and in another with influenza (Gale, 1959, p. 103).

Hardy (1993c, p. 1095) notes that the terms 'whooping cough' and 'chin-cough' first appear as causes of death in the London Bills of Mortality in 1701, and an increasing number of deaths were attributed to them. The toll rose from 119 in the fifteen-year period 1702–17, to 4,252 in the period 1762–77. With the introduction of the civil registration of deaths in 1838, English mortality figures become more reliable. Deaths from whooping cough reached a peak of some 1,500 per million population under the age of fifteen per annum in England and Wales in about 1870. After this, the death rate from the disease began to decline, a fall manifest first in agricultural areas, later in urban and industrial areas. In London during the nineteenth century, the highest mortality from whooping cough was experienced by the children of the working classes, and death was generally due to complications involving the respiratory organs (Hardy, 1993c, p. 1095).

In the early years of the nineteenth century, measles and whooping cough together began to replace smallpox as the principal killing diseases of young children in England and Wales. From 1851 to 1880, the mortality rate from whooping cough altered little, and it was rather higher than the rate for measles. However, it began to decline rather earlier than did the rate for measles, and it fell below the rate for measles in the quinquennium 1886–90.

The causative organism was first isolated by Bordet and Gengou in 1900. The introduction of vaccines against the disease dates from the 1930s and these are discussed in section 7.2.6.

3.3 The cities

3.3.1 Selecting the 100 cities

As described in section 2.4, in excess of 200 foreign cities were included at one time or another in the mortality tables of the *Weekly Abstract* between 1887 and 1912. A further 150 cities appeared in the mortality tables for the United States. The database of mortality from our six marker diseases (see section 3.2) and all causes therefore contains a potential 3.31 million pieces of weekly information (350 cities×7 mortality categories×52 weeks×26 years).

In addition to the logistical difficulties of transcribing such a large amount of data, by no means all cities were reported sufficiently regularly in the *Weekly Abstract* as to warrant detailed statistical analysis. Some consulates were ephemeral establishments, existing for a few years before closure while, as outlined in section 2.5, communications difficulties, war, and natural disas-

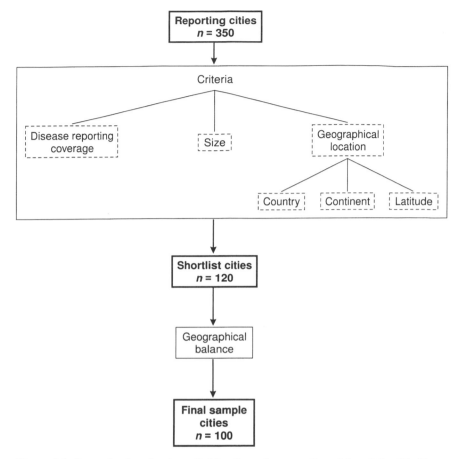

Figure 3.2. Stages in the selection of cities from the mortality tables of the *Weekly Abstract*.

ters severely impeded disease reports from some locations. Epidemics, too, could be so severe as to halt the flow of sanitary information. In these circumstances it was necessary to select those cities for which essentially unbroken data runs were available during the life of the tables.

The process by which we selected cities for analysis is outlined in figure 3.2. The first step consisted of reducing the 350 cities to a 'long shortlist' of cities according to three criteria: (a) reporting completeness as measured by the percentage of weeks in the period from 1887 to 1912 for which mortality data were actually recorded; (b) urban population size; and (c) geographical coverage in terms of countries, continents, and latitude. There is a tension between the three criteria. There would be little point in including a city if the data record was negligible. But application of the reporting criterion alone would have

Table 3.2. *A selection of cities excluded from analysis of the* Weekly Abstract

City	Continent	City	Continent
Algiers	Africa	Manaos	Americas
Barcelona	Europe	Montreal	Americas
Canton	Asia	Nottingham	Europe
East London	Africa	Ottawa	Americas
Florence	Europe	Saigon	Asia
Johannesburg	Africa	Shanghai	Asia
Karachi	Asia	Toronto	Americas
Kingston	Americas	Turin	Europe
Kobe	Asia	Vigo	Europe

resulted in a selection of very large cities drawn almost exclusively from North America and Western Europe. Accordingly, (a), (b), and (c) were used together. In applying the reporting criterion, we looked for cities with high levels of reporting and for which, if gaps were present, the missing observations were concentrated at points in time rather than scattered through the entire time series. The size criterion demanded that cities should be drawn from across the urban size hierarchy, rather than just large cities concentrated in the tail of the size distribution. Finally, the criterion of geographical location urged for as wide a geographical and environmental distribution of cities as possible.

Together, these three criteria enabled us to hone the 350 cities down to a shortlist of 120. A list of some of the 230 or so cities rejected at this stage appears in table 3.2.

A problem remained regarding the geographical balance of our 120 short-listed cities; disproportionate numbers were located in just a few countries (notably, England, Germany, and the United States), continents (Europe and North America) and latitudes (northern temperate latitudes). To ameliorate the problem, the second step of the selection process consisted of reducing the number of cities in overrepresented locations. In the end we eliminated twenty European and North American cities with relatively poor reporting completeness (see section 3.3.3) to leave us with the final set of 100 cities listed alphabetically in table 3.3.

We had originally hoped to study the 100 cities over the whole period for which data were continuously available in the *Weekly Abstract* – that is, the twenty-six years from 1887 to 1912 inclusive. However, as noted in section 2.3, 1887 was the first year in which the original *Bulletins of the Public Health* emerged in their new guise as the *Weekly Abstract*. In that first year, data collection was being restarted by the Marine Hospital Service for the first time in years. As a result, reports were very patchy and, during 1887, the time series

Table 3.3. *Alphabetical list of the 100 world cities used in this study*

City	Country	City	Country
Aix (Aachen)	Germany	Liège	Belgium
Alexandria	Egypt	Liverpool	England
Amsterdam	Holland	London	England
Athens	Greece	Lyon	France
Bahia	Brazil	Madras	India
Baltimore	United States	Manchester	England
Barranquilla	Colombia	Mannheim	Germany
Belfast	Ireland	Melbourne	Australia
Berlin	Germany	Messina	Italy
Birmingham	England	Mexico City	Mexico
Bombay	India	Milwaukee	United States
Boston	United States	Montevideo	Uruguay
Bristol	England	Moscow	Russia
Brussels	Belgium	Munich	Germany
Budapest	Austria-Hungary	Naples	Italy
Cairo	Egypt	Nashville	United States
Calcutta	India	New Orleans	United States
Cape Town	South Africa	New York	United States
Cardiff	Wales	Newark	United States
Cartagena	Colombia	Newcastle	England
Catania	Italy	Nuremberg	Germany
Chicago	United States	Odessa	Russia
Christiania	Norway	Osaka	Japan
Cincinnati	United States	Palermo	Italy
Cleveland	United States	Paris	France
Cologne	Germany	Pernambuco	Brazil
Colombo	Ceylon	Philadelphia	United States
Colon	Colombia	Port au Prince	Haiti
Constantinople	Turkey	Prague	Austria-Hungary
Copenhagen	Denmark	Providence	United States
Denver	United States	Rangoon	Burma
Detroit	United States	Rio de Janeiro	Brazil
Dublin	Ireland	Rotterdam	Holland
Dundee	Scotland	San Diego	United States
Durban	South Africa	San Francisco	United States
Edinburgh	Scotland	Santa Cruz	Spain
Frankfurt	Germany	Sheffield	England
Ghent	Belgium	Singapore	Malaya
Glasgow	Scotland	Smyrna	Turkey
Gothenburg	Sweden	Southampton	England
Guayaquilla	Ecuador	St Petersburg	Russia
Hamburg	Germany	Stockholm	Sweden
Havana	Cuba	Toledo	United States
Honolulu	United States	Trieste	Austria-Hungary
Kansas City, KS	United States	Venice	Italy
Kansas City, MO	United States	Vera Cruz	Mexico
La Guaira	Venezuela	Vienna	Austria-Hungary
Le Havre	France	Warsaw	Russia
Leeds	England	Washington, DC	United States
Leith	Scotland	Zurich	Switzerland

Note:
The city and country names are those current at the start of the study period in 1888.

gradually built up as more and more cities came on stream. To avoid this build-up phase, we decided to finalise our data matrix for each disease and all causes as covering the 100 cities for the 25-year period from 1888 to 1912.

3.3.2 The size distribution

Besides mortality data, the *Weekly Abstract* also gives, on an annual basis, the estimated total population of the cities covered. Such totals are notoriously variable (see the discussion in Davis, 1959). Even with modern census material, specifying the population of a city is fraught with difficulty. The boundaries of a city as given by its legal extent, its continuous built-up area, or its commuting area will invariably include slightly different populations: most cities will be underbounded in the sense that they have outgrown their legal boundaries. If one adds to this the uncertain nature of population counts in the late nineteenth century, the margin for error is very high. In this book, we decided to use the figures as given in the *Weekly Abstract*. The internal consistency that this provides over the twenty-five years outweighs the undoubtedly various ways in which the populations of the 100 cities were counted in different parts of the world. Cross-checking was carried out with national census information wherever possible (see appendix C). As a generalisation, cities in our sample drawn from European regions and North America appear to have their official census populations recorded in the *Abstract*. In developing parts of the world, population totals were undoubtedly estimates provided by the local reporting consul.

Population at 1888: Given this caveat, the total population of the 100 cities at the start of the study period was 35.46 million. The range of populations varied from the ten smallest cities, each of which had populations of less than 50,000 (La Guaira in Venezuela and Colon in Colombia were the smallest) to ten cities of 700,000 or over. The largest city in the 1888 list was London (England) with 5.52 million. There were five millionaire cities: London followed by Paris (2.26) and Berlin (1.41) in Western Europe, and New York (1.53) and Philadelphia (1.02) on the eastern seaboard of the United States. Altogether the top ten world cities summed to 15.76 million, some 44 per cent of the total for all 100 cities.

Population at 1912: By the end of the study period, the total population of the 100 cities had risen to 60 million. La Guaira and Colon remained the smallest, but the number of cities with under 50,000 people had dropped from ten to seven. Growth at the larger end of the spectrum had been spectacular with the populations of twenty-two cities now over 700,000 and ten over one million. The largest remained London (now with 7.3 million), but the rapidly growing New York (4.8 million) had overtaken Paris (2.9 million). Nine of the ten leading cities from 1888 retained their place in the top decile: the only change in membership was the arrival of Moscow at eighth place (previously eleventh) and the displacement of Bombay from ninth to eleventh place. Altogether the top ten cities in 1912 summed to 27.8 million, some 46 per cent of the overall total for all 100 cities.

Population change between 1888 and 1912: Figure 3.3 summarises the population changes that took place between 1888 and 1912. For these years, this plots the population of each of the 100 cities (log scale) against its rank. In ranking the cities, we assigned rank 1 to the largest and rank 100 to the smallest. The upper graph shows the full rank–size distribution at each date, while graphs A–D illustrate segments of the full distributions at a larger scale. The vectors show the movements of cities through the size hierarchy over the period. They show the relative stability of the upper and lower deciles of the distributions, and the dramatic movements both up and down that took place in the centre of the distributions.

The implication of these dramatic movements is that, although the total population of the 100 cities nearly doubled over the twenty-five years, the increases on a city-by-city basis were uneven. These ranged from a few per cent in the case of the Belgian cities of Liège (8.2 per cent) and Ghent (10.8) to Osaka (Japan) and New York (United States) which nearly tripled in size. But, as the vectors in figure 3.3 show, the increase was not related in any very consistent way to population size. Low growth and high growth appeared to occur for small, medium, and large cities (as measured from their 1888 baseline populations). Figure 3.4 confirms this by plotting for each city its percentage change in population over the period 1888–1912 against its population size in 1888. In so far as there is any regularity, the regression line on B shows a very weak downward trend which suggests a slight tendency for the smaller cities to grow marginally faster than the larger cities.

Population shares: Table 3.4 gives, on a country-by-country basis, the percentage of their total population represented by the cities in our sample. National population data c. 1900 have been taken from Showers (1973, Tabular Gazetteer 1, pp. 197–207). The median value is 6 per cent, while values range from 0.2 per cent (Spain) to 30.8 per cent (England). If we calculate the interquartile range, then the middle 50 per cent of countries range from 3.1 to 12.1 per cent in terms of their population representation by our sample cities.

3.3.3 The geographical distribution

(a) Distribution by country
As we noted in section 3.3.1, our choice of the final 100 cities represented a trade-off between (a) disease reporting coverage, (b) urban population size,

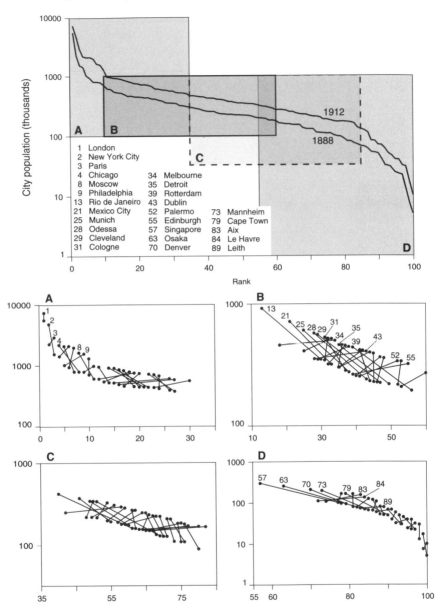

Figure 3.3. Rank–size distributions, 1888 and 1912. City populations (log scale) against rank (1=largest, 100=smallest) for the 100 sample cities,. The upper graph shows the full rank–size distribution at each date, while graphs A–D illustrate segments of the full distributions at a larger scale. The vectors show the movements of cities through the size hierarchy over the period.

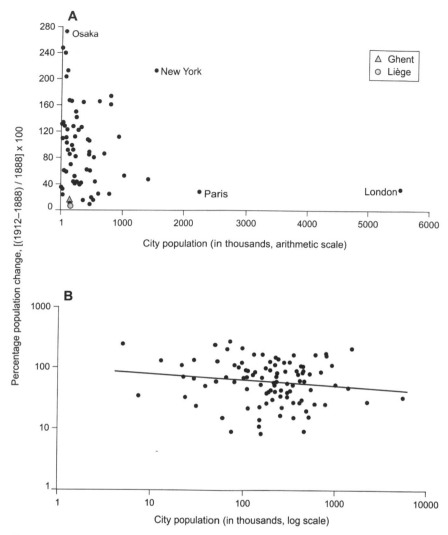

Figure 3.4. Changes in population size of the 100 world cities, 1888–1912. The vertical axis measures percentage increase and the horizontal axis the 1888 baseline population. (A) Arithmetic scales. (B) Logarithmic scales. The regression line shows a weak downward trend which suggests a slight tendency for the smaller cities to grow marginally faster than the larger cities.

Table 3.4. *Geographical distribution of the 100 cities by country*

Country	Number of cities	Percentage of national population 1900	Country	Number of cities	Percentage of national population 1900
Australia	1	12.1	Ireland	2	15.9
Austro-Hungary	4	6.0	Italy	5	3.9
Belgium	3	14.0	Japan	1	0.5
Brazil	3	6.8	Malaya	1	3.3
Burma	1	2.4	Mexico	2	2.7
Ceylon	1	3.6	Norway	1	10.3
Colombia	3	1.7	Russia	4	2.9
Cuba	1	15.3	Scotland	4	28.9
Denmark	1	14.3	South Africa	2	2.9
Ecuador	1	4.7	Spain	1	0.2
Egypt	2	9.3	Sweden	2	7.4
England	9	30.8	Switzerland	1	5.0
France	3	7.9	Turkey	2	4.9
Germany	8	7.4	United States	21	12.2
Greece	1	8.3	Uruguay	1	23.5
Haiti	1	4.6	Venezuela	1	0.5
Holland	2	17.4	Wales	1	6.0
India	3	0.7			

and (c) the geographical range of city locations. Table 3.4 shows the distribution of the 100 cities by country. One-fifth are in the conterminous United States; a further US city (Honolulu) is located in the Pacific and is treated in chapters 4–6 as part of a general Rest of the World region. Two further countries (England with nine and Germany with eight) are the next largest contributors to the sample.

In three countries on the list in table 3.4 (the United States, England, and Germany), a large number of cities was potentially available for analysis. As described in section 3.3.1, an arbitrary decision had to be made to include only those best recorded to avoid swamping the sample with these countries which are all located in the then more economically developed parts of the world; reliance on a data coverage criterion alone would have resulted in picking a surfeit of cities from this narrow geographical and economic spectrum. In the end, the decision was made to omit cities with less complete recording from these overrepresented countries. So Atlanta, Panama, and San Juan were dropped from the United States contingent (two of them in United States territory outside the conterminous United States). Likewise Plymouth, South

Shields, and Sunderland were dropped from England, and Barmen, Bremen, Leipzig, Königsberg, and Stettin from Germany.

If we now discount the United States, England, and Germany, the remaining sixty-two cities were distributed among thirty-two countries. Three (Austria-Hungary, Scotland, and Russia) each contributed four, while a further five (Belgium, Brazil, Colombia, France, and India) contributed three each.

Thus, in overall terms for our 100-city sample, a fifth of the cities are located in a single country and half the cities in six countries. At the other extreme, sixteen countries are represented by a single city and a further seven countries by only two cities.

(b) Distribution by continent
In terms of their distribution by continent, Europe dominates with forty-eight cities, followed by North America (excluding Honolulu) with twenty. Both Latin America and Asia have thirteen cities (Turkey and Russia have been included with Asia for this purpose). Africa has only four cities and Australasia a single city.

Our wish to choose a sample of cities spanning as wide a geographical range as possible has led to three anomalies. Melbourne, the sole Australian city in the sample, has a very incomplete record, with deaths from all causes reported for less than 1 per cent of the total weekly time series. The city was retained because percentage reporting for the individual diseases was somewhat better than that for all causes, and because Melbourne occupies a unique location in an otherwise epidemiologically blank area of our world map. Somewhat similar arguments apply in the case of the two South African cities, although here both Cape Town and Durban have fuller coverage with, respectively, 4 and 12 per cent completeness of the weekly record for all causes of death. Leaving these three anomalies aside, no city in our sample has less than 18 per cent reporting of all causes.

(c) Distribution by environment
From Hippocrates onwards, disease has been seen to be related to the nature of the environment within which it was set, a theme to which we return in some detail in sections 4.5 and 5.4. We look here at the ways in which the 100 cities are positioned in respect to four environmental parameters: latitude, elevation, temperature, and precipitation. Data for these parameters have been taken from Showers (1973, Tabular Gazetteer 2, pp. 321–96).

Latitude: The geographical distribution of the 100 cities is mapped in figure 3.5. The inset histograms show their frequency distributions by latitude and longitude. Seventy-one of the cities lie in the northern hemisphere in the latitudinal range, 35° N to 55° N. Of the 100 cities, nineteen lie in the tropics, four

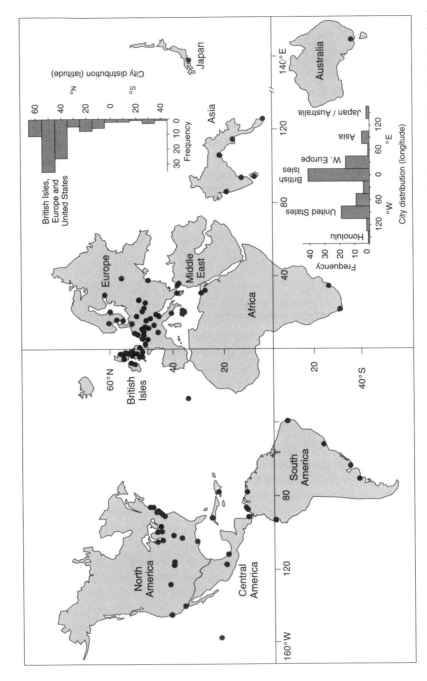

Figure 3.5. Geographical distribution of the 100 cities. The inset bar charts show the frequency distributions of the cities by longitude and latitude.

in the southern hemisphere middle-latitudes, and the remainder (seventy-seven) in the northern hemisphere middle-latitudes. The marked bunching of cities between (a) latitudes 40°–60° N and (b) longitudes 0°–40° E and 90°–100° W is evident. From an epidemiological viewpoint, latitude exerts a critical influence upon the occurrence of disease through its influence upon seasonal patterns of incidence, but the meridional distribution (longitude) is less significant. The implication of figure 3.5 is that there is a stronger representation of temperate northern mid-latitudes than we would have ideally wished, but there is a least one city in every 10° band of latitude from 40° S to 60° N.

While figure 3.5 illustrates the geographical distribution of cities by latitude and longitude in an effective manner, the spatial concentration of cities in certain parts of the globe makes the map projection unsuitable for the purposes of labelling and city recognition. Accordingly, we devised the projection illustrated in figure 3.6 by plotting the cities on the basis of their ranks on longitude and latitude. The most southerly city in the sample was assigned rank 1 on latitude; the most westerly city rank 1 on longitude. The projection preserves the relative geographical locations of the cities while avoiding the spatial 'congestion' that occurs with the British Isles and Western Europe on a conventional map projection like figure 3.5. This slightly special projection is used in a few places in chapters 4–6 where we need to plot all 100 cities with names.

As figure 3.6 shows, the two most poleward cities in the sample occur in the northern hemisphere: the two capital cities of Christiania (Norway) and St Petersburg (Russia) at 60° N. The peculiarities of land/sea and population distribution in the southern hemisphere mean that here the most poleward cities are Melbourne (Australia) and Cape Town (South Africa) at 38° S and 35° S respectively.

Elevation: One indicator of the physical environment of a city is provided by its average elevation above mean sea level. Given the critical economic role of water transport in city growth up to the middle of the nineteenth century, it is not surprising that two-thirds of the 100 cities were on tidewater locations. Of the remainder, most 'inland' cities were also located near the coast or on major inland rivers (for example, Paris on the River Seine) or on lakes (for example, Chicago on Lake Michigan). The three cities with the highest elevations in the sample were Mexico City (5,500 feet), Denver (5,300 feet), and Munich (1,700 feet), each with a mid-continental location.

Temperature: The remaining three environmental measures were climatic. The average annual temperature for the 100 cities was 58 °F, with two of the Russian cities, Moscow and St Petersburg (both averaging 40 °F), as the coldest. At the other extreme, twelve of the cities with tropical locations had

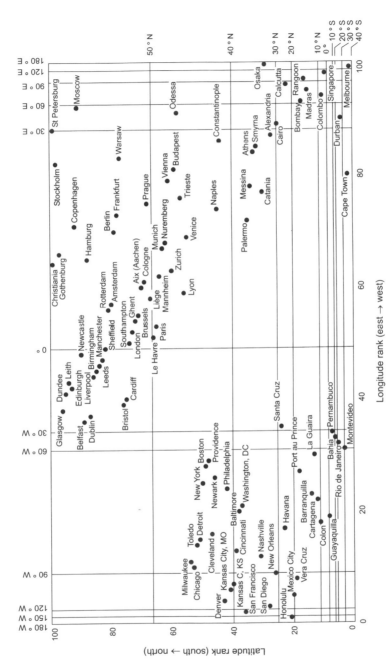

Figure 3.6. Geographical distribution of cities on a map projection constructed on the basis of the ranks of city longitude and latitude. The most southerly city in the sample was assigned rank 1 on latitude; the most westerly city rank 1 on longitude. The projection preserves the relative geographical locations of the cities while avoiding, for plotting purposes, the spatial 'congestion' that occurs with the British Isles and Western Europe on conventional maps like figure 3.5.

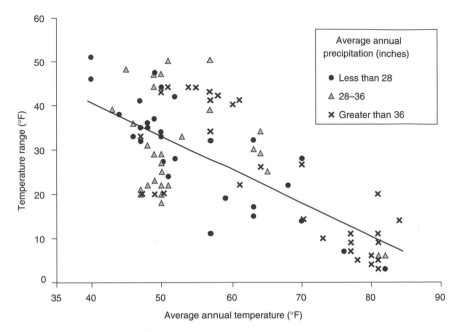

Figure 3.7. Relationship between temperature range and average annual temperature for the 100 cities with regression line plotted. Temperature range is defined as the difference between the average temperatures of the warmest and coldest months. The points have been coded on the basis of the average annual precipitation (in inches) of the cities.

average temperatures of 80 °F and above. The Indian city of Madras and the Venezuelan city of La Guaira were the warmest.

Temperature range is defined as the difference between the temperatures of the warmest and coldest months. As shown in figure 3.7, the range of temperatures is inversely related to average temperature. Cities with high year-round temperatures in the tropics and subtropics tend to have low ranges: thus the near-equatorial cities of Colon, Colombo, Guayaquilla, and La Guaira (in Latin America) and Singapore (in South and East Asia) all have ranges of 5 °F or less. Mid-continental cities tend to have the highest ranges, with Chicago, the two Kansas Cities, and Moscow all having ranges of 50 °F or more. Between the two extremes, most mid-latitude coastal cities have ranges of around 30 °F.

Precipitation: The average precipitation for the 100 cities was 35 inches per year. The twenty wettest cities, with rainfall of over 60 inches, were all located in the tropics or subtropics; Rangoon (104 inches) and Singapore (95 inches) were the wettest. The precipitation figures for the cities have been grouped into three equal classes, and the points in figure 3.7 have been coded on this basis.

(d) Other geographical characteristics

City spacing: Two pairs of 'twin cities' have been included in our sample: Kansas City (Kansas) and Kansas City (Missouri) on opposite banks of the Mississippi, and Edinburgh with its seaport town, Leith, on the banks of the Forth in Scotland. New York and Newark in the United States also serve as comparator cities.

Age of city: Establishing the age of a city depends entirely upon the definition used. The date when a city achieved a particular legal status may be very different from the date at which it passed a particular population threshold. Nonetheless, it is evident that Rome is at least two thousand years older than, say, Melbourne in Australia and a rough characterisation by age may be possible. In this section and later in section 4.6.1, we use the foundation dates given in Showers (1973, Tabular Gazetteer 2, pp. 227–320) as an indicator of age.

The median age for the 100 cities was around 700 years; that is, the median foundation date was around AD 1200. Sixteen of the cities were over two thousand years old, with three settlements (Athens, Smyrna, and Zurich) defined by Showers as over three thousand years old. At the other end of the scale stand the New World cities of North America and Australasia. Nine of the cities were founded post 1800; Denver (1858) and Kansas City, Kansas (1843), in the western United States, and Melbourne (1835) were the youngest.

3.4 The city–disease matrix

3.4.1 The nature of the matrix

(a) Crude mortality
For each of the six diseases and all causes, the data matrix constructed from the records in the *Weekly Abstract* consisted of the weekly reported number of deaths (rows) by city (columns). Each matrix potentially contains nearly 136,000 data points (1,357 weeks between 1887 and 1912, $\times 100$ cities).[3] Since there are effectively no data for 1887, each observed time series is, in practice, reduced to 1,304 weeks from 1888 to 1912 inclusive, leading to the definition of the 25-year time series described in section 3.3.

However, even if we consider the twenty-five years of weekly observations, we still do not have a full matrix of data for each disease. Missing observations are common, sometimes in blocks, but more generally as individual absent reports scattered throughout each disease matrix. As we noted in section 3.3, to reduce the magnitude of the problem, only cities with more than 18 per cent of weeks with reports on deaths from all causes were included in the 100-city set. For the cities with missing observations included in our sample, one approach, rejected here, would have been to interpolate the absent data. If this had been done then, inevitably, the results of any analysis would have reflected in part the interpolation model employed. A second approach, which we have followed, is to take the reported data at face value and then to amalgamate the data in time and space so that the 'holes' in the matrix disappear. This is the method successfully followed by the authors in an earlier study of monthly measles reports for twenty Pacific islands, 1946–81 (Cliff and Haggett, 1985, pp. 70–6).

Experimentation soon showed that, for most cities in the sample, relatively few months were without some data. Accordingly, the decision was taken to combine each city's weekly reports into monthly data. This raised two secondary issues: (i) how to aggregate the weeks into months; (ii) whether to make allowance for the fact that each month's data might comprise one to five weeks of weekly data (depending upon the number of present/absent weekly reports). We consider each issue in turn.

In our study period, the weekly returns were generally made for the week ending on a Friday or Saturday (cf. section 2.4.1). Accordingly, some years (for example 1888) had fifty-three weeks (Fridays/Saturdays), and weeks straddled the boundaries of the calendar months. The simple decision rule was taken to allocate weeks to the month in which the Friday/Saturday of report fell; no attempt was made to 'share' between the months, on a *pro rata* basis, weeks which fell across month boundaries. In the same spirit, no attempt was made to weight the monthly reported deaths on the basis of the number of weeks for which data were reported. For example if, in a given month, reports were available for two of the four weeks, but were missing for the other two, we could have opted to double the observed count to compensate for the missing reports.

It should be apparent from the above discussion that the overarching principle in setting up the basic data matrices was to keep as close as possible to the raw reported data. By avoiding interpolation models, and weighting and sharing of data, we believe that our analyses will have the optimum chance of identifying actual features of the reports rather than a mixture of characteristics that are a complex function of the recorded data and assumptions we have made in patching together the time series. Accordingly, all the analysis to be described in subsequent chapters is derived from the monthly time series of reported deaths (crude mortality) for each of the 100 cities. From these data, dependent matrices for different geographical aggregations were obtained by combining the columns in various ways to define global time series (studied in chapter 4) and series for ten world regions (chapter 5). The matrices were also modelled in their basic 100-city form (chapter 6).

(b) Mortality rates

We used the annual city populations given in the *Weekly Abstract* (see section 3.3.2) as the basis of our rate calculations. Linear interpolation was used to generate monthly population time series from the annual totals. For each city and disease, a monthly death rate per 100,000 population was then readily computed by dividing the crude monthly death rate by the city population (in 100,000s) in the same month.

3.4.2 Data reliability

One of the spectres that haunts all historical research using statistical data is 'What do the numbers actually mean?' In a review of the problems of inter-pretation associated with early mortality data, MacKellar (1993) identifies six basic complications: (a) definition of death, (b) misallocation of deaths by place of occurrence, (c) misallocation of deaths by time of occurrence, (d) age misreporting, (e) completeness of registration, and (f) cause misreporting. Both individually and jointly they can undermine the validity of any general-isations drawn.

MacKellar's complication (a) refers mainly to the way in which stillbirths and neonatal deaths are classified. This can be ignored for data used in this book which deal with infectious diseases and deaths from all causes. Complication (d) is not relevant since analysis by age of death is not under-taken. Complication (b) might well be a major problem for small communi-ties or where fine spatial distinctions are drawn. But for the 100 cities selected, the sheer size of the communities (the average population in 1900 was 469,000) suggests that such effects are likely to be marginal. With respect to misreport-ing by time, complication (c), there would certainly be delays in reporting. The weekly figures returned to Washington that appeared in each *Weekly Abstract* must have included deaths that had actually occurred some weeks earlier but which were reported in the week in question. However, since most of our analysis uses monthly, quarterly, and annual aggregations of the weekly data, this problem is likely to have been partially overcome by averaging over time periods longer than a week.

The two remaining complications are more problematical. As regards (e), completeness of registration, we note that death registration of an entire pop-ulation was rare at our time period. The sources of data drawn upon by the Marine Hospital Service to produce the basic mortality tables have already been described in section 2.5.1. Both explicit exclusions (for example, by reli-gious group) and age exclusions (for example, deaths of infants) varied over time and from country to country. Estimating the completeness of death reg-istration for 100 cities located in thirty-five different countries over a 25-year time period would be a formidable research programme in its own right. We note the two main lines of approach to the difficulty: the *indirect* 'matching' studies of Marks, Seltzer, and Krotki (1974) and of Crimmins (1980), and the *indirect* demographic modelling of William Brass (described in MacKellar, 1993, pp. 211–12).

In tackling (e), we have not tried to emulate these authors. Rather, we have tried to minimise the problem in two ways. First, we use *deaths from all causes* as a baseline against which the rise and fall of specific epidemic diseases can be traced as a proportion. Second, we lay stress in our analysis on broad comparative trends rather than specific estimates and report the crude figures as stated in the *Weekly Abstract*. We hope that, by making the vast data in the *Abstract* available to a wider audience, demographers may be able to rework our findings in subsequent research.

The treatment of complication (f), misclassification of cause of death, must be considered on a disease-by-disease basis.

(a) Deaths from individual causes

Preston, Keyfitz, and Schoen (1972) have produced a comprehensive review of the problems which can occur under (f). Errors can arise from changing conventions of disease nomenclature through to the difficulty of assigning cause when the cause of death is multiple and complex. Biases can also ensue from differential registration: if deaths among the elderly are systematically underreported, the resulting cause-of-death structure will understate the role of chronic and degenerative diseases. Conversely if the deaths of very young children are underreported, infectious diseases afflicting children may be underreported.

In selecting our six indicator diseases, we have tried to choose those infectious diseases which not only produce rather large numbers of deaths (to aid statistical analysis) but also those where diagnosis is fairly robust and cause of death is reasonably secure. Nonetheless, severe problems remain. For example, in the case of enteric fever, the accurate diagnosis of typhoid at the onset of the disease is possible in only a minority of patients. Where fever may be the only complaint, typhoid is easily confused with a host of other diseases that share its geographical patterns (for example, malaria, hepatitis, tuberculosis, brucellosis, and typhus). As early as 1896, Fernand Widal determined that most persons infected with *S. typhi* develop antibodies to its cell wall (O antigen) and flagellae (H antigen) which can be determined through a Widal blood test (LeBaron and Taylor, 1993, p. 1074). In practice, the test was little used in the period covered by the survey and the security of the 'enteric fever' label for mortality must rest largely on the fact that the later and final stages of typhoid and paratyphoid are much easier to diagnose than the earlier.

By contrast, measles is rather more straightforward. Diagnosis of measles will usually follow from the distinctive clinical course of normal measles, depending heavily on the character of the rash, in particular the presence of

Koplik's Spots. These were first described by the New York physician Henry Koplik (1858–1902) in 1896. Koplik observed that: 'On the buccal mucous membrane and the inside of the lips we invariably see a distinct eruption. It consists of small irregular spots of a bright red colour. In the centre of each spot there is noted, in strong daylight, a minute bluish white speck' (Koplik, cited in Bloomfield, 1958, p. 434). Koplik's Spots have been shown by modern electron microscopy to be focal areas of virus proliferation in the oral mucosa.

But even with measles problems remain. Ramsay and Emond (1978) have reviewed the overlap with other conditions. Confusion with *scarlet fever* should not occur if note is made of the state of the tongue and throat, and absence of rash on the face. *Infectious mononucleosis* and occasionally *paratyphoid fever* may be accompanied by eruptions suggestive of measles. Laryngeal stridor and the paroxysmal cough in the prodromal stage of measles are sometimes responsible for an erroneous diagnosis of *pertussis*, as is the paroxysmal cough due to areas of pulmonary collapse following measles. *Drug* eruptions which are frequently morbilliform in appearance do not evolve from above downwards.

Hardy (1993b, p. 991) argues that, by the end of the seventeenth century, the identity of scarlet fever was well recognised, although much epidemiological confusion remained, and still remains, over the respective roles of scarlet fever, streptococcal sore throat, and diphtheria (*cynanche maligna*) in seventeenth-century and eighteenth-century epidemics. But, by the nineteenth century, scarlet fever records were more reliable.

With epidemic diseases we suspect that, during the higher points of epidemic waves, there would be great pressure on physicians and a tendency to ascribe cause of death to the widely prevailing condition. If this is so, the peaks of particular epidemic diseases might well be slightly overrepresented.

In summary, then, the data recorded in the *Weekly Abstract* will be subject to errors of misreporting in time and space as well as errors of misdiagnosis. But, rather than adopt a counsel of despair, we have tried to minimise the chance of error by frequently working with data that have been aggregated in various ways from weeks and cities to, for example, months, countries, and regions. We have also chosen diseases with comparatively low risks of misdiagnosis by our time period. Taken together, these techniques will tend to increase the signal-to-error ratio of the data and give greater confidence in the results of any analysis.

3.4.3 Disease coverage: the basic pattern

(a) Total deaths

The grand totals of deaths over the whole period for the 100 cities are given in table 3.5. Nearly 18.5 million deaths were recorded from all causes. Of these, more than 2 million (11.1 per cent) were caused by the six selected infectious

Table 3.5. *Total number of reported deaths in the 100 world cities, 1888–1912*

Disease	Reported deaths	Share of all six fevers (%)	Adjusted share of all six fevers (%)
All causes	18,456,917		
Tuberculosis	982,752	48.2	61.3
Diphtheria	290,239	14.2	10.5
Measles	268,178	13.1	9.9
Enteric fever	181,795	8.9	6.6
Whooping cough	163,584	8.0	6.1
Scarlet fever	154,002	7.5	5.6
All six infectious diseases	2,040,550	99.9	100.0

diseases used in this study. The leading cause of death within the infectious disease group was tuberculosis which accounted for almost 1 million deaths (48 per cent of the total). Of the remaining five infectious diseases, the two leading causes of death were diphtheria (14 per cent) and measles (13 per cent). The remaining three diseases each resulted in between 7 and 9 per cent of the total deaths from infectious diseases.

In one respect, table 3.5 underestimates the importance of tuberculosis. Reporting for this disease did not begin until the very end of the nineteenth century. It started in the United States in week 49 of 1899. For the rest of the world, the earliest report is for Havana (Cuba) in week 29 of 1896. The next city to commence reporting was Montevideo (Uruguay) in week 30 of 1899. Once generalised tuberculosis recording commenced, its collecting rate was slightly better than that for the other diseases, a reflection of its clinical significance. For the period for which tuberculosis data are available, the average reporting rate over the 100 cities was 74.8 per cent. If the death rates for the six diseases given in column 2 of table 3.5 are scaled to allow for the late start-up for tuberculosis reporting, then the importance of tuberculosis is increased to 61 per cent (see the third column of table 3.5).

In a much smaller degree, the comments for tuberculosis hold also for measles. In the United States, the recording of measles mortality began in week 28 of 1888. For the rest of the world, it was slightly earlier, in week 22 of 1888.

(b) Reporting rates
The completeness of reporting varies by disease. For deaths from all causes, three cities recorded information in more than 90 per cent of the weeks in their

time series (Palermo, 94 per cent; Glasgow, 92 per cent; and Amsterdam, 91 per cent). New York and Nashville (90 per cent) were the best recorded US cities.

For tuberculosis in the 100 cities over the whole period, data were recorded in just over one-third of the total possible weekly time periods (37.6 per cent); the rate for each of the other five diseases was nearly two-thirds. The contrast between tuberculosis and the other five diseases is illustrated in figure 3.8. Diphtheria reporting across the 100 cities has a characteristic skewed distribution about an average coverage rate of 64.7 per cent of all weeks. The modal value lies in the 80 per cent band, but ten cities had over 90 per cent of weeks with reports; Palermo (Italy), Amsterdam (Holland), and Glasgow (Scotland) bettered 95 per cent. The diagrams for enteric fever and scarlet fever (averages 64.8 and 64.6 per cent) are similar to that for diphtheria, with the same three cities achieving better than 95 per cent of their weekly time series with disease reports. Measles (63.3) and whooping cough (62.5) were slightly less well recorded; for these diseases, only three cities (Amsterdam, Palermo, and New York) had records for more than 90 per cent of the weeks.

The late commencement of tuberculosis recording has been allowed for in figure 3.8 by plotting the frequency distribution as per cent reporting from 1888 to 1912 (black bars), and as per cent reporting in the period 1899–1912. This switches the modal class from the 41–50 per cent to the 91–100 per cent.

3.4.4 Disease coverage: the frequency distribution

In this section, we examine the frequency distributions of mortality values in the cities, and apply a statistical analysis to them. We consider first some general issues and then discuss the results of the analysis.

(a) General issues in frequency analysis

Frequency distribution: The concept of a frequency distribution is best illustrated by a particular example. Figure 3.9 plots the monthly time series of crude mortality for each of the six diseases in different cities. If we consider that for tuberculosis in Newark (USA), then the time series plot (graph, upper) may be reduced to a frequency distribution (bar chart, lower) by counting the number of months in the time series in which 1, 2, . . . deaths were reported. This frequency distribution characterises the time series plot. The Newark time series displays relatively regular cycles of mortality, and this type of time series yields a symmetric 'normal' frequency distribution. If we look at the diphtheria time series by way of contrast, we see that, of the months with reports, high mortality was recorded in a few in 1893–4 but that low mortality was reported in the other months. Such a time series pattern yields a sharply peaked and asymmetric frequency distribution. The remaining plots

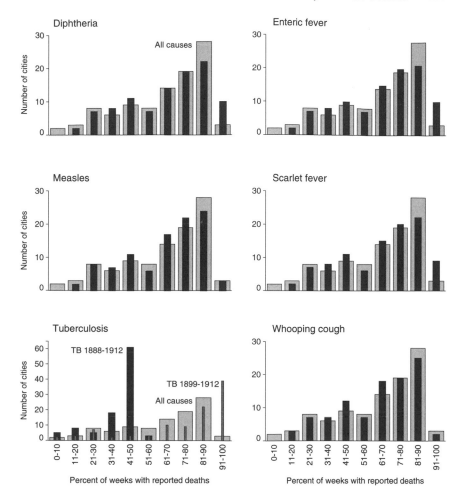

Figure 3.8. The coverage rate for infectious disease reporting. The number of cities in the sample (vertical axis) is plotted against the percentage of weeks in their time series with disease reports (horizontal axis) for the six marker diseases of diphtheria, enteric fever, measles, scarlet fever, tuberculosis, and whooping cough. In all graphs, the bar chart for the named disease (black) is plotted against deaths from all causes (light stipple). For example, for diphtheria, over twenty of the cities studied reported mortality information in 81–90 per cent of the weeks in the time series (the modal class); for all causes, nearly thirty cities achieved the same rate of reporting. Note that for tuberculosis, most cities recorded deaths only from the turn of the century, so that two frequency distributions for that disease are plotted: coverage over the whole period (black) and coverage 1899–1912 (mid-grey).

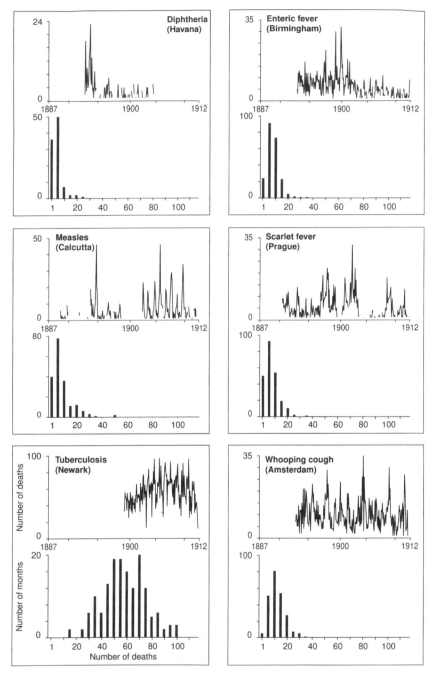

Figure 3.9. Frequency distribution analysis of time series. For each of the six diseases, the monthly time series of reported deaths (graph, upper) is re-plotted as a frequency distribution (bar chart, lower) that gives the number of months in the time series in which 1, 2, . . . deaths were reported. The zero class has been omitted.

in figure 3.9 show how different time series traces alter the shape of the frequency distribution.

Treatment of zero values: In figure 3.9, the frequency distributions have been drawn only for positive counts of deaths (one death or more per month); months with zero values have been ignored. The decision to analyse only positive values was made because the tables in the *Weekly Abstract* do not differentiate unambiguously between 'zero deaths' and 'missing observations'. In the absence of secondary evidence, the choice lay between two assumptions:

(i) Assumption A: The presence of a 'zero', '–', or a gap in a column (the practice varied over the 25-year period) indicated no deaths for a given disease had occurred in that city during the week reported. In some instances, it was clear that this was inherently unlikely – for example, where a break occurred in the middle of a weekly sequence of values that gave every indication of an ongoing intense and sustained epidemic; this was unlikely to have abated suddenly for a single, short period.

(ii) Assumption B: The presence of a 'zero', '–', or gap in a column indicated that there was no information as to whether deaths for a given disease had occurred in that city during the week reported.

For the six diseases, assumption B was adopted on the grounds that it could be unambiguously applied to all the data. Any other approach would have meant uncertain switching between definitions which were unlikely to remain constant either over time or from one city to another. The analysis which follows both in this chapter and in the remainder of the book is therefore based on the number of weeks in which there was positive evidence of a disease being present in a given city as confirmed by one or more deaths being recorded in that week.

For the combined total of deaths from all causes, the question of missing data rarely arose but, on those few occasions when it did, it was treated under assumption A. Even more rarely, the total for all deaths in a given week was *less* than the combined total of deaths reported for the individual diseases. In such cases, an error in either reporting, transcription, or printing was assumed to have occurred (highly likely given the long chain of communication from the death in a given city to the printed table, and the millions of individual figures being transcribed); such entries were discarded, and the cell was treated as a missing observation.

(b) Statistical analysis of the frequency distributions
$S - I$ *characteristics*: One approach to comparing the 100-city time series for each disease is to compute the frequency distributions of all the series as outlined under (a) above, and then to use the so-called $S - I$ *index* as a basis for comparisons.

The theoretical properties of the $S - I$ index are described in Ord (1972). It

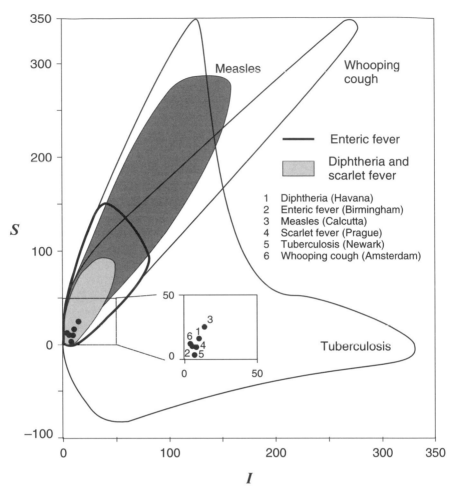

Figure 3.10. *S–I* regions for the 100 cities. Each hull contains the *S–I* values of all 100 cities for each marker disease. The locations in *S–I* space of the sample cities used in figure 3.8 are marked. *S–I* is defined in the text.

has been applied to geographical problems by James, Cliff, Haggett, and Ord (1970), and it is calculated as follows. Let m_1, m_2, and m_3 denote the sample mean, variance, and third central moment respectively of a frequency distribution. Then

$$S = m_3/m_2 \qquad (3.1)$$

and

$$I = m_2/m_1. \qquad (3.2)$$

Using the $S - I$ index, all discrete frequency distributions can be plotted on a chart in such a way that their locations will reflect the shapes of their frequency distributions.

The $S - I$ patterns: The 700 $S - I$ indices (100 cities × 6 diseases and all causes) were computed from the frequency distributions of each time series. Stage 1 was to plot the $S - I$ values for the cities on a disease-by-disease basis. This has been done in figures 3.10 and 3.11. Figure 3.10 shows that, although the hulls overlap, there are substantial differences between the diseases. The hull for tuberculosis has the biggest area, and this implies that variations in the city frequency distributions (and hence in the corresponding time series plots) are greatest for this disease. The other five diseases occupy similar areas of the $S - I$ chart, oriented along a southwest–northeast axis stretching from the origin of the chart. Measles and whooping cough have hulls of similar size, as do diphtheria, enteric fever, and scarlet fever.

The diagram indicates that the time series of these six diseases across the 100 cities fall into three broad groups: group 1 consists of diphtheria, enteric fever, and scarlet fever; group 2 consists of measles and whooping cough; group 3 contains only tuberculosis. Figure 3.1, which shows the lengths of the incubation and communicability periods for each of the diseases, suggests a possible basis for the disease groupings. As discussed in section 3.2.3, five of the diseases (diphtheria, enteric fever, measles, scarlet fever, and whooping cough) have very short incubation periods compared with tuberculosis. This may account for the very much larger hull for tuberculosis. In the same way, the period of communicability of tuberculosis is substantially longer than for the other five diseases, so that this disease is altogether different from the other five in terms of its frequency distributions.

It would be too much to hope that we might account for the patterning of diseases into groups 1 and 2 above on the basis of the total duration of their incubation and communicability periods. But, for this to hold exactly, we would expect scarlet fever and whooping cough to swap groups; this would then enable us to characterise a new group 1 (diphtheria, enteric fever, and whooping cough) as consisting of diseases of relatively long overall duration, and a new group 2 (measles and scarlet fever) as one of short-duration diseases.

Despite these complications, it does appear that the $S - I$ index is drawing our attention to a very important and, in one sense, obvious point: the time series for each of the six diseases will be fundamentally influenced by the duration of their periods of incubation and communicability. Thus we may expect to see the aetiologies of each of these diseases reflected fairly and squarely in the time series plots.

One statistical property of the $S - I$ index that hampers interpretation is the fact that neither S nor I is dimensionless and their values (since we are dealing with discrete frequency distributions) will reflect the magnitude of reported deaths. Accordingly, in stage 2 of our $S - I$ analysis, we looked at the position of individual cities within the disease hulls to determine how location within a hull is influenced by the form of the frequency distribution.

The individual charts in figure 3.11 show the locations of each of the 100 cities within the hulls for deaths both from all causes and from each of the six diseases. The general shapes of the hulls illustrated in figure 3.10 have been redrawn at a smaller scale and plotted as the first chart. Note that the scales of the charts vary to reflect the differing ranges of $S - I$ values obtained for each disease. Where possible, cities have been named.

To assess the relationship between $S - I$ values and the nature of the corresponding frequency distribution, each $S - I$ pair was associated with its frequency distribution plot and the associations were then inspected visually. We found that, as we moved up the diagonal from the origin of the $S - I$ chart to the northeast corner, frequency distributions changed from J-shaped to positively skewed unimodal distributions, through to symmetric, bell-shaped curves. In terms of the original time series, unimodal bell-shaped frequency distributions are characteristic of strongly cyclical time series. Thus it appears that this frequency distribution approach is capturing the degree of regularity in a time series. A well-behaved epidemic with build-up, peak, and fade-out phases will be bell-shaped and yield a bell-shaped frequency distribution (cf. tuberculosis in figure 3.9). Irregular time series will generate J-shaped frequency distributions (cf. diphtheria in figure 3.9). Such time series irregularity is more likely in small cities where epidemic episodes of a disease will be separated by periods when little or no mortality from that disease will occur. It may also be an artefact of reporting, with sudden bursts of deaths because a consulate was especially vigilant, for example; this is an example of MacKellar's complication (c) discussed in section 3.4.2.

Stage 3 of our frequency distribution approach was to use cluster analysis (see Cormack, 1971, for a discussion of clustering methods) to classify the 100 cities on the basis of their $S - I$ values. For each disease, we took the 100 $S - I$ values as the data input and used the complete linkage method to determine groups on the basis of inter-city distances in the $S - I$ space. This method uses the most distant pair of objects in two clusters to calculate between-cluster distances. It tends to produce compact globular clusters and, unlike many other cluster methods, does produce a hierarchical tree with strictly increasing amalgamation distances. The correlation between the assignments of cities to clusters for each disease appears in table 3.6.

All the correlations in table 3.6 are positive and eleven of the twenty-one in the lower triangle are statistically significant at the $\alpha = 0.01$ level (one-tailed test). Thus, although none of the correlations is very large, we conclude that there is some overlap in the classification of cities from one disease to another. Five of the six diseases were significantly correlated with all causes, reflecting

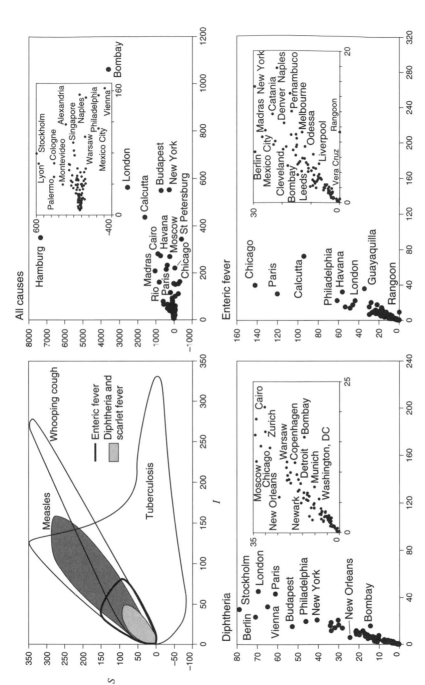

Figure 3.11. City locations in the hulls of figure 3.10 on a disease-by-disease basis. $S–I$ is defined in the text. The general positions of the hulls illustrated in figure 3.10 have been reproduced at a small scale in the first chart. (Figure continues overleaf.)

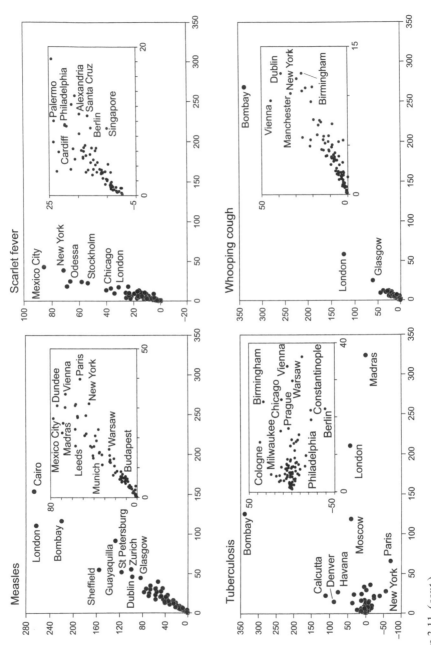

Figure 3.11. (cont.)

Table 3.6. *Correlation between cluster assignments of cities for six diseases and all causes*

	All causes	Diphtheria	Enteric fever	Measles	Scarlet fever	Tuberculosis	Whooping cough
All	1.00						
Diphtheria	0.32*	1.00					
Enteric fever	0.23*	0.15	1.0				
Measles	0.36*	0.29*	0.21*	1.00			
Scarlet fever	0.13	0.22*	0.03	0.08	1.00		
Tuberculosis	0.57*	0.24*	0.14	0.16	0.28*	1.00	
Whooping cough	0.27*	0.18	0.08	0.33*	0.06	0.16	1.00

Note:
* Significant at the $\alpha = 0.01$ level (one-tailed test).

the fact that each disease is, of course, a component of all deaths. For three of the diseases (enteric fever, scarlet fever, and whooping cough), there was significant overlap in the city classification with only one other disease (measles for enteric fever and whooping cough; diphtheria for scarlet fever). There is no simple relationship between (a) duration of the incubation and communicability periods of the different diseases and (b) degree of overlap in the classification of cities. We conclude that, although some cities may have similar time series behaviour across diseases in terms of reported crude mortality, many do not; because one disease behaves in a particular way in a given city, there is no reason to expect that another disease will behave in essentially the same way.

3.5 Conclusions

Between 1888 and 1912, weekly mortality data of one kind or another were published in the *Weekly Abstract* for some eleven diseases and 350 cities scattered around the world. In this chapter, we have rehearsed the reasons for our particular choice of the six diseases and 100 cities that we ultimately selected to form the basis of the analyses to be described in chapters 4–6. Two main criteria were employed in fixing our choice: percentage of weeks in the time series for which reports were made and geographical coverage. We sought time series that were as complete as possible, and cities from a wide range of geographical and economic environments.

For each of the diseases (diphtheria, enteric fever, measles, scarlet fever, tuberculosis, and whooping cough), we described their main aetiological and epidemiological characteristics up to the beginning of our study period. The important issues of data reliability and potential sources of error in our data were discussed. This led us to propose a research design in which most of the data to be analysed have been aggregated from their original weekly–city format to larger units such as months and years in time, or to countries and regions in space. By so doing, we hope to mitigate MacKellar's errors of mis-allocation of deaths by time and location of occurrence. Our handling of the data will not eliminate errors, but we anticipate that the approach will increase the signal-to-noise ratio.

In the final part of the chapter, the time series for each of the diseases and all causes were analysed using the $S - I$ index. This showed that the aetiological characteristics of each disease, especially the duration of the incubation and communicability periods, have a profound impact upon their time series behaviour; and the greater the duration of these periods, the greater was the variety from city to city in their time series characteristics. Further, there was only limited evidence to suggest that, in a given city, different diseases would have similar time series plots despite the fact that the main transmission routes (respiratory and oral) for all six diseases require close interpersonal contact in some form or another.

We have stressed in chapter 1 the special position that our time period from 1888 to 1912 occupies from a medical point of view. It coincides with the golden age of bacteriological studies when the aetiology of many diseases, including five of those selected here, was being systematically understood for the first time; mortality from them still remained high and yet fresh treatments could now be contemplated as a result of the new scientific advances. It was also a special period geographically. The industrial and agrarian revolutions in the advanced economies were past, the fires of urbanisation were burning fiercely everywhere, and the improvements in public health wrought by changes to sanitation and water supply were being felt. With these points as background, we turn in the next three chapters to analyse our data at three different spatial levels – the global in chapter 4, the regional in chapter 5, and the individual city in chapter 6.

4

Epidemic trends: a global synthesis

In England practical sanitation has reduced the annual rate of mortality one-half, and in the metropolis to less than 20 to 1,000 inhabitants, while in Havana, notwithstanding better ventilation and a freer circulation of air in houses, due to the fact that the climate permits of open doors and windows, the rate of mortality is almost double that of London.

Dr Erastus Wilson, *Weekly Abstract of Sanitary Reports*, vol. VI (1891), p. 122

4.1 Introduction

In this chapter, we begin the process of analysing the data that make up the various 'city×disease' matrices described in chapter 3. Using a broad-brush analysis, we look initially for any trends discernible within the figures at the *global* level. The term *global* is employed here in two senses: first, using all 100 cities in our sample as a group, without differentiating them either by identifying an individual city or by geographical region; second, by combining the individual records of the 100 separate cities to generate a single worldwide time series for each disease. Both are utilised here as a prologue to the regional and individual city approaches we follow in chapters 5 and 6 respectively.

We commence the chapter with, as we have already freely acknowledged in the preface, a brief look at the debate over the historical 'mortality decline' in human populations recognised in most demographic–historical writing. We review the range of hypotheses which have been generated to explain the decline (section 4.2). Our analysis then begins in section 4.3 by looking at trends in mortality over the twenty-five years covered by our own data in order to determine how far they typify or depart from the expected long-term picture of mortality decline. From the range of hypotheses proposed to account for such decline, we select three (the crisis hypothesis, the 'big-city' hypothesis, and the environmental hypothesis) and test them against our own data (sections 4.4, 4.5, and 4.6). Finally, we systematically re-examine the time series for the 100 cities to determine how far the patterns we expect on the basis of the hypotheses mesh at the global level across diseases (section 4.7).

4.2 The mortality decline and its causes

Few topics cause as much controversy amongst economic historians, demographers, and historians of medicine as the causes of the long mortality decline which has affected Western Europe over the last three centuries. So far as the available demographic data indicate, the facts of decline are not in dispute, at least in the round. But, outside the broad picture, the detail of the ways in which particular age cohorts or sexes were affected remains an area for active research and argument. Wrigley and Schofield's (1989) monumental *Population History of England, 1541–1871* confirms the extent to which the specific demographic parameters of decline still remain to be unravelled. And, what is true for England, with one of the best recorded and most pored-over demographic histories, is likely to be the more true for most countries around the world.

In an introduction to *The Decline of Mortality* (Schofield, Reher, and Bideau, 1991), the Cambridge demographer, Roger Schofield, succinctly summarises the historical development of mortality in Europe in the following terms:

Pre-decline patterns typical of most *Ancien Régime* societies were characterized by high overall levels, punctuated by periodic bouts with epidemics caused by infectious disease (plague, smallpox, typhus, etc.). During the eighteenth century, and chiefly thanks to ever more efficient government intervention, the incidence of crisis mortality diminished drastically in most of Europe. It was the 'stabilisation of mortality' as Michael Flinn (1974) called it, and was essential to the subsequent spurt in European growth rates. With the reduction of epidemics, endemic infectious diseases became relatively more important and gains in life expectancy slowed considerably. It was not until the latter part of the nineteenth century that mortality once again declined sharply in most areas of Europe. Child mortality and, somewhat later, infant mortality were responsible for much of this decline, though gains in life expectancy affected all age groups. Mortality improvement was due mostly to the decline in diseases such as diarrhoea and tuberculosis. The third period of mortality decline began after World War II, spread throughout the world, and seems inextricably, though not exclusively, linked to the discovery and use of sulpha drugs and antibiotics. (Schofield, Reher, and Bideau, 1991, p. 1)

A useful review of the mortality changes both within and outside Europe is provided by Kunitz (1986).

But, if the facts are slowly becoming clearer, the causes which lie behind the observed decline remain a hotbed of controversy. The range of the debate suggests that any understanding of precisely what happened, both when and where, remains tenuous. In general terms there are six main hypotheses, each with a penumbra of minor variations that lie outside our immediate concern. We term them 'hypotheses' here because most remain speculative and the opportunity for testing them as models remains limited. The complex interactions among the factors underpinning the hypotheses are summarised in figure 4.1.

(a) Crisis hypotheses: These suggest that the background level of mortality in so-called 'normal' years remained roughly constant over long periods of time. Long-term decline in mortality is then attributed to a reduction in the number of 'epidemic years', each with a consequent flare-up of excess mortality. The concept is discussed at length by Landers (1993). Schofield and Reher (1991, p. 3) link the early phase of the mortality transition over a period stretching from the latter part of the seventeenth century to the beginning of the nineteenth to the decline, or even disappearance, of crisis mortality caused by epidemics of plague which had all but vanished from the continent by the early part of the eighteenth century.

(b) Urbanisation hypotheses: To the contemporary mid-Victorian urban observer such as Charles Dickens or Emile Zola, the living conditions in crowded and filthy cities were seen as a major obstacle to any mortality decline. As Schofield and Reher (1991, p. 14) observe: 'Towns had always been characterized by higher mortality rates due mainly to greater population

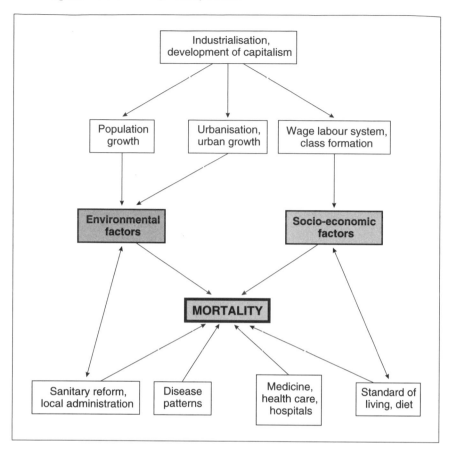

Figure 4.1. Schematic model of factors affecting levels of mortality. Source: Woods and Woodward (1984), fig. 1.1, p. 21; reproduced with kind permission of Professor Robert Woods.

densities which facilitated infection and filth; and during the nineteenth century increasing proportions of the population were living in those urban centres.' In *An Atlas of Victorian Mortality*, Woods and Shelton (1997) use registrar general's records for 614 small districts in England and Wales to test the hypothesis that urbanisation had a profound influence on national mortality because an increasing proportion of the population of England and Wales became concentrated in a relatively small number of urban districts. Generally speaking, the rural districts were the healthy ones, where mortality was at its lowest compared with the urban areas, but not all the groups or causes of death considered in the atlas showed clear urban–rural differentials. In infancy, diarrhoea and dysentery and, in old age, diseases of the lung were especially important in establishing and maintaining the urban–rural mortality differential. Woods and Shelton found that the infectious diseases in early childhood displayed the most sensitivity to differences in population density, with measles and scarlet fever exhibiting a pronounced mortality gradient between town and country. But the maps show a complex pattern. That for scarlet fever mortality in the 1860s picks out some of the largest urban centres and it is these places that benefited most from the lower mortality at the end of the century. But, unlike measles, there are many counter-examples, especially at mid-century, of relatively high mortality in more rural areas. The maps also emphasise the uncertainty concerning the extent to which pulmonary tuberculosis was principally an urban disease, throw doubts on whether urban areas fostered tuberculosis, and challenge the prevailing nineteenth-century explanation that rural life afforded some protection against the disease.

(c) Economic and nutritional hypotheses: Thomas McKeown (1976) in *The Modern Rise of Population* argued forcefully that the fall in mortality was due mainly to improved nutrition, linked to increased levels of economic development. His arguments were largely based on British data for deaths classified by age and certified cause from 1837 onwards. He observed that diseases spread by airborne micro-organisms (especially tuberculosis) had accounted for most of the decline in mortality during the nineteenth and twentieth centuries. From this observation he went on to argue that, since tuberculosis and some of the other airborne diseases like measles were largely unaffected by advances in public health until well into the twentieth century, exposure to them could not have been limited during that part of the mortality transition prior to significant medical intervention. His conclusion – that therefore resistance to them must have grown on account of the improved nutritional status of the population – has been widely criticised. Wrigley and Schofield (1989, pp. 224–48) have demonstrated that the role McKeown attributed to mortality decline in eighteenth-century population change is inaccurate: changes in fertility trends were the key to population growth rates. Szreter (1988) has also shown that social intervention played a much larger part in mortality decline in the period from 1850 to 1914 than McKeown would allow.

(d) Public health and sanitation hypotheses: Expanding on Szreter's critique of McKeown, this explanation stresses the key role of the state in organising public defence against disease, providing basic health facilities, and informing the population of advances in health care. A leading advocate of this view is Preston (1976) who, in his *Mortality Patterns in National Populations with Special Reference to Recorded Causes of Death*, used twentieth-century national data to demonstrate that income, nutrition, and other indicators of the standard of living cannot have been responsible for more than 25 per cent

of the rise in life expectancy. Public health technology is left as the most important residual explanation for declining mortality. Such ideas have been supported by evidence from the developing world since 1950 where mortality has been reduced drastically despite few improvements in the standard of living.

(e) Medical hypotheses: As Schofield and Reher (1991, p. 14) point out, the role of medicine and medical science in the decline of mortality has been belittled by McKeown and many other scholars. Medical advances could not be credited with the decline in mortality since, with the exception of smallpox and diphtheria, most other diseases (whooping cough, measles, scarlet fever) were declining long before effective chemotherapy or other scientific techniques became available. As we show in chapter 7, before the discovery of antibiotics and sulpha drugs during the middle part of the twentieth century, physicians had almost no effective weapons with which to combat disease and infection directly. By and large, hospitals were more places for the spread of contagion than centres of cure. But, as with the other hypotheses, evidence is building up to suggest that the role of the physician may be more important than McKeown's arguments would suggest (see, for example, Kunitz, 1991).

(f) Environmental hypotheses: A few studies have explored the links between climatic variation in determining both long- and short-term fluctuations of mortality in Europe. For example, Galloway (1985, 1986) has associated warmer summers or colder winters with higher-than-average mortality especially among very young children. In the same vein, Caselli (1991) has observed that infant, and especially child, mortality patterns in Europe suggest that, in areas with hot, dry summers, there may be deleterious consequences for food and water purity. Such regions display anomalously high child mortality levels from diarrhoea and other intestinal diseases when compared with other parts of the continent.

With these ideas in mind, we now go on to analyse our own data to see how far they typify or depart from the various model patterns. In section 4.3, we check our twenty-five years of records for evidence of mortality decline. We then take three of the groups of hypotheses proposed to account for decline (crisis hypotheses, urbanisation hypotheses, and environmental hypotheses) that are capable of statistical testing using crude mortality figures, and examine them with our data (sections 4.4, 4.5, and 4.6).

4.3 Testing the mortality decline

As we noted above, there is wide agreement among demographers that, despite many local variations and occasional setbacks, the mortality of the human population has been declining overall for at least the last three centuries. Because of data restrictions, that generalisation has been based upon evidence from countries with well-documented records, mainly but not exclusively in Western Europe and North America. So, for example, figure 4.2 shows schematically the cause-specific influences on mortality decline in England and Wales in the second half of the nineteenth century. In this section, we establish a methodology for identifying the long-term mortality trends in our own worldwide dataset over the 25-year study period (section 4.3.1). In section 4.3.2, the method is used to test for mortality decline in our data, where we also report our findings.

4.3.1 Identification of long-term trends

To examine global long-term trends in mortality, the data for individual cities were pooled as described below to yield seven monthly world time series, 1888–1912, one for each marker disease and all causes.

(a) Measures of mortality

Crude mortality series: Given the monthly city series of section 3.4, generation of a world series was straightforward. For each disease, the corresponding monthly values were summed across the 100 cities, yielding a global crude monthly mortality series.

Deaths weighted by population: Corresponding time series of death rates per 100,000 population at the global scale were obtained by dividing the crude mortality series by the (scaled) total population of all 100 cities combined.

Disease mortality as a share of all deaths: A perennial issue that arises when analysing mortality data is the relative importance of each disease as a cause of total mortality. The most obvious ratio to compute as one answer to this question is the monthly mortality from each marker disease, divided by the monthly mortality from all causes. Less obvious, but equally interesting, is to compute the ratio time series of deaths for all pairs of the six marker diseases (yielding fifteen further time series for study). If both diseases are equally important sources of mortality in a given month, the ratio will be one. These ratio time series enable time trends in the relative importance of, say, respiratory as opposed to intestinal infectious disease to be investigated.

Figures 4.3–4.9 plot the global monthly time series of crude mortality as a percentage of all causes, and as a rate per 100,000 population. Examination of the plots shows that each of the series has a broad shape over the study period, but that each also contains complex patterns of oscillations of varying amplitudes and wavelengths. It is the 'broad shape' of each of the series, technically their time *trend*, that we wish to isolate here and compare with the expected trend under the mortality decline model.

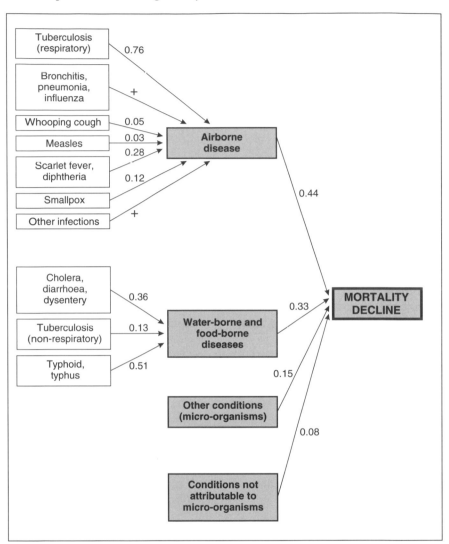

Figure 4.2. Cause-specific influences on mortality decline, England and Wales, 1848–1854 to 1901. Figures give the percentage contribution of factors to the decline. Source: Woods and Woodward (1984), fig. 1.4, p. 29; reproduced with kind permission of Professor Robert Woods.

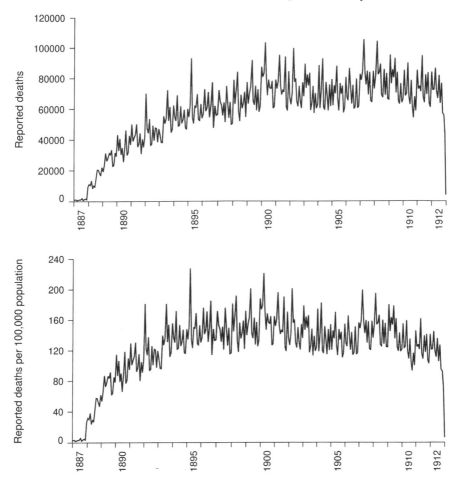

Figure 4.3. World mortality from all causes, 1887–1912. Monthly reported deaths from all causes (upper) and death rate per 100,000 population (lower) constructed from the 100-city sample.

(b) Isolation of global long-term disease trends

The simplest method of isolating the trend in any time series is to fit a linear regression model. Let y_t denote the variate value (number of reported deaths, deaths as a percentage of all causes, or death rate per 100,000 population) in month t of the series. Then a trend model may be specified as

$$y_t = \beta_0 + \beta_1 t + e_t, \tag{4.1}$$

where β_0 and β_1 are model parameters to be estimated from the data and the $\{e_t\}$, are stochastic errors. The coefficient, β_1, provides a direct estimate of the long-term trend (assumed to be linear in equation 4.1). If the trend in the

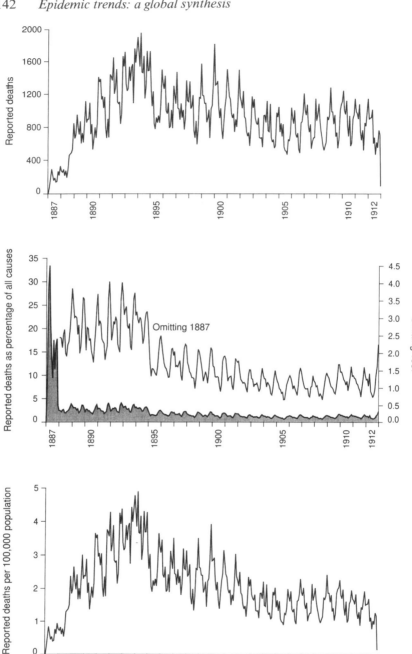

Figure 4.4. World mortality from diphtheria, 1887–1912. Monthly reported deaths (upper), as a percentage of deaths from all causes (centre), and as a rate per 100,000 population (lower). Because of the low level of reporting in 1887, time series have been plotted for 1887–1912 (stippled) and 1888–1912 (line trace).

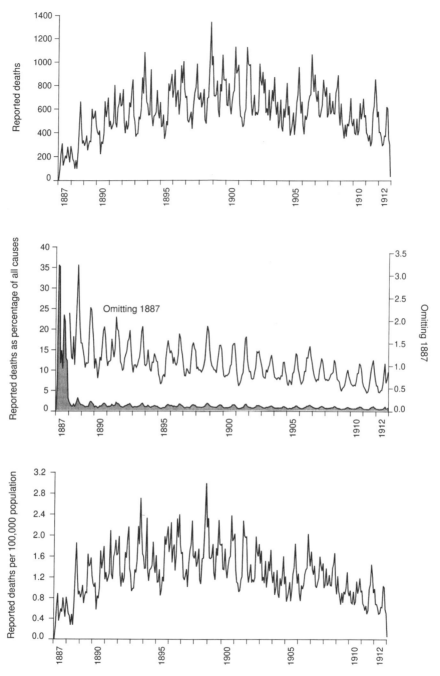

Figure 4.5. World mortality from enteric fever, 1887–1912. Monthly reported deaths (upper), as a percentage of deaths from all causes (centre), and as a rate per 100,000 population (lower). Because of the low level of reporting in 1887, time series have been plotted for 1887–1912 (stippled) and 1888–1912 (line trace).

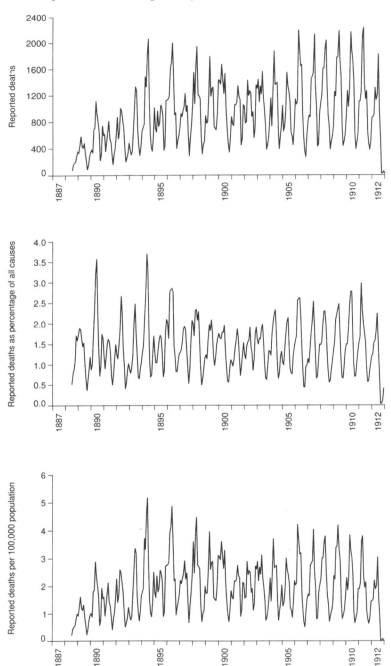

Figure 4.6. World mortality from measles, 1887–1912. Monthly reported deaths (upper), as a percentage of deaths from all causes (centre), and as a rate per 100,000 population (lower).

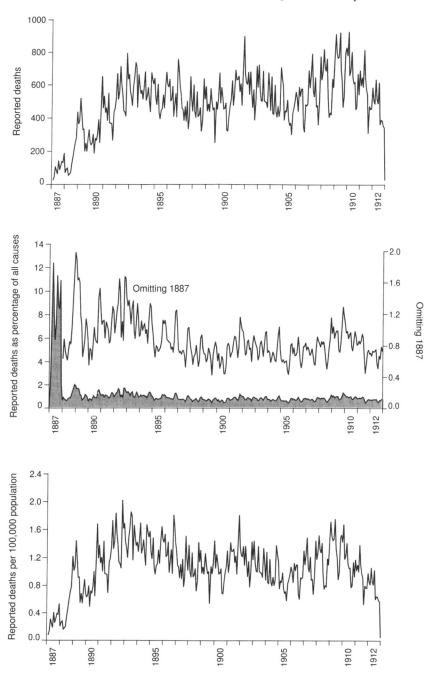

Figure 4.7. World mortality from scarlet fever, 1887–1912. Monthly reported deaths (upper), as a percentage of deaths from all causes (centre), and as a rate per 100,000 population (lower). Because of the low level of reporting in 1887, time series have been plotted for 1887–1912 (stippled) and 1888–1912 (line trace).

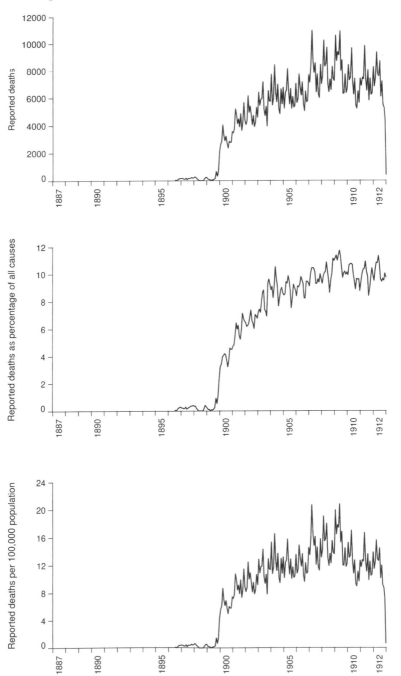

Figure 4.8. World mortality from tuberculosis, 1887–1912. Monthly reported deaths (upper), as a percentage of deaths from all causes (centre), and as a rate per 100,000 population (lower). For most cities, the recording of tuberculosis deaths in the *Weekly Abstract* commenced only from 1899.

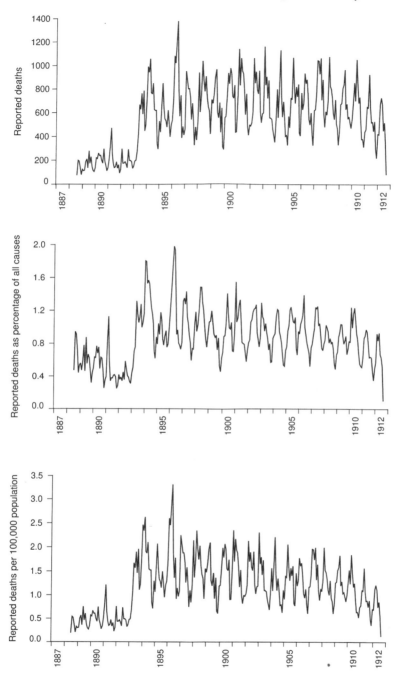

Figure 4.9. World mortality from whooping cough, 1887–1912. Monthly reported deaths (upper), as a percentage of deaths from all causes (centre), and as a rate per 100,000 population (lower).

variable is falling (mortality decline) the sign of β_1 will be negative. A positive value for β_1 indicates a rising trend, while a value of β_1 statistically not significant from zero implies that there is no time trend in deaths.

4.3.2 Testing for decline

Model 4.1 was fitted to all the series plotted in figures 4.3–4.9; table 4.1 gives the critical regression results. For crude mortality, only diphtheria had a declining trend over the period. There was no significant trend for enteric fever while, for measles, scarlet fever, tuberculosis, whooping cough, and deaths from all causes, the time trend was upwards.

Of the measures of mortality described in section 4.3.1, crude mortality is the one most likely to be affected by vagaries of reporting (which cities were reporting, number of cities reporting) and population growth. Expressing reported deaths as a rate per 100,000 population mitigates these effects, and table 4.1 shows that substantially different trend results are then obtained. Significant falling trends, consistent with mortality decline, were found for diphtheria and enteric fever. There was no significant time trend for either measles or scarlet fever. Of the infectious diseases, tuberculosis and whooping cough experienced significant rising trends, as did death rates from all causes.

Global time trends for deaths from each marker disease as a percentage of all causes are especially interesting. As table 4.1 shows, there was a significant declining contribution from diphtheria, enteric fever, and scarlet fever. There was no significant change for measles and whooping cough, but there was a substantial upwards shift in the contribution from tuberculosis.

In summary, therefore, the results of our analysis suggest that, at the global scale, evidence for mortality decline is much more ambiguous than at smaller spatial scales. It was only for diphtheria that a significant falling trend was found with all three measures of mortality we used. In contrast, tuberculosis had a significant rising trend on all three. For measles and whooping cough, significant rising trends were detected for two of the three indices. Significant falling trends on two indices were found for enteric fever. Our conclusions for scarlet fever must remain indeterminate (one rising, one horizontal, and one falling trend).

There is one further caveat. Some of the plots illustrated in figures 4.3–4.9 (for example, reported deaths per 100,000 population from diphtheria in figure 4.4) suggest that trends may have been affected by underreporting in the early months of the *Weekly Abstract*. If we wished, it would be possible to accommodate this complexity in the trend model 4.1 by adding a term in t^2. This revised model was in fact applied to all the series plotted in figures 4.3–4.9 as a check on the impact of this possible reporting problem but, from c. 1890, without altering the substantive conclusions based upon the simple linear trend of equation 4.1.

Table 4.1. *Time trends in global mortality and the mortality decline model*

Results of fitting linear trend models to three indices of mortality.

Disease	Crude mortality			Rate per 100,000 population			As percentage of all causes			Count of falling trend
	β_1	t	R^2	β_1	t	R^2	β_1	t	R^2	
Diphtheria	-0.899	-4.24*	0.06	-0.00531	-10.46*	0.27	-0.00688	-20.77*	0.59	3
Enteric fever	0.188	1.42	0.01	-0.00150	-5.13*	0.08	-0.00284	-13.72*	0.39	2
Measles	2.051	6.53*	0.12	0.00147	2.22	0.02	-0.00015	-0.35	0.00	0
Scarlet fever	0.745	7.75*	0.17	-0.000152	-0.69	0.00	-0.00128	-8.29*	0.19	1
Tuberculosis	41.684	19.12*	0.66	0.0699	15.54*	0.56	0.0582	26.84*	0.79	0
Whooping cough	1.364	7.88*	0.18	0.0013	3.29*	0.04	0.000432	1.97	0.01	0
All causes	155.000	16.73*	0.48	0.137	6.41*	0.12				0

Note:
* Significant at $\alpha = 0.01$ level (one-tailed test).

4.4 The crisis hypothesis

We encountered earlier in this chapter the concept of the progressive thinning out over time of the occurrence of years with epidemiological 'crises' as a possible explanatory factor for mortality decline. In this section, we rehearse the nature of the crisis hypothesis in more detail (section 4.4.1), set up a model for testing the hypothesis on our data (section 4.4.2), and report the results of our tests (section 4.4.3). Finally, we develop a 'world infection series' using data for all six diseases to provide a composite check on the hypothesis.

4.4.1 The nature of the hypothesis

The crisis hypothesis is an alternative model to the mortality decline hypothesis that may be used to account for the declining time series of death rates that many researchers have found in pre-industrial and industrial societies. Following Landers (1993, pp. 14–22), the main assumptions underpinning the hypothesis as it developed from the 1950s to the 1970s were the following:
(1) That a distinction can be made between crisis mortality levels and so-called 'background' levels of mortality characterising 'normal' years.
(2) Secular variations (i.e., time trends) in mortality levels of pre-industrial populations resulted primarily from changes in the incidence and severity of mortality crises, with background levels of mortality varying relatively little in time or space.
(3) The mortality transition (to lower levels of mortality), at least in its initial stages, was caused by a reduction in the incidence and severity of crises, with little change in the background of mortality.

As Landers notes, an implication of the crisis hypothesis is that mortality crises had an essential character of their own; they were not just the extreme right-hand tail of a frequency distribution of death rates. Rather, the notion is that crisis years were qualitatively distinct from the background mortality characterising 'normal' years, and that they stemmed from some external shock. The usual historical approach has been to correlate such crises with environmental triggers (leading to poor harvests, for example). Epidemic mortality crises resulting from the spread of infectious disease, and military crises brought on by war have also been recognised. Equally, there must be instances when aspects of all three combined to create a mortality crisis. Further, as Michael Flinn (1981, p. 53) has pointed out, 'whatever the basic cause of a crisis, epidemic disease generally took over, so that mortality crises of all kinds very commonly appear as great increases in the number of deaths from infectious diseases'.

There are contradictions between the crisis hypothesis and the mortality decline model considered in sections 4.2 and 4.3. Postulates 2 and 3, above, of the crisis hypothesis imply that mortality time series are stationary (constant) in the mean but are non-stationary in the variance; the variance reduces over time. Conversely, mortality decline implies a time series process which is non-stationary (specifically declining) in the mean. Further, Landers (1993, pp. 17–18) suggests historical studies have shown that the relationship between the stability and intensity of mortality has been empirically variable and, contrary to the assumptions of crisis theory, that levels of background mortality have also varied in time and space.

Given these seeming contradictions and our own analyses described above that provide only ambiguous support for mortality decline in our 25-year period, we use the time series plotted in figures 4.3–4.9 to examine the crisis hypothesis on the global scale. We consider first ways of testing the hypothesis and then present the results of our analysis.

4.4.2 Ways of testing the hypothesis

As Landers (1993) notes, the model revolves around the definition of mortality crises themselves; that is, how the background level of mortality should be measured, and of the excess mortality beyond that background which should be recognised as a 'mortality crisis'. In the literature on historical demography, these issues have generally been resolved by defining crisis mortality ratios (CMRs). CMRs can be specified in a number of ways (M. W. Flinn, 1974; Hollingsworth, 1979; Wrigley and Schofield, 1981, pp. 646–9). A common approach is to define a trend (the 'background mortality') by replacing each observed value in a mortality time series with an eleven-point moving average, and then defining 'excesses' by comparing the observed values to the moving average trend (for example, by using the standard deviation).

A parallel problem has been addressed at the United States Centers for Disease Control and Prevention (CDC) in defining 'excess mortality' attributable to influenza in American cities. Early models employed by CDC attempted to establish 'background mortality' by considering mortality only in non-influenza epidemic years (Serfling, 1963; Serfling, Sherman, and Houseworth, 1967); see figure 1.1. This begs the question of how to split a time series into epidemic and non-epidemic years in the first place. However, once the background mortality had been defined, this is used as a benchmark to identify excess mortality attributable to influenza in years when influenza epidemics occurred. Current methodology employed by CDC tackles the problem by fitting autoregressive-moving average (ARIMA) models to a time series, and using the forecasts from these models to generate a 'background' series against which actual deaths may be compared to define excesses (see Choi and Thacker 1981a, 1981b for details).

A further way of separating 'background' from 'crisis' mortality is to split the total variance in the time series into its elementary parts using the methods of time series decomposition (Box and Jenkins, 1976; Chatfield, 1980;

Makridakis, Wheelwright, and McGee, 1983). We now outline this approach and use it as the basis of a method for detecting mortality crises that does not involve calculating CMRs.

(a) Time series decomposition
A time series consists of a set of ordered observations on a quantitative characteristic taken at different points in time. Although it is not essential, it is common for these points to be equidistant from each other. The essential quality of a time series is the ordering of the observations according to the time variable, as distinct from observations which are not ordered at all (for example, chosen simultaneously) or which are ordered according to their own internal properties (for example, by magnitude). The plots shown in figures 4.3–4.9 are thus time series within the definition given.

Four components will be present in varying degrees in an observed time series. These are (a) trend or long-term movement; (b) seasonality; (c) cyclical fluctuations about the trend, over and above any seasonal effects; and (d) a residual, irregular, or random effect.

Identification of trends: We have already encountered the idea of long-term trend when testing for mortality decline in section 4.3.1. The essential idea of trend is that it is the smooth rising or falling of a series and, in section 4.3.2, we have seen how trend may be modelled using regression. From the viewpoint of time series decomposition, the residuals in equation 4.1 represent the detrended time series. Using the global series of reported deaths from diphtheria per 100,000 population as an example, figure 4.10A shows the original values and the linear time trend; the detrended series is plotted in B. Notice that, as compared with graph 4.10A, the detrended values oscillate about a zero mean rather than a declining trend. Since the crisis hypothesis assumes a constant mean process (postulates 2 and 3), observed time series should be detrended prior to checking the model.

Seasonal elements: All the series in figures 4.4–4.9 exhibit fluctuations in the deaths recorded, whether expressed as crude mortality, deaths as a proportion of deaths from all causes, or as a rate. The easiest of these fluctuations to understand are those which are due to some periodic generator associated with recurring astronomical phenomena. Many infectious diseases, for example, exhibit winter peaks and summer minima of incidence in the northern hemisphere (cf. section 5.4). From the viewpoint of the crisis hypothesis, it can be argued that seasonal fluctuations are part of background mortality and, like trend, should be filtered from the mortality series before checking for crises. Such fluctuations are commonly removed by assuming that, over the course of a year, they sum to zero; see Chatfield (1980) or Box and Jenkins (1976) for technical details. Weights reflecting this assumption are then added

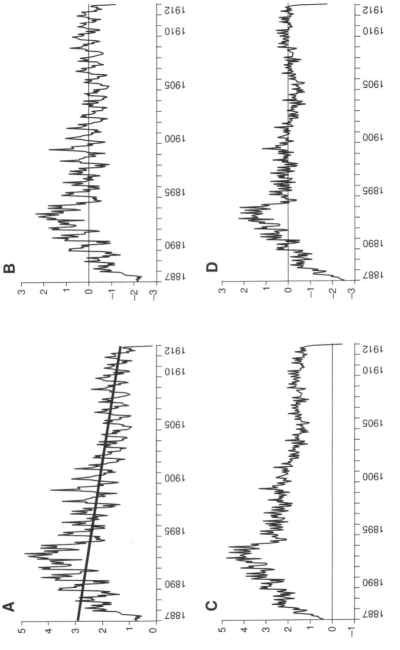

Figure 4.10. Time series decomposition: death rates per 100,000 population from diphtheria, 1888–1912. (A) Original series and linear time trend (heavy line). (B) Detrended series. (C) Deseasonalised data (trend still present). (D) Detrended and deseasonalised series.

to (compensating for seasonal deficits) or subtracted from (compensating for seasonal surpluses) individual values. Figure 4.10C shows the deseasonalised diphtheria series (trend still present). Figure 4.10D plots the detrended and deseasonalised diphtheria series.

Cycles: We must be careful to distinguish between seasonal effects and fluctuations of a cyclical kind unrelated to astronomical phenomena. In the context of the crisis hypothesis, once trend and seasonal elements have been removed from the time series, any remaining oscillations (referred to as *cycles* in the time series literature) will reflect the excess (crisis) mortality, over and above 'normal' background deaths.

Residual effects: If the trend, seasonal, and cyclical components are abstracted from a time series, we are commonly left with a fluctuating series which may, at one extreme, be purely random or, at the other, a smooth oscillatory movement. Usually, it is somewhere between the two. This represents the residual component, (d). Irregular crisis events are likely to find their way into this element of the decomposition.

(b) Decomposition and the crisis hypothesis

To examine the crisis hypothesis at a global scale, we analysed the time series of reported deaths per 100,000 population for each marker disease and all causes plotted in the lower graphs of figures 4.3–4.9. As our discussion above has indicated, the postulates of the crisis hypothesis imply that (a) trend and seasonal components in a mortality time series are part of 'normal' background mortality, and (b) crisis mortality will be reflected in the time series values remaining after removal of these effects. Accordingly, our first step was to detrend and deseasonalise all the reported series. To allow for the possibility of underreporting in the early months of the reported time series, a quadratic trend was fitted (see sections 4.3.1 and 4.3.2). To filter out seasonal effects, an additive, rather than a multiplicative, model was used. The additive model assumes that the amplitudes of seasonal fluctuations are independent of the trend. The multiplicative model assumes seasonal fluctuations damp on a falling trend and increase on a rising trend. We have no *a priori* reason for believing that disease seasonals behaved in this manner during our study period. In addition, the idea of amplified/damped seasonal swings could be confounded with the crisis element we are seeking to isolate (see the discussion below).

From the detrended and deseasonalised series, two new time series were generated as follows:

(1) Crisis peaks: A 25-element series was created by identifying the peak rate in each year, 1888–1912;

(2) Crisis troughs: A equivalent 25-element series was created from the death rate minimum in each year.

To search for long-term trends in these time series of crisis peaks and troughs, linear regression models were fitted to each by ordinary least squares. The model used was (cf. equation 4.1)

$$y_t = \beta_0 + \beta_1 t + e_t, \tag{4.2}$$

where y_t is the value from the time series of crisis peaks/crisis troughs in year t, and the $\{e_t\}$ are stochastic errors. The analysis parallels the identification of long-term trends in mortality described in section 4.3, so that the sign of β_1 indicates whether the trend of peaks or troughs is rising (positive β_1) or falling (negative β_1). The advantage of this methodology is that it sidesteps the issue of identifying 'excesses' over background mortality that arises with the CMR approach.

Figure 4.11 shows schematically the trend combinations possible for peaks (vertical axes) and troughs (horizontal axes). The shaded quadrant corresponds with the crisis model. Here, a long-term decline in death rates would result from damped cycles of crisis peaks and troughs. In the northwest quadrant, a long-term rising trend in death rates would result from increasing crisis swings. In the northeast and southwest quadrants, the overall trend in mortality rates would depend upon the relative angles of the trend lines fitted to peaks and troughs. If the trend lines converge, there will be a long-term fall; if they diverge, there will be a long-term rise.

A further advantage of the decomposition approach we have adopted is that, by separating out trend and seasonal elements ('normal mortality') from cycle and residual ('crisis mortality'), we can make an assessment of the long-term trends in each. This will permit better evaluation of the relative utility of the mortality decline and crisis models in accounting for variations in overall mortality rates; that relative utility may also vary over space and time.

4.4.3 Results of the tests

Figure 4.12 plots the location of each disease in the manner of figure 4.11. The horizontal axis gives the values of the slope coefficients for the linear trend lines fitted to time series of annual troughs; the vertical axis gives the values from the trend lines fitted to annual peaks. For representative diseases, graphs 4.12B and C show the annual maxima and minima, with the linear trend lines fitted to these peaks and troughs.

Tuberculosis and all causes stand apart from the other diseases in terms of their crisis behaviour. Tuberculosis recording began in the *Weekly Abstract* only in the second half of our period. We have already shown in section 4.3.2 that the long-term trend of tuberculosis mortality rose from 1900 to 1912, and that the disease had a rising share of deaths from all causes. The location of tuberculosis in the northwest quadrant of figure 4.12 is consistent with the growing significance of the disease. Comparison with the schematic chart of

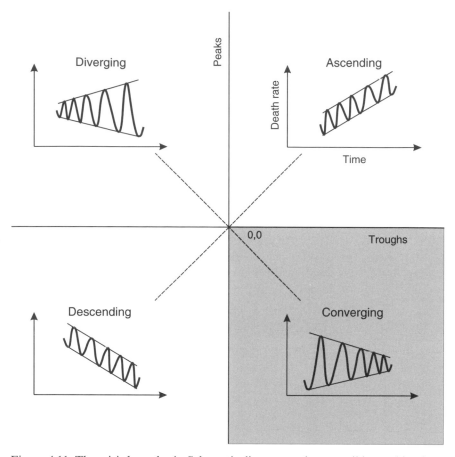

Figure 4.11. The crisis hypothesis. Schematic diagram to show possible combinations of regression slope coefficient values for OLS trend lines fitted to maximum (peaks) and minimum (troughs) monthly death rates occurring in each year of a hypothetical time series. Values for peaks are plotted on the vertical axis, and for troughs on the horizontal axis.

figure 4.11 implies that this increasing importance arose through both a rising trend and greater crisis oscillations (see figure 4.12B). For all causes, the trend line for troughs had a much greater negative slope than that for peaks. This suggests a greater amplitude for swings arising mainly from a downwards trend at the base of cycles.

   Diphtheria, enteric fever, scarlet fever, and whooping cough all appear in the same small area of figure 4.12. Comparison with figure 4.11 shows that diphtheria, enteric fever, and whooping cough lie in the quadrant that is consistent with the crisis hypothesis, while scarlet fever is on the edge. In section

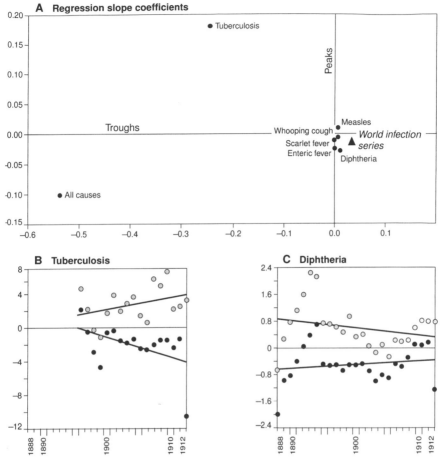

Figure 4.12. The crisis hypothesis: global patterns. (A) Regression slope coefficient values for OLS trend lines fitted to maximum (peaks) and minimum (troughs) death rates occurring in each year of the detrended and deseasonalised monthly rates for six marker diseases and all causes. Values for peaks are plotted on the vertical axis, and for troughs on the horizontal axis. Results are shown for each world series separately, and for a combined world infection series identified by principal components analysis. For tuberculosis (B) and diphtheria (C), graphs show annual series of maxima (shaded circles) and minima (solid circles) with trend lines fitted.

4.3.2, we showed that the long-term trend of mortality over the period for diphtheria and enteric fever was also down; thus there appears to be a consistent story of declining importance as contributors to overall mortality, 1888–1912, for these two diseases in terms of both trends and crises. The results of section 4.3.2 pointed also to the generally declining importance of scarlet fever, and it is compatible to find this disease on the margin of the crisis quadrant. The long-term trend for measles (section 4.3.2) was neutral; the results of this section suggest a similar broadly neutral crisis effect. For whooping cough, the long-term trends in section 4.3.2 indicated that the disease became a more important source of mortality over the period; the test of the crisis hypothesis implies that the cyclical swings for the disease tended to reduce.

4.4.4 A world infection series

For our final examination of the mortality decline and crisis hypotheses at the world scale, we first constructed a combined world infection series using principal components analysis. Let the $(t \times n)$ matrix, $\mathbf{X}$, consist of the monthly global death rates (rows) from 1888 to 1912 for the five marker diseases, diphtheria, enteric fever, measles, scarlet fever, and whooping cough (columns); tuberculosis was omitted because recording commenced only at mid-period. All of the diseases included in $\mathbf{X}$ declined in importance as causes of death in nineteenth-century England and Wales (figure 4.2). We wish to check the mortality decline and crisis hypotheses at the world scale for a composite infection series based on these five diseases.

The composite world infection series was constructed by extracting the first principal component from $\mathbf{X}$, and treating the scores on the component as the infection series. The eigenvalue associated with the leading component was 2.22, and it accounted for 44 per cent of the total variance in the data. All the variables were positively correlated with the component with the following loadings: diphtheria 0.503; enteric fever 0.353; measles 0.376; scarlet fever 0.554; whooping cough 0.417. Thus the component modestly represents in roughly equal measure the variance of each disease.

A linear trend model (equation 4.1) was next fitted to the world infection series to check the mortality decline model. A slope coefficient of –0.00395 was obtained. The associated values of t and R^2 were –3.87 and 0.05 respectively (significant at the $\alpha=0.01$ level in a one-tailed test). Thus the composite series has a gently falling time trend which conforms with mortality decline.

To test the crisis hypothesis, the methodology of section 4.4.2 was followed. The trend line associated with the time series of annual crisis peaks had a slope coefficient of –0.012 ($t=-0.36$, $R^2=0.01$; not significant at the $\alpha=0.01$ level in a one-tailed test); the slope coefficient of the trend line for the annual crisis troughs was 0.037 ($t=1.73$, $R^2=0.12$; not significant at the $\alpha=0.01$ level in a one-tailed test). While the signs of the slope coefficients are consistent with the crisis model, neither was statistically significant.

We conclude that global mortality rates as measured through the composite infection series fell slightly over the period from 1888 to 1912. This fall was effected mainly through a declining trend, with only weak evidence to support the crisis model.

4.5 The 'big-city' hypothesis

We described earlier in this chapter (section 4.2) the role of urbanisation as a factor which played a part in explaining cross-sectional variations in mortality. If larger cities were indeed associated with higher mortality rates for our six diseases, then it would follow that increased urbanisation would act as a brake on any overall mortality decline. Since our data is exclusively made up of city records, then we are not in a position to comment on urban/rural contrasts. However, we can explore the ways in which changes in city size might be implicated in mortality change. We thus select from within the urbanisation debate the 'big-city' hypothesis, testing whether crude death rates are related in any systematic way to city size. We look first at the big-city hypothesis (section 4.5.1), then at the population characteristics of cities in our 100-city sample (section 4.5.2), and finally consider the implications for epidemiological behaviour (section 4.5.3).

4.5.1 The nature of the hypothesis

It is through what we have called the 'big-city' hypothesis that spatial rather than temporal variations in mortality are modelled. It is attributed mainly to the work of McNeill (1977) and is discussed in Landers (1993, pp. 28–31) whose account we summarise here.

The *'high potential' model of metropolitan mortality*, as Landers (1993, p. 90) describes McNeill's formulation, derives from the extreme contrasts in population density found between large metropolitan areas (high density), their rural hinterlands (low density), and smaller cities (intermediate density). Metropolitan centres were large enough to act as perennial reservoirs of infection, they were characterised by high levels of retention of pathogens in the environment, and, given crowded populations and poor sanitation, they encouraged the rapid interpersonal spread of disease. McNeill argued that people born into such populations suffered high mortality in childhood but acquired a corresponding level of immunological resistance if they survived to adult life. Accordingly, the pool of susceptibles to infections was largely restricted to children and to recent immigrants. In these circumstances, McNeill suggested, death rates would be high, especially among the young, but also fairly stable since the scope for epidemics was restricted. By way of contrast, hinterland and small-city populations would be too thinly distributed for serious endemic infections to persist and they would accordingly experience lower secular mortality levels. But these populations would also suffer from reduced immunological resistance and be more vulnerable to the recurrent epidemics of metropolitan infections.

McNeill's observations were based upon the apparent behaviour of many of the simple infectious crowd diseases of man like diphtheria and measles. It represents a substantive interpretation of the well-known models of bio-mathematicians that relate the size and spacing of epidemics of infectious diseases to the densities of susceptible populations; this literature strand is encapsulated in the threshold theorems of Kermack and McKendrick (1927) developed, among others, by Bartlett (1957, 1960), Kendall (1957), and Black (1966).

However, accounting for spatial variations in death rates is likely to be much more complex than the McNeill model implies. Rates will be affected by a complex of factors, many of which are summarised in figure 4.1. They are likely to be especially high among three population subgroups: (i) infants after weaning when mother-conferred immunity disappears. Such infants are especially vulnerable to gastric disease (represented in this book by enteric fever) spread by contaminated food and water; (ii) children who initially lack a wide spectrum of immunity and thus experience high mortality from infectious disease (represented in this book by diphtheria, measles, scarlet fever, and whooping cough); (iii) recent immigrants who through lack of exposure will behave epidemiologically like children.

4.5.2 City size distributions

As we have seen in section 3.3.2, the 100 cities in our sample vary enormously in size from the smallest (in 1887), Colon (Colombia) with a population of 5,000, to the largest, London (England), with a population of 5.42 million, a thousand times larger. Figure 4.13 shows the full size distribution of cities in the sample by plotting, on the vertical axis, the cumulative population of the cities against rank (1=smallest) for the first and last year of the study period. In 1887, the cumulative population of the cities was c. 30 million, and this had doubled to c. 60 million in 1912. The graphs show that, at both dates, the size distributions were exponential in form and that roughly two-thirds of the total population was concentrated in the twenty-five largest cities. We thus have a wide variation in city sizes against which to examine the big-city hypothesis.

4.5.3 City size and epidemic behaviour

To examine the relationship between city size and death rates, we first computed two simple time-invariant indices of mortality, namely:
(1) *Absolute mortality*: This was defined as the median death rate taken over the 300 months from 1888 to 1912 inclusive.
(2) *Relative mortality*: This was defined as the mean death rate over the 300

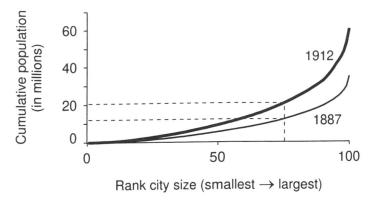

Figure 4.13. Rank–size distributions, 1887 and 1912. Cumulative population curves against rank (1=smallest, 100=largest) of cities. Pecked lines show two-thirds of the cumulative population is concentrated in 25 per cent of the cities.

months as a percentage of the mean death rate from all causes over the same period.

Variables 1 and 2 were calculated for the time series of each marker disease in each city (6 diseases×100 cities×2 variables).

Next, the 100 cities were ranked in terms of their death rates on variables 1 and 2. Their mean ranks were then calculated as the average of their individual ranks on the two variables to define a measure of death rate intensity. In ranking, rank 1 was assigned to the city with the smallest variate value and rank 100 to the city with the largest. For each of the six marker diseases, figure 4.14 graphs the result of this analysis by plotting as a scattergram average rank (death rate intensity) against the logarithm of the 1900 population (that is, mid-period) for each city. Because of the way in which ranks were assigned, death rate intensity increases away from the origin on the vertical axis. Regression lines were fitted to the scattergrams using ordinary least squares. The best-fit lines are plotted as the heavy solid lines ('All' in figure 4.14; the significance of the regression lines for 'Developed' and 'Developing' is explained later in section 4.6). The striking feature of the graphs is that, contrary to our expectations from the McNeill model, greater death rate intensity is found in smaller cities; this interpretation is reinforced by the fact that city populations have been plotted on a log scale. Table 4.2 gives the regression results. Each of the best-fit lines for all cities has a negative slope and, except for tuberculosis, is significant at the $\alpha=0.05$ level (one-tailed test).

These results do not support the conventional wisdom of the urbanisation hypotheses outlined in section 4.2, paragraph (b). Like the results of Woods and Shelton outlined there, they suggest a more complex relationship between city size and intensity of disease.

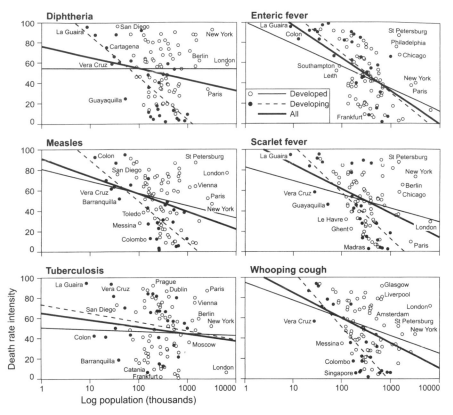

Figure 4.14. Six marker diseases: global variations in disease intensity. Average rank
on absolute and relative mortality (death rate intensity) against logarithm of the
1900 population (mid-period) for 100 world cities. Death rate intensity increases
away from the origin on the vertical axis. Regression lines for all cities and for
developed and developing cities are shown.

To check whether our findings were solely an artefact of levels of reporting,
Pearson correlation coefficients were calculated between average rank and
percentage of months in which cases were reported. These correlations appear
in table 4.3. To define a reporting rate across all six marker diseases, the
median of the reporting rates for the six diseases separately was taken. As table
4.3 shows, a negative correlation between death rate intensity and percentage
reporting (implying high intensity is a function of low rates) was found only
for all six diseases together and enteric fever, and none of the seven correlations in table 4.3 is significant at the $\alpha=0.01$ level (two-tailed test). We conclude that intensity is not just a function of reporting.

Table 4.2. *The 100 world cities: regression analysis of death rate intensity (dependent variable) against log population in 1900 (independent variable)*

Disease	Number of cities	Intercept	Slope	R^2
All six markers	99	156.4	–19.9	0.34*
Diphtheria	98	110.7	–11.3	0.04*
Enteric fever	99	223.0	–31.9	0.30*
Measles	95	145.5	–17.9	0.11*
Scarlet fever	96	177.1	–23.6	0.17*
Tuberculosis	95	85.3	–6.9	0.02*
Whooping cough	94	179.6	–24.2	0.17*

Note:
* Significant at $\alpha = 0.05$ level (one-tailed test). Sample sizes are less than the maximum possible because of missing data.

Table 4.3. *The 100 world cities: Pearson correlations between average rank for death rate intensity and percentage of months with cases recorded*

Disease	r(intensity, % reporting)
All six diseases	–0.127
Diphtheria	0.219
Enteric fever	–0.136
Measles	0.065
Scarlet fever	0.051
Tuberculosis	0.256
Whooping cough	0.213

4.6 Environmental hypotheses

One of the less commonly invoked ways of accounting for mortality variations has been to link them to environmental variables. A schematic model of possible causes has already been illustrated in figure 4.1, while McKeown's interpretation of the reasons for the decline of mortality in late nineteenth-century England and Wales is plotted in figure 4.15. The dominant factors in figures 4.1 and 4.15 can be divided into two groups: environmental and cultural (socio-economic). The latter group of co-factors have not been analysed at all thus far in this chapter. In this section, we tackle the problem of explanation at the world scale without prejudging the issue of mortality decline. A number of variables that reflect both cultural and environmental factors are specified,

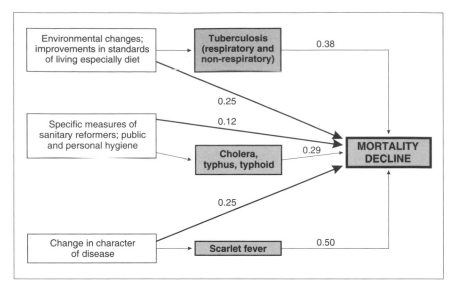

Figure 4.15. A generalised model of McKeown's interpretation of the reasons for the decline of mortality in late nineteenth-century England and Wales. Figures give the percentage contribution of factors to the decline. Source: Woods and Woodward (1984), fig. 1.5, p. 30; reproduced with kind permission of Professor Robert Woods.

and their correlation with rates of mortality is examined. In our analysis, we work with the 100 cities rather than the global series used in sections 4.3 and 4.4.

4.6.1 Measurement of cultural and environmental variables

(a) Cultural

With 100 cities, any cultural variables chosen are likely to be at best correlates of the local economic and social factors that influenced rates of mortality in individual cities.[1] The 'big-city' hypothesis described in the previous section provides the rationale for variables 1 and 2.

(1) City size: Cities were ranked from largest (rank 1) to smallest (rank 100) on the basis of their mid-period population sizes.

(2) City growth: The percentage growth in the size of each city was calculated as

100[(1912 *population* – 1888 *population*)/1888 *population*].

As we have seen in section 2.2, the *Weekly Abstract* originated as part of the US quarantine system, and special importance was attached to outbreaks of disease in port cities with strong trade links to the USA. Variable 3 captures this aspect.

(3) Coastal: A dichotomous locational variable was defined by identifying cities with coastal (1) and non-coastal locations (2).

Old World cities might be expected to possess more sophisticated public health systems than those of the developing world. Variables 4 and 5 are designed to reflect this possibility.

(4) Development: Cities were divided into developed (coded 1) and developing (coded 2), with the cities of Europe, North America, and European Asia constituting the bulk of the developed set.

(5) City age (date of foundation): Dates of foundation of cities are often ambiguous, especially for Old World cities; we have used data from Showers (1973) to define this variable. Using date of foundation implies 'young' cities will have large positive values and 'old' cities will have negative (BC) or small positive values on the variable.

Climatic variables have a mixture of effects upon viruses and bacilli; broadly speaking, they are adversely affected by high temperatures and ultraviolet light. In addition, there is the indirect effect that poor weather tends to cause crowding of susceptibles indoors which enhances the probability of person-to-person transmission of infectious agents. To try to capture this complex of factors, a number of climatic and positional variables were defined.

(6) Latitude.

(7) Elevation (in feet above sea level).

(8) Average annual temperature (in degrees Fahrenheit).

(9) Average temperature, warmest month (in degrees Fahrenheit).

(10) Average temperature, coldest month (in degrees Fahrenheit).

(11) Precipitation (in inches).

4.6.2 Disease intensity and economic development

As a simple example of the way in which variations in death rates can be affected by cultural variables, we re-examine the 'big-city' hypothesis of section 4.5. To check whether the explanatory power of this hypothesis is affected by levels of economic development and population size, the regressions of figure 4.14 (which plot intensity of mortality against log of population) were recomputed using the developed/developing split defined by variable 4. The best-fit lines obtained are graphed in figure 4.14. Regression details appear in table 4.4. As with the undivided city set, tuberculosis was the only disease for which statistically non-significant regressions were obtained. The death rate intensity/city size relationship is substantially stronger for the developing than for the developed cities (larger R^2 values in table 4.4). We conclude that, although the 'big-city' hypothesis remains unsupported in both developed and developing city groups, the mortality/city size relationship is affected by level of economic development. Among developing cities, there is

Table 4.4. *Impact of economic development upon mortality in the 100 world cities*

Regression analysis of death rate intensity (dependent variable) against log population in 1900 (independent variable).

Disease	Number of cities	Intercept	Slope	R^2
All six markers	70 (developed cities)	111.7	−11.4	0.12*
	29 (less developed cities)	239.2	−36.9	0.80*
Diphtheria	70 (developed cities)	54.9	−0.2	0.00
	28 (less developed cities)	253.8	−41.7	0.57*
Enteric fever	70 (developed cities)	166.5	−22.1	0.12*
	29 (less developed cities)	265.1	−39.1	0.56*
Measles	69 (developed cities)	117.0	−12.0	0.04
	26 (less developed cities)	247.3	−39.6	0.57*
Scarlet fever	70 (developed cities)	123.1	−13.4	0.05*
	26 (less developed cities)	284.8	−45.4	0.55*
Tuberculosis	68 (developed cities)	56.6	−2.0	0.00
	27 (less developed cities)	99.1	−8.7	0.04
Whooping cough	69 (developed cities)	147.7	−17.5	0.10*
	25 (less developed cities)	317.4	−53.2	0.71*

Note:
* Significant at $\alpha=0.05$ level (one-tailed test). Sample sizes are less than the maximum possible because of missing data.

strong evidence to suggest that greater death rates are found in smaller than in larger cities. Among the developed cities, this relationship is still found but in a weaker form.

Figure 4.16 summarises the death rate intensity/city size relationship by plotting intensity, averaged across the six marker diseases, against city size. Pooling the data in this way highlights the inverse relationship found for the marker diseases separately.

4.6.3 Disease intensity and multiple cultural and environmental variables

As figures 4.1 and 4.15 indicate, any explanation of temporal and spatial variations in death rates must be multifactorial. Accordingly, to handle the joint effects of the cultural and environmental variables specified above, the global data were analysed by two multivariate methods: principal components and canonical analysis. Principal components analysis was used to identify the significant components of variability first in death rates and second in the set of cultural and environmental variables. Canonical correlation was then

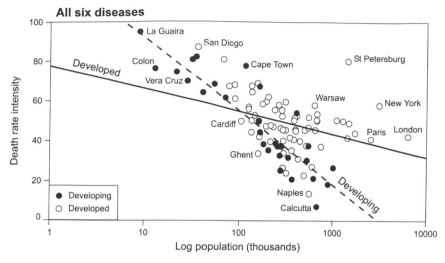

Figure 4.16. Death rates and level of economic development in the 100 world cities. Average rank on absolute and relative mortality (death rate intensity) against logarithm of the 1900 population (mid-period). Death rate intensity increases away from the origin on the vertical axis. Regression lines for developed and developing cities are shown.

employed to cross-correlate the components of variability identified among death rates with the components extracted from the explanatory variables.

(a) Principal components analysis

Disease intensity: To capture the different aspects of the global time series of death rates from the six marker diseases, we used the two variables already defined in section 4.5.3, namely *absolute* and *relative mortality*, to which a third, *variability in mortality*, was added. By construction, relative and absolute mortality are time-invariant variables. *Variability in mortality* is designed to capture the temporal variability in each time series, and is defined as:

Variability in mortality: The coefficient of variation, *CV*, was used where

$$CV = 100(s/\bar{x}) \tag{4.3}$$

and $\bar{x}$ and s are the arithmetic mean and standard deviation respectively of the reported monthly death rates in each time series over the 300-month period.

Principal components were extracted from the (100 city×18 variable) matrix in which the columns consisted of the three variables defined above for each of the six diseases. Because of missing observations, components were

Table 4.5. *Eighty-five world cities: loadings for three principal components based on measures of intensity and variability of mortality for six marker diseases*

Disease	Variable	Loadings		
		Component 1	Component 2	Component 3
Diphtheria	Absolute mortality	0.224	0.216	−0.183
	Relative mortality	0.199	0.418	0.059
	Variability in mortality	−0.086	0.341	0.289
Enteric fever	Absolute mortality	0.259	−0.381	0.145
	Relative mortality	0.300	−0.248	0.134
	Variability in mortality	−0.071	−0.135	0.187
Measles	Absolute mortality	0.352	−0.161	0.049
	Relative mortality	0.258	−0.076	0.443
	Variability in mortality	−0.137	−0.236	0.485
Scarlet fever	Absolute mortality	0.367	0.126	−0.104
	Relative mortality	0.252	0.352	0.130
	Variability in mortality	−0.205	0.222	0.314
Tuberculosis	Absolute mortality	0.136	−0.324	−0.215
	Relative mortality	0.109	−0.082	−0.222
	Variability in mortality	0.069	0.057	−0.054
Whooping cough	Absolute mortality	0.372	−0.019	0.080
	Relative mortality	0.337	0.201	0.131
	Variability in mortality	−0.063	0.073	0.352
Eigenvalue		4.68	2.86	2.25
Cumulative variance		0.26	0.42	0.54

extracted from a subset of 85 of the 100 cities. The first six components had eigenvalues greater than 1. Of these, components 1–3 had relatively clear empirical interpretations and accounted for 54 per cent of the variance in the data; the variable loadings on these components are recorded in table 4.5. To aid interpretation, biplots (Gabriel, 1971; Gabriel and Odoroff, 1990) for component 1 against component 2 and for component 2 against component 3 appear in figure 4.17. A biplot is interpreted as follows, using figure 4.17A as an example. The original variables are represented by arrows which graphically indicate the proportions of their variances accounted for by each component (upper and right axes for components 1 and 2 respectively). The variables are scaled by λ, where λ is the singular value of the data. The directions of the arrows indicate the relative loadings and retain sign information. The lower x-axis represents the scores of the cities on the first principal component, the left y-axis the scores on the second component. The locations of the cities in the space, fixed by their scores on the components, are marked by the shaded circles.

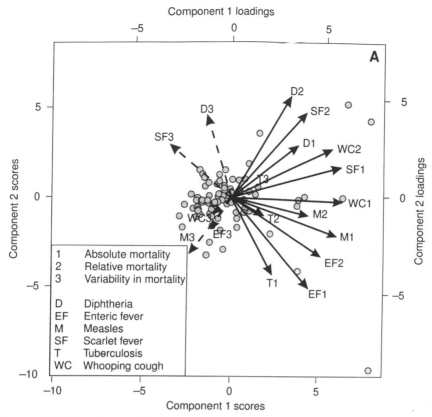

Figure 4.17. Eighty-five world cities: biplots of principal component scores and loadings for disease mortality rates and variability of six marker diseases, 1888–1912. (A) Component 1 against component 2. (B, overleaf) Component 2 against component 3.

For *component 1*, all the loadings are modest in size but, for each of the marker diseases, the correlation between the component and variability of mortality is smaller than that for either absolute or relative mortality. For all the diseases, absolute and relative mortality have positive loadings with the component while, with the exception of tuberculosis, variability (*CV*) has a negative loading. The component may be interpreted as a measure of disease intensity.

Component 2 discriminates between types of diseases. The variables for diphtheria and scarlet fever have exclusively positive loadings. The variables for enteric fever and measles have exclusively negative loadings. The variables for tuberculosis and whooping cough have two negative and one positive loading. The epidemiological/biological basis for this split is unclear.

Whereas component 1 appears to measure size, *component 3* indexes

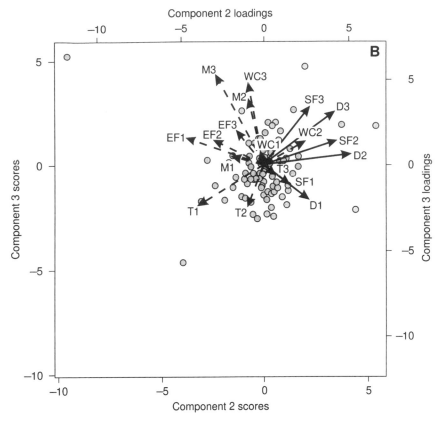

Figure 4.17. (*cont.*)

variability. With the exception of tuberculosis, *CV* has the largest of the variable loadings for each disease (usually by a significant margin), and is positively correlated with the component.

Cultural and environmental variables: There were no missing observations, and so the analysis was performed on all 100 cities. Three principal components had eigenvalues greater than 1. The loadings of the variables on these components appear in table 4.6. The biplots are shown in figure 4.18, and the components may be interpreted as follows:

   Component 1 (climate/economic development): There is a consistent pattern of moderate positive loadings between all the climate variables and this component. The positive loadings of these dominantly temperature variables go with a negative correlation with latitude (high temperatures are correlated with low latitudes). The development/coastal variables are also positively associated with this component.

Table 4.6. *The 100 world cities: loadings for three principal components based on eleven possible variables selected to account for variations in global rates of mortality*

Variable	Loadings		
	Component 1	Component 2	Component 3
City size (rank 1=large, 100=small)	0.197	0.060	0.444
City growth	−0.003	0.544	−0.381
Coastal/non-coastal (1/2)	0.256	−0.406	0.023
Developed/non-developed (1/2)	0.390	0.174	−0.189
City age (date of foundation)	0.077	0.266	0.763
Latitude	−0.373	−0.196	−0.092
Elevation	−0.093	0.622	0.005
Annual average temperature	0.444	0.002	−0.067
Temperature, warmest month	0.369	0.065	−0.114
Temperature, coldest month	0.427	−0.051	−0.028
Precipitation	0.272	−0.048	−0.111
Eigenvalue	4.75	1.37	1.07
Cumulative variance	0.43	0.56	0.65

Component 2 (population growth/elevation): The substantial correlations of the growth and elevation variables with this component are the main features. A number of the cities in our sample, like Mexico City, are at high elevations and grew rapidly over the study period.

Component 3 (city size/age): The high positive correlations of city age and city size, along with the significant negative correlation with city growth, suggest a component that is discriminating between 'old' and 'new' cities.

(b) Canonical correlation

Canonical correlation was used to associate the component scores of the cities on the three disease components with the scores on the three explanatory variable components. Canonical correlation is a special case of the multivariate general linear model,

$$Y = X\beta + E \tag{4.4}$$

where X is a matrix of continuous right-hand side variables (city scores on the explanatory variable components), Y is a matrix of continuous measures (city scores on the disease components), β (estimated from the data) is a matrix of coefficients linking Y and X, and E is a matrix of random errors (Cooley and Lohnes, 1962, pp. 31–45). Table 4.7 gives the coefficients and summary statistics.

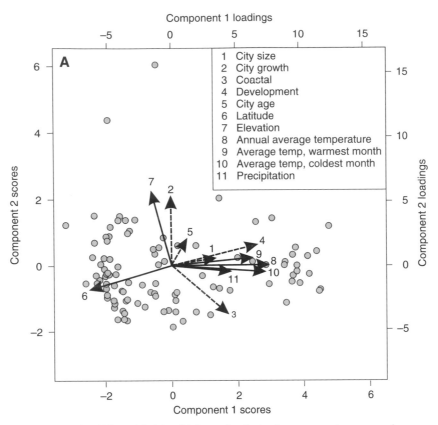

Figure 4.18. The 100 world cities: biplots of principal component scores and loadings for eleven possible explanatory variables to account for mortality rates and variability of six marker diseases, 1888–1912. (A) Component 1 against component 2. (B, right) Component 2 against component 3.

Table 4.7 shows that the climate/economic development and city age components are significantly positively correlated with disease intensity as measured through size of death rates over the time series. Given the codings of the categorical variables in section 4.6.1 from which the explanatory components have been derived (see table 4.6), these positive correlations imply that greater intensity of the six marker diseases is found in the smaller, younger cities of the less economically developed world; rates also increase in more equable climes. The climate/economic development component is also significantly negatively correlated with the disease type component. Again, variable codings imply a negative association with intensity of deaths from diphtheria and scarlet fever and a generally positive association with the other marker

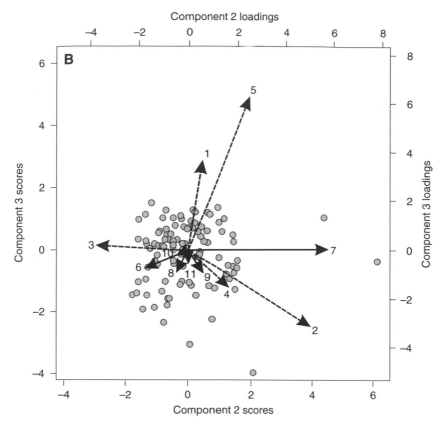

Figure 4.18. (*cont.*)

diseases (enteric fever, measles, tuberculosis, and whooping cough). No other statistically significant relationships exist in table 4.7.

In summary, the results of the canonical analysis put a more detailed gloss upon the findings of figures 4.14 and 4.16. Contrary to expectations, greater disease intensity is found in smaller cities, and rates are higher in less economically developed parts of the world.

4.6.4 *Time trends in disease intensity*

Let y_t be the reported death rate per 100,000 population and t be a time index from January 1888 ($t=1$) to December 1912 ($t=300$). To examine the relationship between time trends in death rates and our selected cultural and environmental variables, the linear trend model used in section 4.3.1, namely

$$y_t = \beta_0 + \beta_1 t + e_t, \tag{4.5}$$

Table 4.7. *Eighty-five world cities and six marker diseases: canonical correlation weights between component scores for disease variables (dependent variables) against component scores for environmental and cultural variables (explanatory variables)*

	Disease components			
Explanatory variable components	*1* Size of death rate	*2* Disease type	*3* Variability of death rate	Multiple correlation
Constant	0.164	−0.202	−0.055	
1 Climate/economic development	0.311*	−0.374*	−0.096	0.381*
2 Population growth/elevation	0.031	0.066	−0.086	−0.046
3 City size/age	0.634*	−0.046	−0.032	−0.032*

Note:
* Significant at $\alpha=0.05$ level (one-tailed test).

was first fitted to each of the 700 time series (6 marker diseases and all causes$\times$100 cities). The model was estimated using ordinary least squares. The coefficient, β_1, measures the time trend, giving the average change in death rates per unit change in time. Negative coefficients imply falling rates, positive coefficients rising rates. To facilitate inter-disease and inter-city comparisons, the estimated coefficients, $\hat{\beta}_1$, were standardised. We denote these standard-ised values by $\hat{\beta}_1$, where

$$\hat{\beta}_1^* = \hat{\beta}_1 \frac{S_t}{S_y} \tag{4.6}$$

and s_x and s_y are the standard deviations of the $\{t\}$ and $\{y_t\}$ respectively.

For each disease, the $\{\hat{\beta}_1^*\}$ were cross-tabulated against variables 1–11 described in section 4.6.1, but with each of these variables reduced to cate-gories to form the main effect variables in an analysis of variance (ANOVA). The ANOVA model is discussed in many books on multivariate statistics. See, for example, Hand and Taylor (1987), Mardia, Kent, and Bibby (1979), and Seber (1984). The categorical variables were constructed so as to yield roughly equal numbers of cities in each class without doing injustice to any natural breaks in the data. The class boundaries used were:

(1) Rank–size: The rank–size distribution was divided into three parts on the basis of the mid-point population 1888–1912. Large cities were defined as greater than 400,000 population, medium size 200,000–400,000, and small as less than 200,000 population.

(2) City growth: The percentage growths in city sizes were ranked and the distribution was split to give high-, medium-, and low-growth cities.

(3) Coastal: The dichotomous locational variable was defined by identifying cities with coastal and non-coastal locations.

(4) Development: Cities were divided into developed and developing.

(5) City age: A fourfold age classification was used: old cities founded prior to 150 BC; 150 BC–AD 1199; AD 1200–1700; and young cities founded after 1700.

(6) Latitude: A threefold division separated out tropical and subtropical cities (less than 30° north/south of the equator), from mid-latitudes (30°–50°), and colder regions (above 50° north/south of the equator).

(7) Elevation: Three elevation categories were used (in feet above sea level): < 51; 51–200; > 200.

(8) Average annual temperature: The class boundaries used were (in °F): < 50; 50–59; > 59.

(9) Average temperature, warmest month: The class boundaries were (in °F): < 65; 65–76; > 76.

(10) Average temperature, coldest month: The class boundaries were (in °F): < 33; 33–43; > 43.

(11) Precipitation: The class boundaries were (in inches): < 28; 28–36; > 36.

Figure 4.19 illustrates the main effects plots. These show the mean (y-axis) of the standardised regression coefficients ($\hat{\beta}_1^*$ in equation 4.6) of the cities in each class of the categorical variables defined above (x-axis). The means are all negative, indicative of the falling death rates found over our study period for these diseases.

A fixed-effects ANOVA was carried out for each disease and all causes. Using a schematic notation for simplicity, the general form of the model fitted was, for disease Y:

Y=constant+rank–size+city growth+(rank–size×city growth)+development+city age+(development×age)+latitude+ elevation+(latitude×elevation)+average annual temperature+ precipitation+(temperature×precipitation)+coldest month temperature+error. (4.7)

The model was designed to examine main and intuitively plausible interaction effects (the crossed terms appear in parentheses in equation 4.7). Because of collinearity of the coastal variable with elevation and of warmest month with average temperature and coldest month, we omitted the coastal and warmest month variables. Because only selected interaction effects were included, estimation was via the general linear model rather than as a fully factorial ANOVA. As a result of fitting the model, effects with low probabilities of occurrence under the null hypothesis of no effect (F-test) are marked in figure 4.19; significant interaction effects are linked with arrows.

With the exception of tuberculosis, the chief effect on trends is exerted through two interaction terms: level of economic development/age of

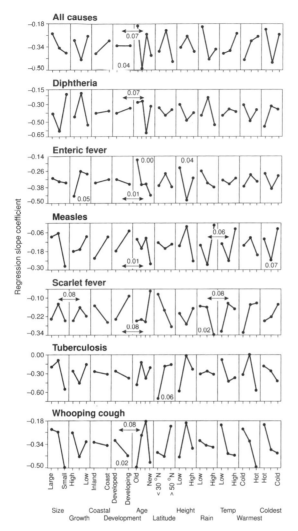

Figure 4.19. The 100 world cities: main effects plots for analysis of variance of regression trend coefficients for all causes and six marker diseases against eleven categorical variables. The vertical axis gives the mean coefficient value (solid circle) for cities in each class of the categorical variables. Categorical variable classes are: rank-size (1=large, 2=medium, 3=small); % growth (1=high, 2=medium, 3=small); coastal (1=inland, 2=coast); development (1=developed, 2=developing); latitude (1=<30° N/S, 2=30°–50° N/S, 3=>50° N/S); city age (1=founded before 150 BC, 2=150 BC–AD 1199, 3= AD 1200–1700, 4=after AD 1700); elevation (1=<51 feet OD, 2=51–200, 3=>200 feet OD); average annual temperature (1=<50 °F, 2=50–9 °F, 3=>59 °F); average temperature, warmest month (1=<65 °F, 2=65–76 °F, 3=>76 °F); average temperature, coldest month (1=<33 °F, 2=33–43 °F, 3=>43 °F); precipitation (1=<28″, 2=28″–36″, 3=>36″). Effects with low probabilities of occurrence under the null hypothesis are recorded.

settlement among the cultural variables and, additionally, for measles and scarlet fever, through the climatic variables, annual average temperature/ annual precipitation. Individual main effects were significant for all causes (development), enteric fever (city growth, age, and elevation), measles (coldest month), scarlet fever (precipitation), and tuberculosis (latitude). For enteric fever, the steepest negative trend lines were found in high-growth young cities.

To explore the crossed effects more fully, figure 4.20 was constructed. The solid circles give the means of the regression coefficients (*y*-axis) for cities in each class of the classificatory variables (*x*-axis). The results are instructive. City age had little impact upon trends in death rates in the economically developed regions of the world; in so far as it is possible to generalise, rates fell less rapidly in younger cities. But among the developing cities, age had a substantial and varying impact. For diphtheria, enteric fever, measles, and whooping cough, the greatest decline in death rates was found in newer cities. For scarlet fever, age had no significant impact. For tuberculosis, older cities experienced a more rapid decline in death rates than newer cities. For all causes, the oldest cities witnessed the slowest decline in rates, and the youngest the most rapid.

In comparison with the two cultural variables, interaction effects of temperature and precipitation appeared to have relatively little impact upon time trends in death rates. This is a reassuring finding. In the absence of major climatic shifts over our 25-year study period, we would expect such variables to exert their main influence by shaping the seasonal distribution of mortality. Seasonal effects are discussed in section 5.4.

4.7 Phase relationships in the global series

While it is reasonably obvious that a wide range of social, economic, and environmental variables will affect death rates at any particular moment in time and space, a less obvious effect might be exerted through the phase relationships of the diseases themselves. We have seen in figures 4.3–4.9 and section 4.4.2 that the global time series for each marker disease and for all causes are made up of complex mixtures of trend, seasonal, and cyclical effects. The extent to which these elements coincide (their *phase relationships*) across diseases will influence overall mortality. For example, if cycles are in phase, so that the diseases all peak in the same year, especially high overall mortality will be recorded in that year, and this will be followed by years of relatively 'flat' mortality. If, on the other hand, the cycles are out of phase, the reinforcing effect of coincident cycles will be diminished.

Comparison of figure 4.3 (deaths from all causes) with figures 4.4–4.9 (the six diseases) appears to suggest that the time series for individual diseases are not fully in phase. The very strongly developed wave forms in the series for the individual diseases largely disappear in all causes where shorter-wavelength, lower-

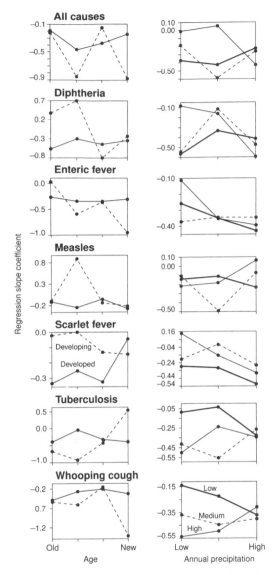

Figure 4.20. The 100 world cities: interaction plots for analysis of variance of regression trend coefficients for all causes and six marker diseases. Vertical axis gives mean of coefficients (solid circle) for cities falling in different classes of the categorical variables. Categorical variable classes are: development (1=developed, solid line; 2=developing, pecked line); city age (1=founded before 150 BC, 2=150 BC – AD 1199, 3=AD 1200–1700, 4=after AD 1700); average annual temperature (1=<50 °F, heavy solid line; 2=50–9 °F, pecked line; 3=>59 °F, light solid line); precipitation (1=<28″, 2=28″–36″, 3=>36″).

amplitude oscillations are the norm. But we must remember that the six marker diseases are only part of overall mortality, albeit a highly significant part.

To explore phase relationships between the diseases adequately, the time series techniques of autocorrelation, partial autocorrelation, and cross-correlation analysis must be employed. Autocorrelations and partial autocorrelations permit identification of the wavelengths of the cyclical peaks in individual time series, while cross-correlations check the extent to which these peaks coincide. These techniques are described in the next subsection. In section 4.7.2, they are applied to the global disease time series.

4.7.1 Identifying phase relationships

Autocorrelation functions (ACFs): To compute the ACF, the degree of correlation between all pairs of observations which are 1, 2, 3, . . ., k time periods apart in the series is calculated. Let x_t denote the value of the variable (deaths per 100,000 population) at time t and x_{t-k} its value at time $t-k$. Then the kth lag autocorrelation, r_k, can be computed from

$$r_k = \frac{\left[\sum_{t=k+1}^{T}(x_t-\bar{x})(x_{t-k}-\bar{x})\right]}{\sum_{t=1}^{T}(x_t-\bar{x})^2}, \tag{4.8}$$

where $\bar{x}$ is the mean of a T-element time series. The greater the degree of association between all pairs of observations k lags apart, the bigger will be the correlation. Perfect positive association yields a value of 1.0, a perfect inverse relationship a value of –1.0, while no association yields a value of zero. The number of months separating any pair of observations is termed the *lag*. This is plotted on the horizontal axis of an ACF, while the correlation, r_k for lag k, appears on the vertical axis.

Partial autocorrelation functions (PACFs): Whereas the ACF makes no allowance at lags greater than 1 for interaction effects between time periods which intervene between the lag of interest, the PACF filters out such effects. As a result, overall levels of correlation are reduced, and only the lags corresponding to any periodic events are emphasised. Put formally, the partial autocorrelations, b_{kk}, denote the correlation between x_t and x_{t-k} given x_{t-1}, . . ., x_{t-k+1} where

$$b_{k+1.k+1} = \frac{\left(r_{k+1}-\sum_{j=1}^{k}b_{jk}r_{k+1-j}\right)}{\left(1-\sum_{j=1}^{k}b_{jk}r_j\right)} \tag{4.9}$$

and

$$b_{k+1,j} = b_{kj} - b_{k+1,k+1} b_{k,k+1-j}, \qquad j = 1, 2, \ldots, k, \qquad (4.10)$$

In addition to previously used notation, $b_{11} = r_1$.

Cross-correlation functions (CCFs): Cross-correlation analysis proceeds by computing the correlation coefficient, r_k, between any pair of time series to determine the value of k at which the maximum correlation occurs. This value of k is conventionally taken as the lead or lag of the one series with respect to the other. Let x_{it} denote the death rate for disease i in time period t and x_{jt} denote the corresponding value for disease j. Then the cross-correlation at lag k, r_k, is given by

$$r_k = \text{corr}[x_{it}, x_{j,t+k}] = \frac{\sum \left[(x_{it} - \bar{x}_i)(x_{j,t+k} - \bar{x}_j) \right]}{\left[\sum (x_i - \bar{x}_i)^2 \sum (x_j - \bar{x}_j)^2 \right]^{1/2}} \qquad (4.11)$$

where $\bar{x}_i$ and $\bar{x}_j$ are the mean of the time series.

4.7.2 Interpreting phase relationships

In the work to be described, the global time series of monthly death rates per 100,000 population, illustrated in figures 4.3–4.9, are analysed rather than those for the group of 100 cities. A basic assumption of ACF, PACF, and CCF methodology is that the data are time-stationary. Accordingly, the series were detrended (quadratic trend) and deseasonalised using the decomposition methodology of section 4.4.2, and the calculations were performed upon the time series values with these elements removed.

ACF and PACF results: Figure 4.21 plots the ACFs (left-hand column of graphs) and PACFs (right-hand column of graphs). Black columns denote significance correlations at the $\alpha = 0.05$ significance level (one-tailed test).

All causes: In the ACF, the largest correlations are at lags 3, 23, and 49 months. Given that the value at lag 2 is also statistically significant, the high value at lag 3 probably reflects similar death rates in adjacent months of the time series. The high values at lags 23 and 49 suggest two- and four-year cycles in the data. This interpretation is confirmed by the PACF which, by cutting out interaction effects, emphasises the high values at lags 3, 23, and 49.

Diphtheria: The slowly damping ACF implies a non-stationary process, despite detrending and deseasonalising. The PACF cuts off at lag 3, so that a MA(3) model is implied. There is also weak evidence for a two-year cycle.

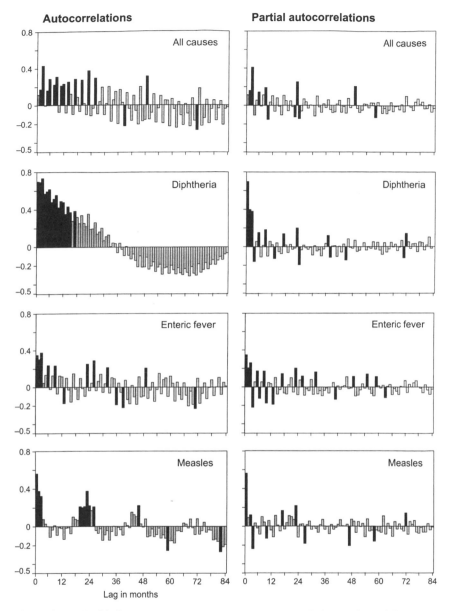

Figure 4.21. World disease patterns, 1888–1912: autocorrelation and partial autocorrelation functions for monthly time series of reported deaths per 100,000 population from all causes and six infectious diseases. Significant values at the $\alpha=0.05$ level (one-tailed test) are shaded black. (Figure continues overleaf.)

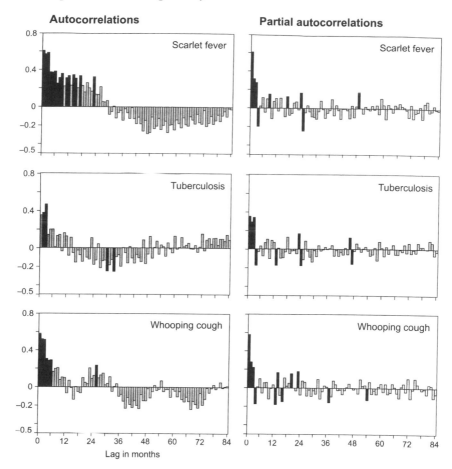

Figure 4.21. (*cont.*)

Enteric fever: The ACF and PACF are similar to diphtheria, with significance correlations to lag 3. The cyclical components appear at about two to two and a half years. There is only weak evidence of a cycle at four to four and a half years.

Measles: The ACF for measles picks out the likelihood of similar death rates in adjacent months, with significant correlations at lags 1–3. There is a strong cyclical component at two years. The PACF confirms this interpretation, and implies that the four-year cycle suggested by the ACF is simply a multiple of the basic and well-known two-year cycle present in many measles time series (see section 6.2.4).

Scarlet fever: Like diphtheria, the ACF bears witness to a non-stationary process best modelled using a MA. The PACF suggests this should be of order 3. There is some evidence from the PACF of two- and four-year cyclical components modellable using AR terms.

Tuberculosis: The overriding feature of both the ACF and the PACF is the strong correlation over short lags suggestive of an AR(3) model. Again there is weak evidence from the PACF for including an AR(23) term to handle a two-year cycle.

Whooping cough: The process is weakly non-stationary; the ACF damps only slowly over short lags. The ACF peaks again around lag 24. With the evidence of the PACF, a similar model to that for tuberculosis appears appropriate. There is evidence for a two-year cycle.

There are two features common to all diseases: (i) the high correlations at short lags implying similar death rates in adjacent months; (ii) a two-year cycle. In addition, enteric fever also has a weak four-year cycle. Point (i) is consistent with (ii) because cyclical series commonly vary smoothly over time.

We now turn to cross-correlation methods to establish the degree to which the cycles in death rates identified in this subsection are in phase.

CCF results: With six diseases and all causes, there are twenty-one CCFs to compute to cover all pairwise comparisons. Figure 4.22 illustrates the leading CCF values for these pairs; the maximum cross-correlation is plotted on the y-axis and the second biggest on the x-axis. With the exception of scarlet fever/whooping cough, the maximum cross-correlation value for all other disease pairs occurred at lag zero (i.e., the series were in phase). This implies that high death rates from the marker diseases are likely to be found in the same year. The second highest CCF values occurred at either ±3 months or c. ±24 months, and the circles in figure 4.22 have been coded to show the disease pairs to which these lags apply. These secondary results suggest that, although the diseases may peak in the same year, the peaks are not perfectly coincident but may often vary within three months. The high CCF values at about two years reflect the reinforcing effect of the two-year cycles noted in the ACF and PACF diagrams.

4.8 Conclusions

In this chapter, we have analysed the data contained in the *Weekly Abstract* at a global level. Worldwide time series based on the 100 cities have been constructed, and the overall trends in mortality from our six diseases – diphtheria, enteric fever, measles, scarlet fever, tuberculosis, and whooping cough

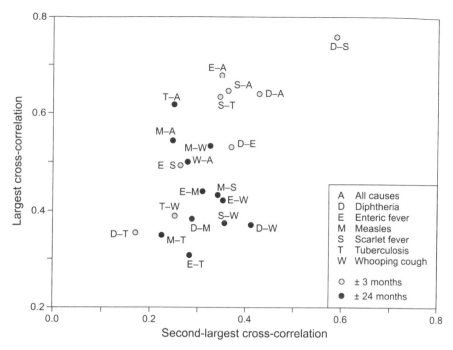

Figure 4.22. World disease patterns, 1888–1912: time series cross-correlations. Largest and second-largest cross-correlation values and lag of occurrence for reported deaths per 100,000 population from all causes and six infectious diseases.

(plus deaths from all causes) – have been examined in the context of some of the prevailing ideas about mortality decline used to account for patterns of mortality in pre-industrial and early industrial societies. So far as mortality decline is concerned, the results of our analysis suggest that, over our 25-year period, evidence for mortality decline is much more ambiguous than at smaller spatial scales (cf. figure 4.2). It was only for diphtheria that a significant falling trend was found with all three measures of mortality we used.[2] In contrast, tuberculosis had a significant rising trend on all three. For measles and whooping cough, significant rising trends were detected for two of the three indices. Significant falling trends on two indices were found for enteric fever. Our conclusions for scarlet fever must remain indeterminate (one rising, one horizontal, and one falling trend).

When we turn to the various hypotheses used to account for decline, an equally complex picture is found. The *crisis hypothesis* attributes declining mortality not to changes in the trend but to the reduced amplitude of cyclical swings in mortality. Diphtheria, enteric fever, and whooping cough appear to have time series behaviours consistent with the hypothesis; tuberculosis and deaths from all causes clearly do not; for measles and scarlet fever, there was no persuasive evidence either way. The *big-city hypothesis* argues that death rates are higher in great cities than in small cities and rural areas. For our 100 cities we found the reverse, and we have shown that the model is more tenuous in developing than developed economies. The third group of hypotheses we examined suggest that variations in mortality will reflect environmental variables. A number of multivariate statistical techniques (principal components analysis, canonical correlation, and ANOVA) were used to relate global variations in death rates to a range of cultural and environmental variables. Greater intensity of the six marker diseases was found in the smaller, younger cities of the economically developing world; death rates also increased in equable climes.

Finally, we tested a more subtle influence upon time–space variations in mortality rates, namely the regularity with which major epidemics recur to cause repeated cyclical upturns in mortality. If such cycles are coincident across diseases, especially high levels of overall mortality may be witnessed in some years. Use of autocorrelation and partial autocorrelation analysis identified two features common to the marker diseases: (i) similar death rates in adjacent months and (ii) a two-year cycle. Cross-correlation analysis suggested that the disease cycles were broadly in phase on a biennial basis. This implies that the diseases studied here made an especial contribution to global mortality every other year (cf. the plots for deaths as a percentage of deaths from all causes in figures 4.4–4.9 where the seasonal element is still present).

Our analysis in this chapter has been entirely at the world scale. The extent to which both the models we have explored and the conclusions we have drawn hold at smaller geographical scales remains to be investigated. It is therefore to an examination of these ideas at the meso-scale of ten world regions that we move in the next chapter.

5

Comparing world regions

Statement of acute infectious diseases in the State of Hamburg, Germany

MEASLES.

In comparison with the figures of the preceding year the number of cases in 1895 was extraordinarily small. The same is true of the years 1888 and 1889, an epidemic season being followed by a favourable season. It is a striking instance of the tendency of measles to recur in force every sixth year.

Public Health Reports, vol. XI (1896), p. 950

5.1 Introduction

In this chapter, we explore patterns of mortality attributable to each of our marker diseases and all causes over the period 1888–1912 at the meso-scale of ten world regions. The analyses described in chapter 4 which were based upon the time series for the 100 individual cities (as opposed to the global series built from the separate city records) showed that spatial differences in mortality were to be found – as between cities in developed and developing regions and across cultural and environmental variables, for example. One problem is to decide how we may best capture such geographical variations in more detail. As we shall see in chapter 6, given seven diseases and 100 cities, any study of the behaviour of disease in the separate cities can only realistically sample from the minimum of 700 time series that might be considered. Confronted with this wealth of data, examination of patterns at the intermediate level of world regions achieves several ends: it eliminates the need to sample; ten regions is manageable and yet presents us with sufficient spatial detail to identify regional contrasts; and it forms a regional context for the examination of selected individual city series in the next chapter.

We begin by describing the ten world regions which we used. We then go on to examine the three models of time trends in mortality tested at the world scale in chapter 4 – mortality decline, the crisis hypothesis, and the 'big-city' hypothesis – to see what regional contrasts are to be found.

An understanding of time–space fluctuations in transmissible diseases must consider possible seasonal variations and regionally varying environmental controls upon rates of incidence. These issues are examined in the second half of this chapter. Conventional mapping and charting methods are used to look at seasonality on a regional basis. But, to study geographical and temporal variations in the non-seasonal intensity of disease, the less commonly used methods of biproportionate scores and multidimensional scaling are employed. As the quarantine basis for publishing the *Weekly Abstract* implies, diseases move between areas at an international scale, and so the chapter is concluded with an application of cross-correlation analysis to establish geographical leads and lags among regions for our marker diseases.

5.2 Creating ten world regions

Ten geographical regions were identified. The regional names with their abbreviations are: British Isles (BI), Eastern Europe (EE), Middle America (MA), North America (NA), Northern Europe (NE), Rest of the World (ROW), South America (SA), South and East Asia (SEA), Southern Europe and the Mediterranean (SEM), and Western Europe (WE). The allocation of the cities to the regions is shown in table 5.1. Assignment of cities to regions was on a

Table 5.1. *Alphabetical list of the 100 cities by world region*

City	Country	World region	City	Country	World region
Belfast	Ireland	BI	Christiania	Norway	NE
Birmingham	England	BI	Copenhagen	Denmark	NE
Bristol	England	BI	Gothenburg	Sweden	NE
Cardiff	Wales	BI	Hamburg	Germany	NE
Dublin	Ireland	BI	Stockholm	Sweden	NE
Dundee	Scotland	BI	Cape Town	South Africa	ROW
Edinburgh	Scotland	BI	Durban	South Africa	ROW
Glasgow	Scotland	BI	Honolulu	United States	ROW
Leeds	England	BI	Melbourne	Australia	ROW
Leith	Scotland	BI	Santa Cruz	Spain	ROW
Liverpool	England	BI	Bahia	Brazil	SA
London	England	BI	Guayaquilla	Ecuador	SA
Manchester	England	BI	Montevideo	Uruguay	SA
Newcastle	England	BI	Pernambuco	Brazil	SA
Sheffield	England	BI	Rio de Janeiro	Brazil	SA
Southampton	England	BI	Bombay	India	SEA
Budapest	Austria-Hungary	EE	Calcutta	India	SEA
Moscow	Russia	EE	Colombo	Ceylon	SEA
Odessa	Russia	EE	Madras	India	SEA
Prague	Austria-Hungary	EE	Osaka	Japan	SEA
St Petersburg	Russia	EE	Rangoon	Burma	SEA
Vienna	Austria-Hungary	EE	Singapore	Malaya	SEA
Warsaw	Russia	EE	Alexandria	Egypt	SEM
Barranquilla	Colombia	MA	Athens	Greece	SEM
Cartagena	Colombia	MA	Cairo	Egypt	SEM
Colon	Colombia	MA	Catania	Italy	SEM
Havana	Cuba	MA	Constantinople	Turkey	SEM
La Guaira	Venezuela	MA	Messina	Italy	SEM
Mexico City	Mexico	MA	Naples	Italy	SEM
Port au Prince	Haiti	MA	Palermo	Italy	SEM
Vera Cruz	Mexico	MA	Smyrna	Turkey	SEM
Baltimore	United States	NA	Trieste	Austria-Hungary	SEM
Boston	United States	NA	Venice	Italy	SEM
Chicago	United States	NA	Aix (Aachen)	Germany	WE
Cincinnati	United States	NA	Amsterdam	Holland	WE
Cleveland	United States	NA	Berlin	Germany	WE
Denver	United States	NA	Brussels	Belgium	WE
Detroit	United States	NA	Cologne	Germany	WE
Kansas City, KS	United States	NA	Frankfurt	Germany	WE
Kansas City, MO	United States	NA	Ghent	Belgium	WE
Milwaukee	United States	NA	Le Havre	France	WE

Table 5.1. (*cont.*)

City	Country	World region	City	Country	World region
Nashville	United States	NA	Liège	Belgium	WE
New Orleans	United States	NA	Lyon	France	WE
New York	United States	NA	Mannheim	Germany	WE
Newark	United States	NA	Munich	Germany	WE
Philadelphia	United States	NA	Nuremberg	Germany	WE
Providence	United States	NA	Paris	France	WE
San Diego	United States	NA	Rotterdam	Holland	WE
San Francisco	United States	NA	Zurich	Switzerland	WE
Toledo	United States	NA			
Washington, DC	United States	NA			

Notes:
The city and country names are those current at the start of the study period in 1887.
The regional abbreviations are: BI, British Isles; EE, Eastern Europe; MA, Middle
America; NA, North America; NE, Northern Europe; ROW, Rest of the World; SA,
South America; SEA, South and East Asia; SEM, Southern Europe and
Mediterranean; WE, Western Europe.

geographical basis, but subject to the statistical constraint that no region had
fewer than five cities.

Table 5.2 summarises the principal features of the reporting record for the
ten regions. All regional populations grew substantially over the study period,
ranging from the largest rate of 130 per cent in Eastern Europe, down to 42
per cent in the British Isles. European regions grew less rapidly (average 71 per
cent) than the Americas (101 per cent). There was a marked contrast between
the developed world (Europe and North America) and regions in the developing world on percentage of months with disease reports. In broad terms, the
average percentage of months with reports in the developing world was down
about 25 per cent as compared with Europe and North America. This devel-
oped/developing split carried over into the completeness of the data record for
individual diseases. It is perhaps unsurprising that deaths from all causes had
the fullest coverage. Bearing in mind that the reporting of tuberculosis commenced only in the second half of our study period, the coverages of around
50 per cent imply a very full set of reports once recording started. In Europe
and North America, reporting coverage was uniformly high for all diseases.
Whooping cough had the lowest average recording rate over the ten regions,
while the percentage of months with scarlet fever reports was relatively low in
the regions of the developing world.

The burden of disease showed stark regional contrasts. If we focus upon the

Table 5.2. *Summary characteristics for all causes and six marker diseases in ten world regions, 1887–1912*

Attribute	Region	British Isles	Northern Europe	Western Europe	Eastern Europe	S. Europe & Med.	North America	Middle America	South America	S.&E. Asia	Rest of World	Average
N of cities		16	5	16	7	11	20	8	5	7	5	10.00
Population (millions)	1887	9.63	1.27	6.57	3.56	2.90	6.61	0.65	0.87	2.09	0.50	3.48
	1912	13.64	2.18	10.17	8.20	4.58	14.02	1.19	1.80	3.52	0.91	6.02
	% change	41.59	71.89	54.80	130.19	57.98	112.24	83.67	107.62	67.95	50.61	77.84
% months reporting	All causes	96.15	95.83	99.68	96.15	96.47	94.55	98.40	99.04	96.79	73.40	94.65
	Diphtheria	99.36	98.08	99.36	97.12	99.36	94.55	59.94	66.35	55.45	46.47	81.60
	Enteric fever	99.36	95.51	99.36	88.14	97.44	94.55	78.21	92.63	78.21	56.09	87.95
	Measles	90.71	75.64	92.95	84.94	80.13	94.23	51.60	59.94	80.45	13.46	72.40
	Scarlet fever	99.36	97.12	99.36	97.12	98.72	94.55	41.03	23.40	10.26	15.06	67.60
	Tuberculosis	49.04	48.40	50.96	50.00	50.96	50.32	59.62	46.79	51.28	44.87	50.22
	Whooping cough	85.58	78.85	92.95	84.94	76.60	86.54	44.23	57.05	31.73	10.90	64.94
Average		88.51	84.20	90.66	85.49	85.67	87.04	61.86	63.60	57.74	37.18	
Total deaths	All causes	4448550	597230	3174742	2264344	1088150	4027656	394128	408204	2034852	19061	1845691.70
	Diphtheria	62882	11555	46508	52056	10862	103202	1041	828	669	636	29023.90
	Enteric fever	31472	2474	22380	29969	15430	63407	3612	6470	5413	1·68	18179.50
	Measles	112062	5416	41732	51699	9202	30637	1840	1763	13748	79	26817.80
	Scarlet fever	36452	6461	17268	48219	4493	39315	1289	203	134	168	15400.20
	Tuberculosis	73783	33235	220110	193875	44989	288456	27517	34331	64793	1663	98275.20
	Whooping cough	87350	7358	22444	16532	1621	25032	1266	1107	766	108	16358.40
Average (excl. all causes)		67333.5	11083.2	61740.3	65391.7	14432.8	91674.8	6094.2	7450.3	14253.8	637.0	

Average annual deaths per 100,000 population	1508.68	1413.97	1501.68	1447.89	1165.87	1758.85	1937.29	1130.30	2732.51	103.75	1470.08
All causes											
Diphtheria	21.74	28.28	22.46	36.25	11.59	48.07	5.23	2.22	1.00	3.76	18.06
Enteric fever	10.84	6.24	10.27	19.48	16.55	29.01	19.24	19.86	7.00	6.99	14.55
Measles	38.01	12.37	19.90	32.82	9.39	13.56	8.71	5.53	18.53	0.41	15.92
Scarlet fever	12.50	15.77	8.02	31.57	4.56	17.66	5.87	0.76	0.20	0.90	9.78
Tuberculosis	23.08	67.18	93.30	109.63	44.06	104.99	136.38	84.74	82.25	8.37	75.40
Whooping cough	29.30	16.69	10.52	10.50	1.84	11.74	6.02	2.82	1.06	0.62	9.11
Average (excl. all causes)	22.58	24.42	27.41	40.04	14.66	37.51	30.24	19.32	18.34	3.51	

average annual death rate per 100,000 population, the rate for all causes in South and East Asia was almost double that in the next largest region, and some twenty-seven times greater than that in the region with the lowest rate, Rest of the World. The average annual death rates across the six marker diseases were highest in Eastern Europe (forty) and North America (thirty-eight). The next highest was Middle America (thirty), and the average fell as low as fifteen in Southern Europe and the Mediterranean, and four in the Rest of the World. Rates were lowest for scarlet fever and whooping cough, and highest for tuberculosis.

5.3 Comparing regional time series

5.3.1 Trend comparisons: mortality decline revisited

As we noted in section 4.2, the long-term decline in mortality discussed in the demographic–historical literature is based primarily upon European evidence. With the ten world regions defined in section 5.2, we now have the opportunity to look at regional variations in that decline. The model is tested here using reported death rates per 100,000 population (70 time series; 6 diseases and all causes ×10 regions) and, for each marker disease, reported deaths as a percentage of deaths from all causes (60 time series; 6 diseases ×10 regions). For each time series, the linear model given in equation 4.1 was fitted using ordinary least squares.

Death rates: The seventy coefficients split almost exactly 50–50 in terms of rising (thirty-four) and falling (thirty-six) trends in rates of mortality; at the $\alpha=0.05$ level (two-tailed test), twenty-one (30 per cent) of the time series had significantly rising trends in death rates over the period, twenty-seven (39 per cent) had significantly falling rates, and twenty-two (31 per cent) had no significant trend.

Deaths as a percentage of all causes: Declining time trends were more common than rising. Of the sixty time series, thirty-six (60 per cent) had negative regression slope coefficients; twenty-four (40 per cent) had positive trend coefficients. At the $\alpha=0.05$ level (two-tailed test), thirty-two time series (53 per cent) had significantly declining trends over the period in deaths as a percentage of all causes, eighteen (30 per cent) had significantly rising trends, and ten (17 per cent) had no significant trend.

Figure 5.1 summarises our findings. For each marker disease, it plots, on the *y*-axis, the regression coefficients for time trends in deaths as a rate per 100,000 population against, on the *x*-axis, the coefficients for time trends in deaths as a percentage of deaths from all causes. The main story is clear. At the world region level, deaths from tuberculosis were on a rising trend almost every-

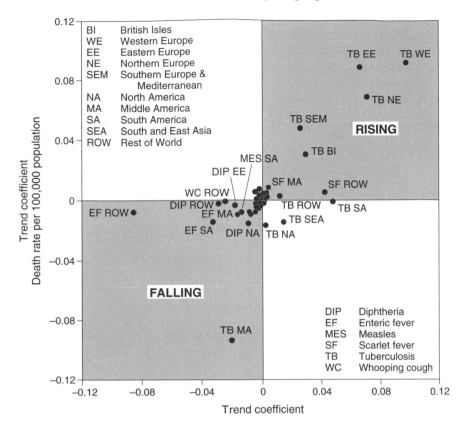

Figure 5.1. Mortality decline: world regions. For each marker disease, the regression coefficients for time trends in deaths as a rate per 100,000 population are plotted against the coefficients for time trends in deaths as a percentage of deaths from all causes.

where, whether expressed as a rate or as a percentage. The other marker diseases were on long-term decline in many areas. This finding is broadly the same as that reported in section 4.3 at the global level, and confirms the increasing importance over this period of tuberculosis as a cause of death at different geographical scales.

5.3.2 Cyclical comparisons: the crisis hypothesis revisited

In section 4.4, the so-called *crisis hypothesis* was examined at a global scale. The notion underpinning the hypothesis is that the background level of mortality in 'normal' years remains roughly constant over time, and that any long-term decline in mortality may be attributed to a reduction of excess mortality occurring, for whatever reason, in periods of episodic flare-up. The model therefore stands in contrast to the mortality decline model discussed in the previous subsection.

In section 4.4.2, a method for checking the crisis hypothesis was outlined and tested using the global time series defined there. In this section, the same methodology is applied to the regional time series of death rates for the six marker disease and all causes. The regional series were first detrended and deseasonalised by fitting a quadratic trend and additive seasonals. The annual maxima (peaks) and minima (troughs) in the residual series were identified, and linear trend lines were fitted to the resulting 25-point time series using OLS regression. The slope coefficients were used to specify regional positions on a graph (figures 5.2–5.3), with the x-axis representing the slope coefficient of the minima (troughs) and the y-axis the slope of the maxima (peaks) for each regional time series. Figure 4.11 shows schematically the various combinations possible. The graphs in each quadrant of that diagram give illustrative time series of death rates against time, with trend lines for peaks and troughs marked. The lower right quadrant represents the crisis hypothesis as defined in section 4.4.

The results of the analysis are summarised on a disease-by-disease basis in figure 5.2, and on a regional basis in figure 5.3. With the exception of all causes, the scale of each diagram is the same. From figure 5.2, the following points are evident:

(1) Perhaps unsurprisingly, the spread of values is much greater for all causes than for the marker diseases individually.

(2) With the exception of tuberculosis, regions are generally clustered close to the (0,0) origin of each graph, implying relatively gentle gradients to the peak and trough trend lines.

(3) For all causes and for each of the marker diseases, regions lie dominantly on a northwest–southeast line, implying either converging (shaded quadrant) or diverging (northwest quadrant) trends for peaks and troughs. For diphtheria and enteric fever, most regions lie in the 'converging' quadrant, thus supporting the crisis hypothesis; for tuberculosis, regions are mainly in the 'diverging' quadrant; for all causes, measles, scarlet fever and whooping cough, there is generally a 50–50 split.

The analysis by regions summarised in figure 5.3 shows that regional behaviour is as complex as that for the diseases. Variability between diseases is least for South and East Asia, and most in the Americas.

Our findings suggest that the temporal behaviour of mortality from these diseases is very much more complex than is suggested by the crisis hypothesis. The diverging trend lines generally found for tuberculosis are consistent with the growing importance of tuberculosis as a cause of death over the study period (see sections 4.3 and 4.4).

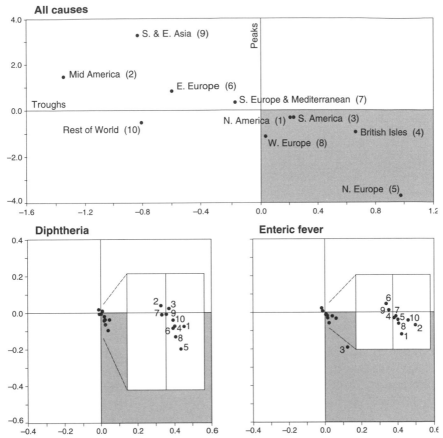

Figure 5.2. The crisis hypothesis at the scale of world regions, I: time trends, 1888–1912, in death rates per 100,000 population for all causes and six marker diseases. Values of regression slope coefficient values for OLS trend lines fitted to maximum (peaks) and minimum (troughs) monthly death rate occurring in each year, 1888–1912. Values for peaks are plotted on the vertical axis, and for troughs on the horizontal axis. The shaded quadrant is consistent with the crisis hypothesis. (Figure continues overleaf.)

5.3.3 The 'big-city' hypothesis revisited

In section 4.5, the *'big-city' hypothesis* (the notion that death rates are proportionately higher in large metropolitan areas than in their rural hinterlands and smaller cities) was tested at the global scale. This was done by plotting the average rank of the 100 cities in terms of their death rates on two variables (absolute and relative mortality) against the log of their 1900 populations. Little evidence was found to support a 'high potential model' of metropolitan mortality at the world scale.

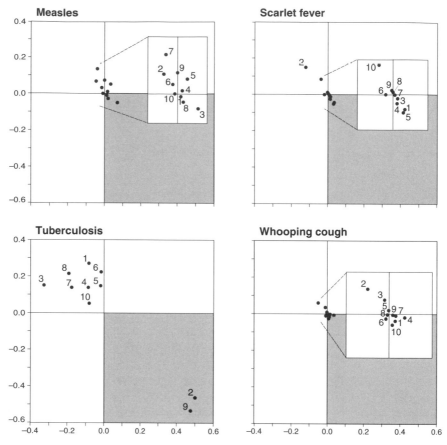

Figure 5.2. (*cont.*)

To re-examine the hypothesis at a regional scale, the 100 cities were allocated to the regions described in section 5.2, and the ranking was carried out for each region separately. Regressions were fitted to the data for each region and marker disease. The sixty slope and intercept coefficients generated were used as *xy* coordinates to plot each region/disease combination on a scattergraph (figure 5.4). Given the ranking method described in section 4.5, a 'high potential' model of metropolitan mortality would produce regression lines with positive slope coefficients. As part A of the diagram shows, only nine of the sixty had positive gradients; of these nine, six were for developed regions of the world. The evidence strongly confirms our findings at the world scale; the 'high potential' model is only weakly supported by these data, and the main evidence for the model is found in developed economies.

Given the allocation of cities to regions shown in table 5.1, sample sizes for

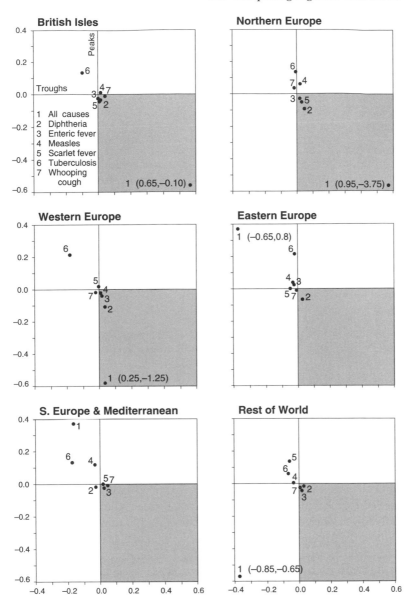

Figure 5.3. The crisis hypothesis at the scale of world regions, II: time trends in ten world regions, 1888–1912, in death rates per 100,000 population for all causes and six marker diseases. Values of regression slope coefficient values for OLS trend lines fitted to maximum (peaks) and minimum (troughs) monthly death rates occurring each year, 1888–1912. Values for peaks are plotted on the vertical axis, and for troughs on the horizontal axis. Values falling in the shaded quadrant are consistent with the crisis hypothesis. (Figure continues overleaf.)

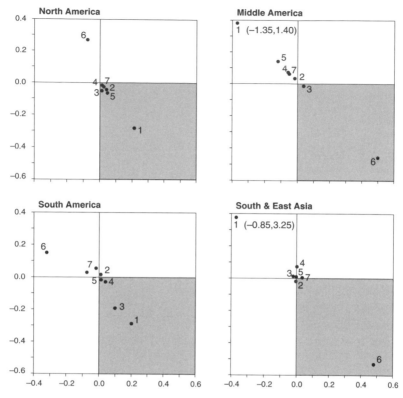

Figure 5.3. (*cont.*)

individual regressions varied greatly, from five (ROW) to twenty (NA). To give an idea of average behaviour, figure 5.4 also plots the mean intercept and slope values for each region irrespective of disease (graph B), and for each disease irrespective of region (graph C). In B, Eastern Europe is the only region with a positive average slope coefficient. Most of the regions have very similar averages, with only Southern Europe and the Mediterranean substantially out of line. In this region, very steep negative slope coefficients were consistently found. In C, tuberculosis had the shallowest average gradient but no disease had the positive average implied by the 'big-city' hypothesis.

Many of the great cities in our sample had already made substantial progress in public health reform (improved sanitation, water supply, for example) by the beginning of our study period (see section 6.2). For these cities, the sobriquet 'filthy dirty' was less relevant than it had been a generation before. One possible explanation of the gradient reversal we have found is that such large cities had made more progress than smaller cities in public health reform by the end of the nineteenth century, leading to a replacement

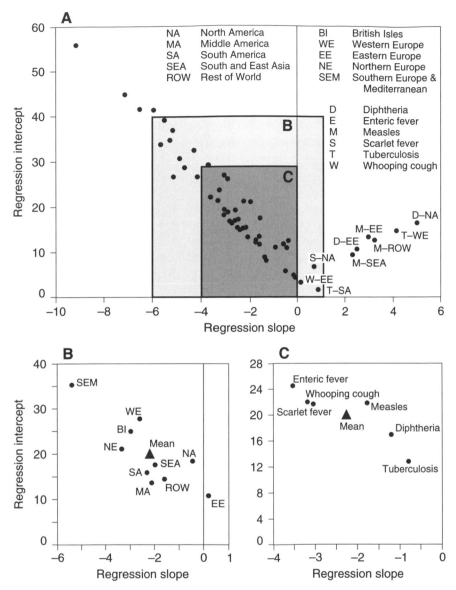

Figure 5.4. The 'big-city' hypothesis: world regions. (A) Intercept (vertical axis) and slope (horizontal axis) coefficient values from simple linear regressions of disease intensity against logs of 1900 city populations. (B) Average coefficient values for world regions. (C) Average coefficient values for each marker disease.

of large cities by smaller cities as the main locations of excess mortality from disease.

5.4 Regional contrasts in seasonality

5.4.1 *Mapping seasonal variation*

It is well known that many infectious diseases exhibit strong seasonal patterns of both morbidity and mortality (see sections 4.4.2, 6.2.2, and 6.2.4). There are a number of ways of identifying geographical patterns of seasonal variation. One of the simplest is illustrated in figure 5.5 for measles. To construct this map, we first calculated the median reported deaths per 100,000 population in each month of the year over the period, 1888–1912, for each of the 100 cities. Next, the month of the year with the largest median rate was identified for each city. Circles were coded black if the peak fell in the northern hemisphere winter (here defined as October–March), and coded white if the peak fell in the northern hemisphere summer (April–September). To avoid plotting problems, the circles are shown on a map constructed on the basis of the ranks of the latitudes and longitudes of cities taken from the bottom left-hand corner of the map. Critical latitudes and longitudes have been marked, along with hulls to mark the rough positions of the world regions (except for the dispersed region, Rest of the World).

A test for spatial autocorrelation among first nearest neighbours using Moran's I yielded a standard Normal deviate of $z=2.47$ (see section 6.3.2 for a discussion of the method), significant at the $\alpha=0.01$ level in a one-tailed test. This implies clustering of black and white circles on the map – cities in the same region of the world tend to have peak death rates in the same month of the year. While this seems an obvious statement, inspection of the map shows that, even for measles where we would expect, on the basis of the discussion in section 6.3.2, to find strong seasonal contrasts, the seasonal concentration is not simply a flip over on the basis of the winter months in each hemisphere. If that were so, the black circles should be concentrated in the northern hemisphere and the white in the southern. In fact, regions in the same latitudes may display starkly different patterns (South and East Asia, northern winter peak; Middle America, northern summer peak, for example). In so far as general statements can be made about figure 5.5, it appears that more cities coded black are found south of latitude 40° N, and more cities coded white are found north of that latitude. This implies that, in warmer climes, the peak month may be earlier in the year. Thus, although geographical contrasts in seasonal patterns are to be seen, they are more subtle than is implied by the naïve model of peaks in the winter season because of an indoor crowding effect, and more complex methods are needed to identify the main features. It is to such methods that we now turn.

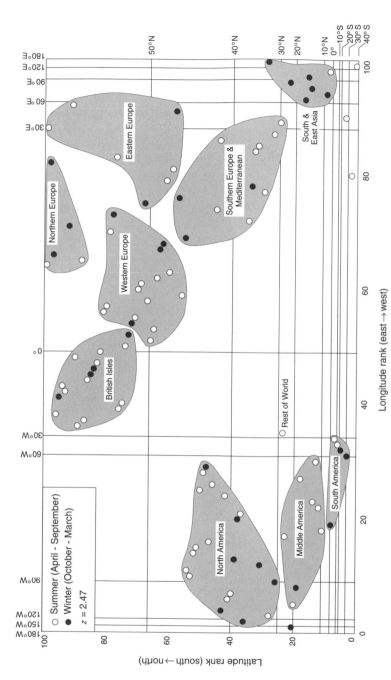

Figure 5.5. Ninety-one world cities: hemispherical contrasts in measles seasonality. Geographical distribution of cities whose monthly median reported deaths per 100,000 population from measles, 1888–1912, peaked in the northern summer (white circles) and the northern winter (solid circles). Map projection characteristics are discussed in the text. The value of the spatial autocorrelation statistic (z) is also given as a standard Normal deviate.

5.4.2 Cobweb charts

Figures 5.6 and 5.7 use cobweb graphs to investigate seasonal distributions. For each marker disease, figure 5.6 plots as black bars the number of cities in the sample of 100 with their peak median death rate in each month of the year against a backcloth (stippled) giving the same information for deaths from all causes. There are marked differences between the diseases. Whooping cough shows the least variability from month to month; diphtheria and enteric fever display the greatest contrasts with marked peaks in the second half of the year. Measles, tuberculosis, and whooping cough peak most strongly in the period March–May (the northern spring). Scarlet fever has a bimodal peak (in May and November). Deaths from all causes is markedly bimodal, with clear peaks in March and July. Like figure 5.5, figure 5.6 again highlights the complexities to be found when analysing seasonal variations in death rates. But, bearing in mind that most of the cities in our sample are in the northern hemisphere, there is still some evidence in figure 5.6 to suggest that peaking may be related to the winter season of the year (the bimodal distribution for all causes and scarlet fever, the northern spring peak for measles, tuberculosis, and whooping cough).

To investigate this possibility more fully, figure 5.7 plots for each marker disease the seasonal distribution of peak death rates on a broadly hemispherical basis. Taking the northern tropic as the dividing line, we conventionally defined 'southern' cities as those located south of 23 1/2° N, and 'northern' cities as those to the north of this tropic. The percentage of cities in each of these groups peaking in each month of the year is plotted as a lightly stippled cobweb for the southern cities, and as a dark stipple for the northern cities. The labelling around the circumference of the cobweb plots indicates the quarters of the year on a hemispherical basis.

For enteric fever, tuberculosis, and whooping cough, there are distinct hemispherical contrasts. Enteric fever and tuberculosis peak in the third quarter of the year (autumn) of each hemisphere; whooping cough peaks in the second quarter (summer) of each hemisphere. Diphtheria is a disease of the winter in the northern hemisphere, and of the second and fourth quarters in the southern. In the northern hemisphere, measles peaks in its second quarter; in the southern hemisphere, the peak is in its third quarter. Scarlet fever is bimodal in both hemispheres, with peaks in the second and fourth quarters of each.

Taken together, figures 5.6 and 5.7 show that, while there are seasonal contrasts in the marker diseases which reflect the regional locations of the cities, these contrasts vary greatly from disease to disease. Peak incidence does not simply 'follow the sun' in any simplistic way. Accordingly, in the remainder of this section, we move from mapping and charting methods for examining seasonality to some statistical techniques that may be used to uncover seasonal contrasts. The contrasts discovered are then related to climatic factors.

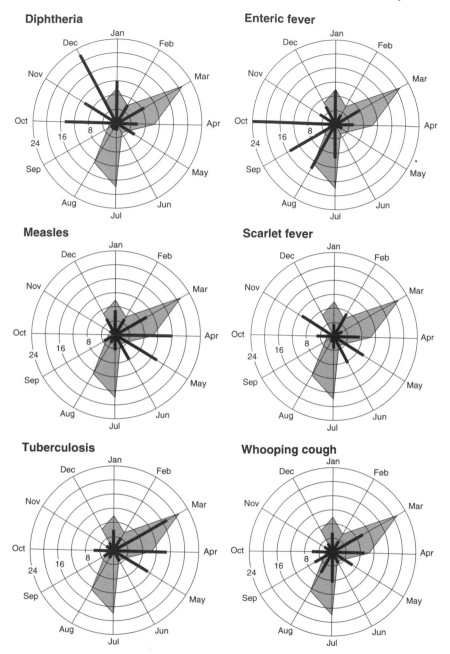

Figure 5.6. Monthly variations in deaths per 100,000 population for six marker diseases (solid bars) and all causes (stippled), 1888–1912. Number of cities in the sample of 100 with their peak median death rate in each month of the year.

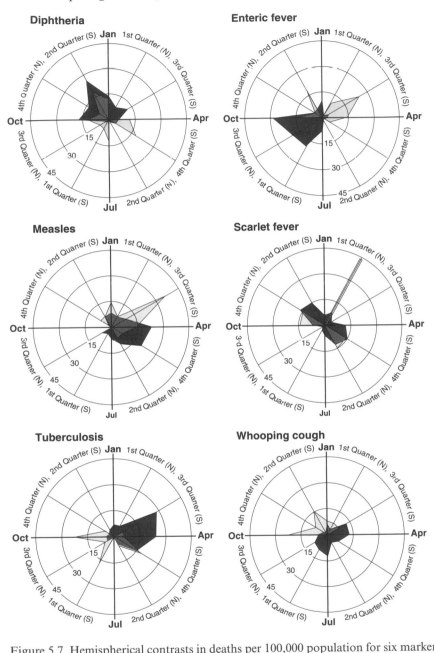

Figure 5.7. Hemispherical contrasts in deaths per 100,000 population for six marker diseases, 1888–1912. Percentage of cities north of 23 1/2° N (dark stipple) with their peak median death rate in each month of the year. Light stipple gives percentage of cities south of 23 1/2° N with their peak median death rate in each month of the year.

5.4.3 Indices of seasonality

As before, the basic data consisted of the median reported deaths per 100,000 population in each month of the year over the period 1888–1912 for each of the 100 cities. From these values, three indices were computed.

(1) *Peak concentration*: Peak concentration was defined as the ratio of the month with the maximum median rate to the overall median rate over the period, 1888–1912.

(2) *Median range*: This was defined as the ratio of the month with the maximum median rate to the month with the minimum median rate.

(3) *Variability*: The coefficient of variation, *CV*, was used where

$$CV = 100(s / \bar{x}) \tag{5.1}$$

and $\bar{x}$ and s are the arithmetic mean and standard deviation respectively of the twelve median monthly death rates.

In cities where there is little or no variation in rates over the year, both 1 and 2 will be close to unity; as deaths become more and more concentrated in a few months of the year, the ratios will increase. For *CV*, increased seasonal contrasts will yield larger values.

Taking diphtheria as an example, figure 5.8 illustrates the geographical variability in each of these indices over the 100 cities by plotting the values as shaded contour surfaces. Surface values were estimated by fitting quadratic polynomials to the observed values of the indices, 1–3, using distance weighted least squares. The algorithm is described in McLain (1974). Denote the surface by $z = f(x,y)$. Suppose we wish to estimate the surface height $f(a,b)$ at a point (a,b). Our aim is to fit a polynomial $P(x,y)$ which will fit as accurately as possible in the least squares sense the data points (x_i, y_i), where

$$P(x,y) = c_{00} + c_{10}x + c_{01}y + c_{20}x^2 + c_{11}xy + c_{02}y^2 \tag{5.2}$$

for a quadratic polynomial. We require those data points (x_i, y_i) close to (a,b) to carry more weight than distant points. More precisely, we choose the coefficients c_{rs} to minimise the quadratic form

$$Q = \sum_{i=1}^{u} \left[P(x_i, y_i) - z_i \right]^2 \bullet w \left[(x_i - a)^2 + (y_i - b)^2 \right] \tag{5.3}$$

where w is a weight function such as $w(d^2) = 1/d^2$, which is large when (a,b) is close to (x_i, y_i) and small when it is remote.

Figure 5.8 shows two main features. First, a similar spatial pattern of values is found for all three indices. Second, higher values are found mainly in tropical and subtropical regions, implying that seasonal contrasts in diphtheria rates are more marked in these areas. The coefficient of variation appears to detect local variations more effectively than either peak concentration or median range. This feature was repeated for the other five marker diseases and

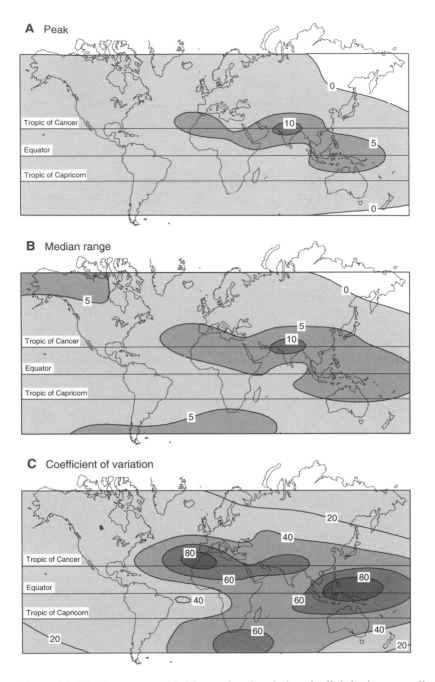

Figure 5.8. Ninety-seven world cities: regional variations in diphtheria seasonality. Shaded contour maps of measures of seasonal variability in reported deaths from diphtheria per 100,000 population, 1888–1912. (A) Peak concentration. (B) Median range. (C) Coefficient of variation, *CV*.

Enteric fever

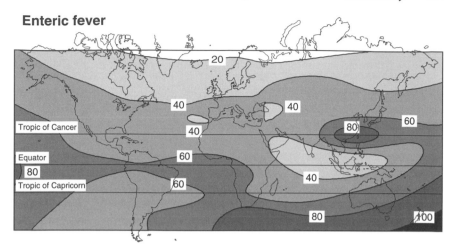

Scarlet fever

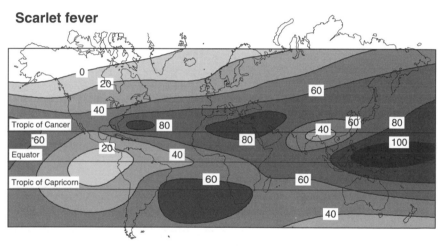

Figure 5.9. The 100 world cities: regional variations in the seasonal incidence of enteric and scarlet fevers. Shaded contour maps of coefficient of variation, *CV*, for seasonal variation in reported deaths per 100,000 population, 1888–1912, from enteric fever and scarlet fever.

all causes. Accordingly, we have used *CV* as our best measure of seasonal contrasts in disease rates, and figure 5.9 maps *CV* for two other diseases, enteric fever and scarlet fever.

Figure 5.9 shows some striking similarities in the seasonal patterns of the two diseases. There is evidence of raised *CV* values in tropical and subtropical regions, with especially high values found in South and East Asia. This feature of raised *CV* values in the tropics and subtropics was found for all the marker diseases.

5.4.4 *Environmental controls on seasonality*

Seasonal patterns are commonly a response to environmental factors. As we have already noted, in general terms, many of the diseases considered here are conventionally held to peak in the colder period of the year. While this may be attributed in part to the effect of increased crowding indoors (and therefore higher transmission rates through greater mixing of susceptible and infectious individuals) during the cold part of the year, there is also the adverse effect of ultraviolet light upon virus and bacilli survival rates (which tend to be lower during longer summer days). For these reasons, figures 5.8 and 5.9 seem to produce counterintuitive results, with greater seasonal contrasts apparently found in lower latitudes. But a further factor may be intervening, namely the relative distributions of land and water. The more continuous land masses of the northern hemisphere may result in less variability in seasonal patterns of mortality rates between its cities than among the cities of the southern hemisphere; there, the relatively fragmentary intermixing of land and water can result in a greater variety of local environmental controls, particularly because many of the cities in our sample occupy coastal locations (section 4.6.1).

To capture the impact of environmental factors upon seasonality, the variables already defined in section 4.6.1 (elevation above sea level; annual average temperature; average temperature in the warmest month of the year; average temperature in the coldest month; average annual precipitation; latitude) were re-employed in this subsection. For each disease and all causes, Pearson product moment correlation coefficients were calculated between the CV values of the 100 cities and the values of each of the environmental variables. The strongest correlations were obtained with annual average temperature (table 5.3); sample sizes fell below the maximum of 100 because of missing observations. Except for tuberculosis, the correlations in table 5.3, although modest, were all significant at the $\alpha = 0.01$ level (one-tailed test). The fact that the correlations were positive implies greater variability in seasonality of the diseases in warmer climates; this is consistent with figures 5.8 and 5.9.

For three of the marker diseases (enteric fever, scarlet fever, and tuberculosis), figure 5.10 illustrates the scattergrams between CV and annual average temperature. The OLS regression lines are also marked, along with the correlation coefficients between the variables. To tie this diagram into seasonal contrasts, box and whisker plots (Tukey, 1977) for the distribution of reported death rates per 100,000 population in each month of the year, 1888–1912, have been added for three cities for each disease. In a box and whisker plot, the following features are illustrated. The continuous line joins the median rate reported in each month of the year, where the median has been calculated from the twenty-five rates recorded in that month in each year, 1888–1912. The variability in the monthly values is shown by plotting as the outer limits of the shaded box the first and third quartiles, and Q_1 and Q_3 respectively, of the

Table 5.3. *Impact of temperature upon regional variations in the seasonality of disease*

Pearson correlation coefficients between coefficient of variation (CV) for seasonal distribution of death rates and annual average temperature.

Disease	Number of cities	$r(CV$, average temperature)
All causes	97	0.25
Diphtheria	97	0.33
Enteric fever	98	0.41
Measles	93	0.30
Scarlet fever	90	0.41
Tuberculosis	94	0.14
Whooping cough	90	0.44

twenty-five values. The whiskers extend from the box edges to encompass all monthly values that satisfy the following limits:

Lower limit: $Q_1 - 1.5(Q_3 - Q_1)$;
Upper limit: $Q_3 + 1.5(Q_3 - Q_1)$.

In figure 5.10, CV is positively correlated with annual average temperature for all diseases. This again confirms the shaded contour plots of figures 5.8 and 5.9; seasonal contrasts appear on average to be greater in warmer latitudes. But, although seasonal variability does increase with the temperature variable, figure 5.10 again illustrates the complexities of the relationship. For example, for tuberculosis, the month-by-month median for Cartagena (latitude 10° N) scarcely varies as compared with Mannheim (49° N) and San Francisco (38° N), but displays greater variability in one month (December) than either of the other two cities. For enteric fever, Melbourne (38° S) shows greater variability in the median than either St Petersburg (60° N) or Havana (23° N). For scarlet fever, the three cities have similar annual average temperatures, are well outside the tropics (Warsaw 52° N, New York 42° N, Paris 48° N), and yet have marked differences in their median and interquartile ranges on the box and whisker plots.

It is possible that the positive relationship we have uncovered between CV and annual average temperature is partly an artefact of the data. Many of the cities for which our time series have fewest observations (and are likely to yield less reliable results) are located in low latitudes. But this is not true for all such cities. For example, in figure 5.10, Havana reported information on deaths from enteric fever in 45 per cent of months, 1888–1912, and Cartagena in 70 per cent of months for tuberculosis (the median rates across all cities were 57 and 76 per cent for enteric fever and tuberculosis respectively).

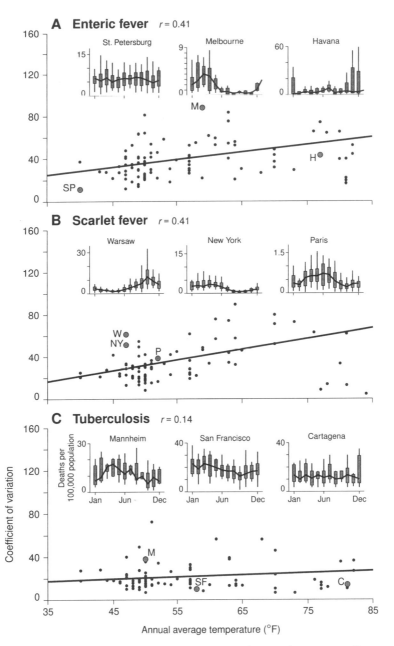

Figure 5.10. The 100 world cities: environmental controls on seasonality. Scattergraphs and OLS regression lines for coefficient of variation (*CV*) of monthly deaths per 100,000 population, 1888–1912, against average annual temperature. (A) Enteric fever. (B) Scarlet fever. (C) Tuberculosis. For each disease, box and whisker plots, defined in the text, have been added to show the considerable variability in median death rates (solid line) and interquartile ranges (limit of shaded boxes) within the general positive relationship between *CV* and temperature.

A facet of this problem is that, *ceteris paribus*, we would expect smaller cities (which tend to have fewer observations) to display greater fluctuations than larger cities. The Bartlett model (see section 7.5.1) implies that great cities will have predictable, large, and regularly spaced epidemics; small cities will miss some epidemics completely and, after such a 'miss', have occasional very large epidemics. This more erratic epidemic behaviour will affect the seasonal distribution of cases, even though we are dealing with death rates. The evidence of figure 5.10 is also ambiguous on this point as a possible explanation. For enteric fever, Havana is half the size of Melbourne, and yet it has a substantially smaller CV value. Similarly for tuberculosis, Cartagena (population 25,000 in 1900) is much smaller than either Mannheim (131,000) or San Francisco (300,000), and yet it has a CV value only marginally larger than that for San Francisco.

If we seek a substantive rather than a data recording explanation of the conundrum we have reported, then three possibilities are most likely:

(i)   Used alone, a single index of seasonality (here CV) and a single environmental variable (annual average temperature) may not adequately capture the variations in the data.

(ii) Seasonal contrasts in the incidence of disease are indeed more complex than has been thought on the basis of studies which have focused principally upon mid-latitude cities.

(iii) A third possibility is an 'epidemiological isolation' effect. Under this hypothesis, we might argue, in terms of the prevailing transport technology of the 1888–1912 period, that the mid-latitude cities (coincidentally located in more developed countries) were better connected both internally by rail and externally by sea links. Under these conditions, disease could be readily exchanged between cities and there might be constant replenishment of disease by movements of infectives. Cities located in lower latitudes (coincidentally located in developing countries) were probably less well interconnected internally and externally. With less free movement of infectives, susceptibles could accumulate to allow occasional explosive epidemics. This would generate the strong temporal contrasts in the time series of infections consistent with the trends observed in figures 5.8–5.10.

To try to eliminate (ii) as a possibility we resorted, as in section 4.6.3, to principal components analysis.

Principal components analysis

(a) Indices of seasonality: For each disease and all causes, the three indices of seasonality defined in section 5.4.3 were subjected to a principal components analysis. The first principal component was the only, and highly significant, axis; the loadings of the variables appear in table 5.4. The striking features are

Table 5.4. *The 100 world cities: variable loadings on leading principal
component for indices of seasonality*

Disease	Variable	Loadings Component 1
All causes	Peak concentration	0.58
	Median range	0.59
	CV	0.58
	Variance explained (%)	92
Diphtheria	Peak concentration	0.58
	Median range	0.59
	CV	0.56
	Variance explained (%)	94
Enteric fever	Peak concentration	0.56
	Median range	0.57
	CV	0.60
	Variance explained (%)	86
Measles	Peak concentration	0.59
	Median range	0.58
	CV	0.57
	Variance explained (%)	94
Scarlet fever	Peak concentration	0.58
	Median range	0.59
	CV	0.56
	Variance explained (%)	93
Tuberculosis	Peak concentration	0.53
	Median range	0.57
	CV	0.64
	Variance explained (%)	79
Whooping cough	Peak concentration	0.58
	Median range	0.54
	CV	0.62
	Variance explained (%)	81

the high levels of explanation and, for each disease, the very similar positive
loadings of the variables on the component. This suggests that the three indices
are measuring congruent features of the seasonal distribution of the city time
series. We will refer to this component as a seasonal variability component.

(b) Environmental variables: The principal components analysis was then
repeated for the environmental variables described at the head of this section
to create a single environmental index. Table 5.5 shows the loadings for components 1 and 2, although only component 1 had an eigenvalue greater than

Table 5.5. *The 100 world cities: loadings of environmental variables on first two principal components*

	Loadings	
Variable	Component 1	Component 2
Elevation	0.109	0.967
Average annual temperature	−0.513	0.047
Average temperature, warmest month	−0.442	−0.001
Average temperature, coldest month	−0.483	0.054
Average annual precipitation	−0.341	−0.111
Latitude	0.425	−0.220
Eigenvalues	3.61	0.99
% of variance explained	60.2	16.5

1. Component 1 reveals two clusters of variables: one main group consisting of the temperature variables and precipitation, and a second consisting of latitude and (weakly) elevation. Component 2 reflects almost wholly the effect of elevation. For convenience, component 1 will be referred to as a temperature component.

The final stage was to combine the results of the two component analyses by plotting the scattergrams of component scores of the cities on the seasonal variability component against the scores on the environmental component. Echoing figure 5.10, figure 5.11 shows these plots for enteric fever, scarlet fever, and tuberculosis. Comparison of figures 5.10 and 5.11 reveals no major differences. Seasonal variability is again seen to be weakly positively correlated with temperature effects.

5.5 Biproportionate analysis

5.5.1 The method

The conventional way of studying the changing temporal incidence of disease for geographical areas is to plot the values on a graph on a region-by-region basis. This is illustrated in the main part of figure 5.12A, where some hypothetical values are shown for two areas, A and B, at five different points in time. Incidence starts at a very much higher level in A than in B, but falls more rapidly so that, by time period 5, both display similar levels of infection.

In making this interpretation we must remember that the data for each area have been plotted independently of each other, so that absolute changes are being compared. While this is reasonable with the global time series of chapter 4 (figures 4.3–4.9, for example), once the geographical dimension of a set of

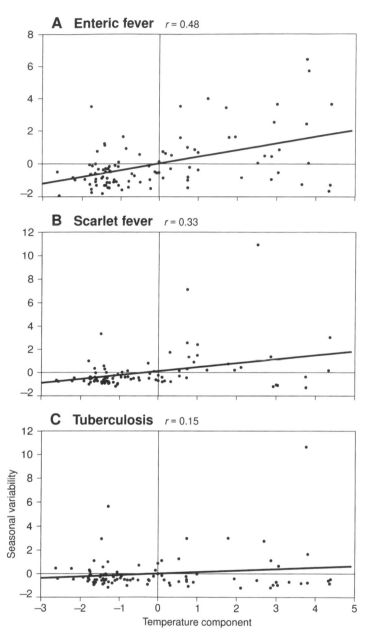

Figure 5.11. The 100 world cities: principal components analysis of environmental controls on the seasonal incidence of mortality. Scattergraphs and OLS regression lines for city scores on a seasonal variability component constructed from monthly deaths per 100,000 population, 1888–1912, against city scores on a temperature component. (A) Enteric fever. (B) Scarlet fever. (C) Tuberculosis.

regions is introduced (as in this chapter), we will wish to comment upon the degree of temporal change which has taken place in one region as compared with the amount of change experienced in others. Or we may want to establish which of the time periods in the time–space data matrix exhibits the most change over the set of areas.

A variety of methods exist for standardising a matrix so that relative change may be assessed. One of the most common is to use row and column totals to generate expected values in each area in each time period and then to examine departures of the actual values from these expectations. A particularly powerful alternative method is to use biproportionate scores and we illustrate the computational procedures involved by examining the data plotted in figure 5.12A. The raw data appear in part A of table 5.6.

Suppose a matrix of observations $\{x_{ij}\}$ is available in which m areas form the rows (denoted by i) and n time periods form the columns (denoted by j). The quantity in any cell of the matrix gives the value of the variable of interest (for example, deaths or death rate per 100,000 population from any disease) in a particular area in a selected time period. In step one of the standardisation procedure, the values are scaled so that each row sum is equal to the number of columns in the matrix, here five. This is achieved by calculating the row sums in the original data (for example 1,550 in the case of area 1) and then dividing these totals by five to give a scaling factor for each row of the data matrix. For the first row, this procedure yields $1550/5=310$, and for the second row, $155/5=31$. The adjusted scores are then obtained by taking the values in each row of the original data matrix and dividing them by their corresponding scaling factor. This step produces the matrix given in table 5.6B where, to eliminate decimal points, all values have been multiplied by 100.

The standardisation process then continues by scaling the columns of the matrix given in part B so that each column sum is equal to the number of rows in the matrix, here two. This yields the matrix given in table 5.6C where again all values have been multiplied by 100. The process of adjustment is continued, operating alternately on rows and columns until the adjusted matrix converges; that is, the values in the matrix cease, within some margin of error set by the researcher, to change. We can express this process formally as

$$
\begin{bmatrix}
x_{11} & x_{12} & x_{13} & \cdots & x_{1n} \\
x_{21} & x_{22} & x_{23} & \cdots & x_{2n} \\
\vdots & \vdots & \vdots & \vdots & \vdots \\
\vdots & \vdots & \vdots & \vdots & \vdots \\
x_{m1} & x_{m2} & x_{m3} & \cdots & x_{mn}
\end{bmatrix}
\begin{bmatrix}
n+e \\
n+e \\
\vdots \\
\vdots \\
n+e
\end{bmatrix}
=
\begin{bmatrix}
n+e \\
n+e \\
\vdots \\
\vdots \\
n+e
\end{bmatrix}
\tag{5.4}
$$

$$
=
$$

$$
[m+e \quad m+e \quad m+e \quad \cdots \quad m+e]
$$

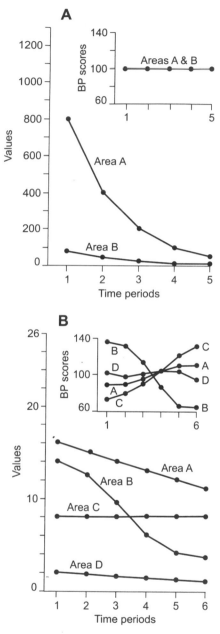

Figure 5.12. Construction of biproportionate scores. (A) Scores for two exponentially declining trends in two areas. (B) Scores for contrasting time trends in four areas.

Table 5.6. *Biproportionate scores: hypothetical data for two regions and five time periods*

	Time periods					
Areas	1	2	3	4	5	Total
PART A Original data						
1	800	400	200	100	50	1550
2	80	40	20	10	5	155
Total	880	440	220	110	55	
PART B First iteration scores						
1	258	129	65	32	16	500
2	258	129	65	32	16	500
Total	516	258	130	64	32	
PART C Second iteration scores						
1	100	100	100	100	100	500
2	100	100	100	100	100	500
Total	200	200	200	200	200	

Note:
The procedure for calculating the scores is described in the text.

where e is an allowable tolerance term. In the simple example given in table 5.6, convergence has already occurred by the end of the second cycle but, in large matrices with irregular relationships between the areas, a substantial number of iterations may be required.

In the matrix recorded in part C of table 5.6, reading across the rows gives the relative change in each area over time, while reading down the columns gives the relative change in each time period over the set of areas. If the time series for both areas change exponentially (either both upwards or both downwards) over time, as in the example used here, then the adjusted or standardised values will be unity (100). These standardised values have been plotted on the inset graph of figure 5.12A. A value of unity (100) in the biproportionate matrix is the expected value if an area is changing exponentially over time, so that cells with values greater than unity have experienced relatively greater change; cells with values less than unity have experienced relatively less change. In figure 5.12A, the line graphs for the raw data show that disease incidence in both areas has declined exponentially over time, while the biproportionate scores confirm that their relative behaviour is the same.

A more complex example appears in figure 5.12B involving four areas and six time periods. The time trends for the raw data in each of the four areas have been

Biproportionate score

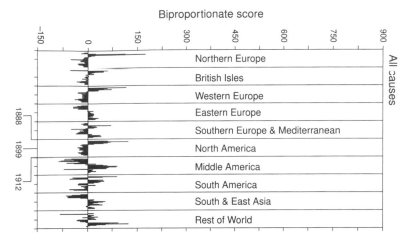

Figure 5.13. Biproportionate scores, 1888–1912, based on reported deaths per 100,000 population: temporal contrasts in intensity of deaths from all causes across ten world regions. The vertical axis within each regional block gives the biproportionate score in each year from 1888 (top) to 1912 (bottom). A score of zero corresponds to average intensity.

plotted on the main graph, along with the biproportionate scores on the inset graph. Thus in terms of the original data, where each area is being examined in isolation and independently of every other area, we see that area A starts at a high initial level in the first time period and exhibits a steady decline in disease intensity. Area B shows a rapid decline from high levels of intensity. Area C appears to have been steady throughout the period at an intermediate level of intensity. Area D is always at a low level of intensity but with a slight decline over time. In terms of the biproportionate scores, however, which enable us to look at the performance of each area, not in isolation but as a part of a changing system of areas where individual behaviour is compared with that of the others, we see that A and D are relatively stable over time, but that the changes in areas B and C are dramatic. Area B has, relatively speaking, experienced a marked decline in intensity over time whereas area C has increased equally clearly.

5.5.2 Application to world regions

There are two ways biproportionate scores can be computed from the data recorded in the *Weekly Abstract*: (i) for each disease across all regions and (ii) for each region across the diseases. We consider each in turn.

Analysis by disease: Figures 5.13 and 5.14 chart the biproportionate scores by disease on a regional basis. Figure 5.13 shows all causes; figure 5.14 plots the

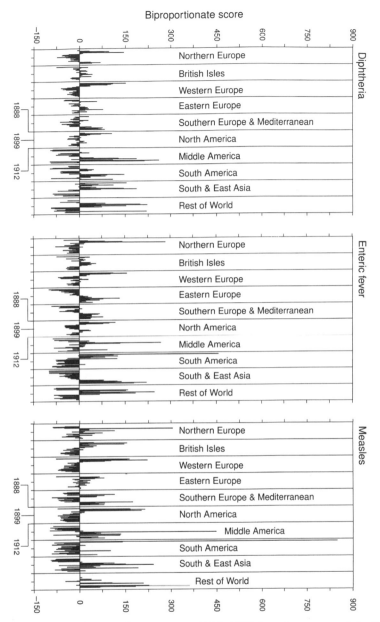

Figure 5.14. Biproportionate scores, 1888–1912, based on reported deaths per 100,000 population: temporal contrasts in intensity of deaths from each of six marker diseases across ten world regions. The vertical axis within each regional block gives the biproportionate score in each year from 1888 (top) to 1912 (bottom). A score of zero corresponds to average intensity. (Figure continues overleaf.)

Biproportionate score

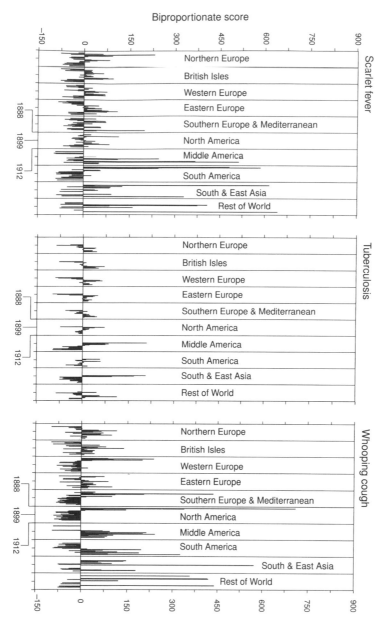

Figure 5.14. (*cont.*)

remaining six diseases. Within each regional block, scores have been plotted as a time series histogram from 1888 (top) to 1912 (bottom). In plotting, a base of 100 has been subtracted from the original scores so that positive scores represent disease concentration in time and space, while negative scores represent a deficit. All scores were calculated on the basis of death rates per 100,000 population.

As shown in figure 5.13, there are striking regional contrasts in deaths from all causes. In the first quarter of the period, rates were highest in the more highly urbanised areas (Northern Europe, British Isles, Western Europe, North America). In the second half of the period after 1900, the less urbanised regions of Eastern Europe, Middle America, South and East Asia, and the Rest of the World dominated. The Mediterranean lands peaked early and late. Of the developing world, only South America peaked early. Whether the broad geographical switch in concentration of mortality rates from the developed to developing world over the period reflects more rapid improvements in medical care (as a result of the public health movements) and nutrition in the old industrial nations remains to be explored.

Figure 5.14 shows that there is a marked contrast between tuberculosis and the other five marker diseases. The range of scores for tuberculosis, like all causes, is much smaller than for any other disease. This may reflect the both the more geographically ubiquitous nature of tuberculosis as a cause of death at this time and its partly non-epidemic character. As we have seen from the time series analysis of section 4.7, the remaining five benchmark diseases are strongly cyclical and epidemic in character and so, *ceteris paribus*, we would expect starker regional contrasts – reflected here in the much bigger range of scores for these diseases.

The time series of biproportionate scores for tuberculosis are the simplest (recall that mortality data for tuberculosis are recorded in the *Weekly Abstract* only during the second half of our study period). They were highest in the European areas (Northern Europe, the British Isles, Western Europe, Eastern Europe, the Mediterranean) and the Rest of the World after 1906, and in the Americas and Asia before 1906.

The biproportionate scores for the other five diseases show complex patterns, but there are some generalisations that can be made. First, the biggest scores (and therefore the greatest within-region contrasts) are usually found in the three American regions and the Rest of the World. A smaller range of scores is found in European regions. Whether this is a reporting artefact or whether it reflects bigger epidemic/non-epidemic contrasts in more susceptible populations (virgin soil) remains to be explored. Second, regions in the Old World generally had higher scores in the first half of the study period than in the second, whereas in Middle and South America, the Mediterranean, and South and East Asia, the reverse prevailed.

Analysis by region: All the graphs in figure 5.15 have been plotted on the same scale. There are stark contrasts between (i) the European regions and North

Biproportionate score

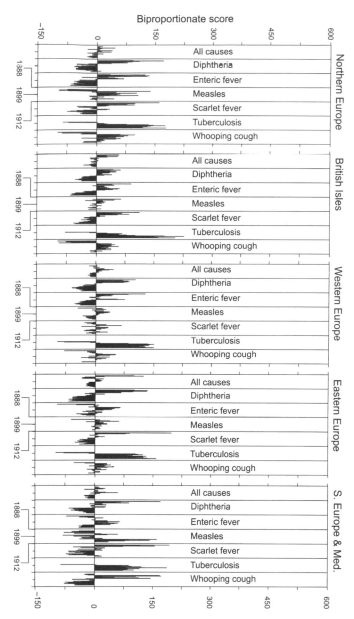

Figure 5.15. Biproportionate scores, 1888–1912, based on reported deaths per 100,000 population: temporal contrasts on a regional basis in the intensity of deaths for six marker diseases and all causes. The vertical axis within each disease block gives the biproportionate score in each year from 1888 (top) to 1912 (bottom). A score of zero corresponds to average intensity.

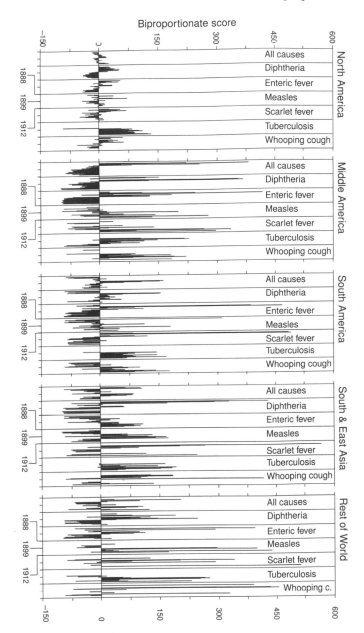

Figure 5.15. (*cont.*)

America (relatively small variance in their time series of biproportionate scores) and (ii) the other regions of the world (high variance in scores). In the five European regions and North America, the epidemic diseases were the signal diseases of the early part of our period, whereas tuberculosis was the disease of the second. It is noticeable in all these regions that tuberculosis began with scores less than zero, indicative of regional deficit rather than concentration, and then switched to positive scores. These patterns are also evident, but somewhat less distinctively, in the remaining world regions.

5.6 Multidimensional mapping

5.6.1 The method

An alternative way of examining regional patterns of mortality and, in particular, temporal behaviour is to employ multidimensional scaling (MDS). MDS refers to a family of statistical methods by which the information contained in a dataset is represented by a configuration of points in multidimensional space, such that the geometrical relationships between the points reflect the empirical relationships in the data. The term *multidimensional* denotes the fact that the space into which the points are fitted may vary from low-order spaces (for example, one-dimensional scales or two-dimensional 'maps') up to higher-order spaces (for example, three-dimensional 'cubes' or four- or more dimensional hyperspaces).

Although the mathematical groundwork for multidimensional scaling was laid as early as the 1930s by Young and Householder as part of the general development of principal component and factor models (Harman, 1960), the classic development of the method came in psychology two decades later in the work of the Gulliksen–Torgerson group at Princeton (Torgerson, 1958) and the Shepard–Kruskal group at the Bell Telephone Laboratories (Shepard, 1962; Kruskal, 1964a, 1964b; Kruskal and Wish, 1978). More recently, the basic mathematics has attracted renewed interest from Kendall (1971, 1975) and Sibson (1978, 1979). Reviews of the literature appear in Schiffman, Reynolds, and Young (1981), Coxon (1982), and Cliff, Haggett, Smallman-Raynor, Stroup, and Williamson (1995).

To date, applications of MDS in epidemiology have been very limited (D'Andrade, Quinn, Nerlove, and Romney, 1972), although two of the present authors have used the method to examine the space–time characteristics of influenza epidemics in Iceland from 1945 to 1970 (Cliff, Haggett, and Ord, 1986). In this section, MDS is used to study the non-linear temporal behaviour of our six benchmark diseases and all causes in the ten world regions. Monthly reported death rates per 100,000 population are used throughout.

(a) The MDS mapping concept

The essential ideas behind MDS are most readily illustrated using a geographical analogy. When a conventional map of a portion of the earth's surface is drawn, some distortion results in transforming a curved segment of the globe onto a flat piece of paper. The particular map projection used will determine the nature and extent of the scale or directional distortion introduced. But, subject to these known errors, all the map projections in common use attempt to ensure that the locations of points on the map systematically reflect their relative positions on the globe.

When MDS is used to represent points on the globe, a map is constructed in which the locations of the points on the map correspond not to their (scaled) geographical locations but to their degree of similarity on some variable measured for them. If the variable is (as here) the death rate per 100,000 population from some disease, then points with similar rates will be located close to each other on the MDS map even though they may be far removed geographically. The greater the degree of similarity between places on the variable measured, the closer together the places will be in the MDS space. Conversely points which are dissimilar on the variable will be widely separated in the MDS space, irrespective of their geographical location. Thus, broadly stated, the problem of MDS is to find a configuration of n points in m-dimensional space such that the interpoint distances in the configuration in some sense match the experimental dissimilarities of the n objects. This may be viewed as a problem of statistical fitting.

(b) The dissimilarity matrix

MDS uses a *dissimilarity matrix*, which defines the degree of correspondence between locations in terms of a variable measured for them over time. For example, let $\mathbf{X}(i \times j)$ be the matrix of death rates from a disease reported by location i in month j. Then define $\mathbf{A}$ by $a_{ij} = 1$ if x_{ij} is greater than the mean rate in area i and $a_{ij} = 0$ otherwise. Let the matrix $\mathbf{S} = \mathbf{A}\mathbf{A}^T$. Then $\mathbf{S}$ is a symmetric matrix in which the ikth element, s_{ik}, is the number of months in which the death rate in both areas i and k exceeded their respective mean rates. We conventionally set $s_{ii} = 0$. It might be argued that, the larger the value of s_{ik}, the greater the similarity between the time series of i and k. Other measures of similarity among the time series might be defined. In the analysis described below, we have used the Pearson product moment correlation coefficient, r, calculated between all pairs of time series of reported deaths per 100,000 population; that is, $s_{ik} = r_{ik}$.

Thus $\mathbf{S}$ is a similarity matrix, reflecting the similarity between locations in terms of their patterns of death rates from a given disease. From $\mathbf{S}$, a matrix $\mathbf{D}$ $(= \{\delta_{ij}\})$ of dissimilarities ($\delta_{ij} = K - s_{ij}$ for some constant K) can be obtained. This matrix of dissimilarities serves as the basis for MDS. The dissimilarities are fixed given quantities and we wish to find the m-dimensional configuration whose distances 'fit them best'. The final locations of the points in the config-uration are selected to preserve the rank ordering of the relative distances of the experimental dissimilarities. Mathematical details of the various fitting options appear in Lingoes and Roskam (1973).

The final distance metric may be regarded as a monotone transformation of the rank ordering. By adopting as our central goal the requirement of a monotonic relationship between the observed dissimilarities and the distances in the configuration, the accuracy of a proposed solution can be judged by the degree to which this condition is approached. For a proposed configuration, we perform a monotonic regression of distance upon dissimilarity and use the residual sum of squares as a quantitative measure of fit, known as the *stress*. We seek to minimise stress. The stress is invariant under translation and uniform stretching and shrinking of the configuration. We therefore nor-malise each configuration by first placing its centre of gravity or centroid at the origin and then stretching or shrinking so that the mean squared distance of the points from the origin equals 1.

If we are to move from statistical fitting to an understanding of the epi-demiological implications of the fitted configuration, then the interpretability of the coordinates of the n points in the m-dimensional space becomes impor-tant. By construction, stress will fall as m increases, but comprehending empir-ically point locations in general hyperspaces as opposed to spaces with $m \leq 3$ is difficult. The analysis to be described is carried out in two dimensions ($m = 2$). From the latter, we will obtain an MDS map upon which the relative locations of points defined in terms of similarity of their time series of death rates from a particular disease may be compared with their locations on a con-ventional geographical map. Indeed, by starting each MDS run with the geo-graphical areas (='individuals') in their natural geographical positions as defined by some cartesian coordinate system such as latitude and longitude, it is possible to track the progressive adjustment from the geographical map to a best-fit epidemiological space.

5.6.2 Results by world region

(a) Spatial cross-sections

The model was first applied to the monthly death rates per 100,000 popula-tion, 1888–1912, from all causes and the six marker diseases. In some regions (for example, South America and Rest of the World) there were substantial numbers of missing observations on some diseases and, where this occurred, the regions concerned were omitted from the analysis. MDS solutions were started from initial configurations where the position of each region was set to the average longitude (x) and average latitude (y) of the cities from which the regional time series was constructed.

To check the degree to which similarity in disease behaviour was driven by

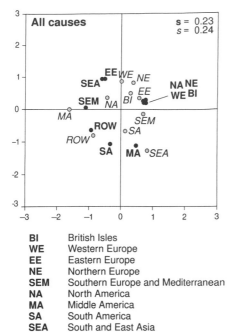

BI   British Isles
WE   Western Europe
EE   Eastern Europe
NE   Northern Europe
SEM   Southern Europe and Mediterranean
NA   North America
MA   Middle America
SA   South America
SEA   South and East Asia
ROW   Rest of the World

Figure 5.16. Regional multidimensional scaling (MDS) for all causes. Final configurations and stresses *s* for regional disease time series based upon reported death rates per 100,000 population (roman, solid circles) and detrended/deseasonalised rates (italic, grey circles). BI=British Isles; EE=Eastern Europe; MA=Middle America; NA=North America; NE=Northern Europe; SA=South America; SEA=South East Asia; SEM=Southern Europe and Mediterranean; ROW=Rest of World; WE=Western Europe.

trend and seasonal effects, the MDS was carried out using, first, the raw rates and then, second, the rates after detrending with a quadratic model and deseasonalising with an additive model as described in section 4.4.2. The resulting normalised MDS spaces are illustrated in figure 5.16 for all causes and in figure 5.17 for the six marker diseases. Regional positions based upon the raw data are plotted with a roman font and, for the detrended/deseasonalised data, in italics. The average correlations across the time series for each disease, as well as the means and standard deviations of the distances of the regions from the origin of the MDS space (0,0) are given in table 5.7.

As table 5.7 shows, the average correlations among the time series are low. The table also indicates that, for enteric fever, measles, scarlet fever, and tuberculosis, detrending and deseasonalising the data prior to scaling reduced the average correlations among the time series leading, as it should, to an increased average distance of points from the origin of the space in the MDS

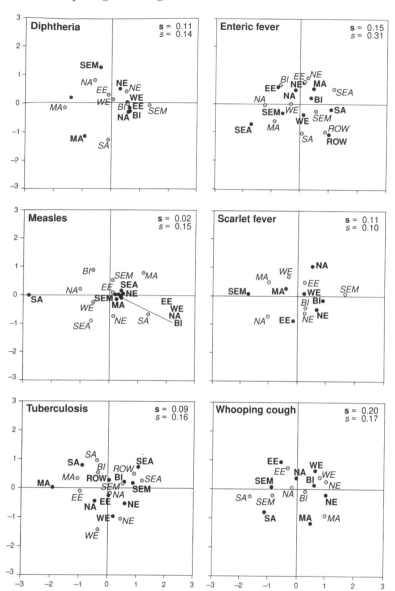

Figure 5.17. Regional multidimensional scaling (MDS) for six marker diseases. Final configurations and stresses *s* for regional disease time series based upon reported death rates per 100,000 population (roman, solid circles) and detrended/deseasonalised rates (italic, grey circles). BI=British Isles; EE=Eastern Europe; MA=Middle America; NA=North America; NE=Northern Europe; SA=South America; SEA=South East Asia; SEM=Southern Europe and Mediterranean; ROW=Rest of World; WE=Western Europe.

Table 5.7. *Regional MDS scaling*

Average time series correlations, means, and standard deviations of distances in MDS spaces. Data are death rates per 100,000 population reported (raw) and detrended and deseasonalised.

Disease	Average correlation ($\bar{r}$)		Mean		Standard deviation	
	Raw data	Detrended and deseasonalised data	Raw data	Detrended and deseasonalised data	Raw data	Detrended and deseasonalised data
All causes	0.288	0.286	0.985	0.930	0.185	0.387
Diphtheria	0.289	0.367	0.924	0.864	0.408	0.538
Enteric fever	0.153	0.110	0.896	0.956	0.472	0.310
Measles	0.160	0.049	0.635	0.913	0.821	0.436
Scarlet fever	0.118	0.139	0.894	0.918	0.484	0.430
Tuberculosis	0.322	0.277	0.879	0.936	0.402	0.371
Whooping cough	0.121	0.174	0.949	0.890	0.334	0.490

configurations for these diseases. Figure 5.17 shows that this effect is especially striking for measles. As well as 'spreading' the configuration of points, detrending and deseasonalising also reduced the standard deviation of distances in the MDS spaces for these diseases. We may conclude that, for these diseases, the similarity in regional time series of death rates is partly driven by the trend and seasonal characteristics of the time series and that, when these features are eliminated, similarity is diminished. As noted above, this is seen most starkly in figure 5.17 in the MDS plot for measles.

For all causes, diphtheria, and whooping cough, detrending and deseasonalising the data had little impact; figures 5.16 and 5.17 indicates that this prewhitening resulted in only modest shifts in the positions of regions in the MDS spaces as compared with their raw data positions. This is best illustrated in the plot for whooping cough.

To define an MDS configuration that reflected regional similarities over the six benchmark diseases and all causes combined, two further analyses were carried out. In these, the measure of similarity between each pair of regions was defined as the average of their individual correlations for the seven separate disease time series. MDS spaces based upon both raw and detrended/deseasonalised data were calculated and, as before, the MDS scaling was seeded with the (x, y) geographical coordinates of the regions. The resulting MDS final configurations are plotted in figure 5.18. To check the extent to which the initial geographical structure was preserved in these final configurations, cluster analysis using complete linkage was carried out. The dendrograms are plotted in figure 5.19, and the basic clusters have been shaded

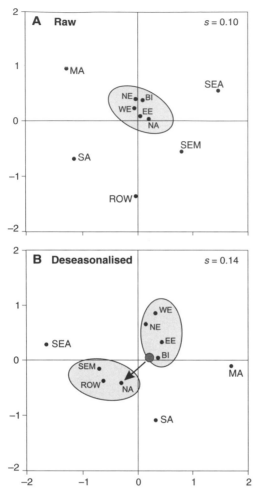

Figure 5.18. Regional multidimensional scaling (MDS) for average disease behaviour on deaths from all causes and six marker diseases combined. Plots show final configurations and stresses *s* based upon reported death rates per 100,000 population (A), and detrended/deseasonalised rates (B). Basic regional groupings defined by complete linkage cluster analysis (see figure 5.19) have been shaded. BI=British Isles; EE=Eastern Europe; MA=Middle America; NA=North America; NE=Northern Europe; SA=South America; SEA=South East Asia; SEM=Southern Europe and Mediterranean; ROW=Rest of World; WE=Western Europe.

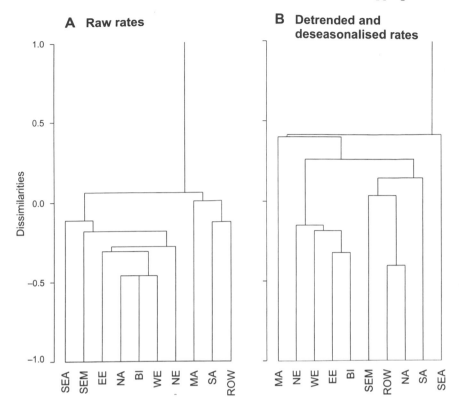

Figure 5.19. MDS clusters for average disease behaviour. Dendrograms from complete linkage analysis applied to final configurations of ten world regions in MDS spaces of figure 5.18. (A) Raw rates. (B) Detrended/deseasonalised rates. BI=British Isles; EE=Eastern Europe; MA=Middle America; NA=North America; NE=Northern Europe; SA=South America; SEA=South East Asia; SEM=Southern Europe and Mediterranean; ROW=Rest of World; WE=Western Europe.

on the MDS plots. As shown, a core European block persists with both types of data. Detrending and deseasonalising the data had the effect of pushing North America out of this European block in A, into a non-geographical grouping with Southern Europe and the Mediterranean and the Rest of the World in B. For both types of data, other regions float loosely around the central core, and there is no evidence of an American block. We conclude that geographical proximity and similar behaviour of disease time series is the norm for a core of European regions, but neither geographical proximity nor trend and seasonal factors markedly influence the MDS positions of other regions.

(b) Temporal variations

To study changes in the regional behaviour of the diseases over time, the study period was divided into two halves: 1888–99 and 1900–12. To define a measure of time series similarity among regions, a two-step procedure was followed in each time block: (1) the correlation matrix between the time series of reported deaths per 100,000 population in each of the ten world regions was computed for each of the index diseases and all causes (note that tuberculosis was omitted because recording of deaths only began in 1899 in our dataset); (2) the average correlation for each regional pair was then calculated, where the average was taken over the six correlations obtained in step 1. Put formally, let r_{ijd} denote the correlation between the time series of regions i and j on disease d. Then $s_{ij} = \bar{r}_{ij}$ where $\bar{r}_{ij} = \sum_{d=1}^{6} \bar{r}_{ijd}$. This similarity matrix, $\mathbf{S} = \{s_{ij}\}$, formed the basis of the MDS and, as before, each solution was seeded with the geographical coordinates of the regions. The analysis was carried out using both the raw rates and rates which had been detrended and deseasonalised.

The results obtained are summarised in figure 5.20. Regional positions based on the 1888–99 data are shown by the solid circles, and their corresponding positions, 1900–12 (grey circles), are pointed to by the direction vectors. For the raw data (figure 5.20A), there is a general 'bolting up' of epidemic behaviour. Western Europe, Northern Europe, and North America move into the main cluster of points, and the only long-distance moves are by regions for which missing observations on one or more of the diseases meant sample sizes were reduced. Examplar regions are South America, Southern Europe and the Mediterranean, and South and East Asia. Figure 5.20B, based on detrended and deseasonalised data, shows several critical differences. There is a main group of British Isles, Western Europe, Northern Europe, Eastern Europe, and Southern Europe and the Mediterranean which remains as a cluster from the first time period to the second. There is a second core group of Middle and South America which is also unchanging. Between the two time periods, this American core is joined by North America from the European group, while South and East Asia moved from the American group to join the European cluster.

Together, figures 5.20A and B imply again that trend and seasonal features in the data drive the epidemic behaviour of regions together. If these characteristics are allowed for, then distinct geographical groupings of mortality behaviour arise, splitting into a European pattern and an American pattern. South and East Asia became more like the European model over time.

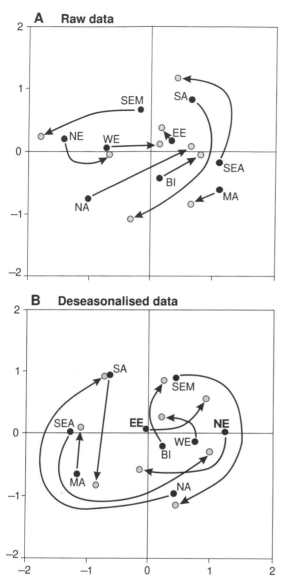

Figure 5.20. MDS analysis of time changes in average disease behaviour of ten world regions between 1888–1899 (solid circles) and 1900–1912 (grey circles). Vectors point from 1888–99 location to 1900–12 location in the final configuration MDS spaces. (A) Using raw rates. (B) Using detrended/deseasonalised rates. BI=British Isles; EE=Eastern Europe; MA=Middle America; NA=North America; NE=Northern Europe; SA=South America; SEA=South East Asia; SEM=Southern Europe and Mediterranean; ROW=Rest of World; WE=Western Europe.

5.7 Lags between world regions

5.7.1 The method

As we have seen in figures 4.3–4.9, the time series for the marker diseases analysed in this book have a temporal waveform, with recurrent peaks when high numbers of deaths were reported. These peaks are separated by periods during which relatively low numbers of deaths were recorded. The marker diseases we have considered are infectious and are passed from person to person, so that the inter- and intra-regional propagation of infection by trade, travel, and migration is likely. This can lead to pulse-like epidemic waves of morbidity from which the cyclical raised mortality seen in charts like figures 4.3–4.9 can result. The classic nineteenth-century example of recurrent disease spread on a global scale is provided by cholera (see, for example, Cliff and Haggett, 1988, for a review) and, as discussed in section 2.2, it was fear of the spread of infection from the world's great ports into the United States that was one of the reasons for establishing the 'early-warning' international surveillance of disease on a regular basis in the *Weekly Abstract*.

There are two aspects to geographical spread. The first, at a local level, is within regions, from city to city and from city and town into rural hinterlands. The second, at a regional level, is between continental areas of the globe. The detection of local spread is considered in section 6.5, using the concept of average time-lag maps. In this section, we search for the inter-regional propagation of infection for two of our marker diseases, enteric fever (an intestinal disease – cf. cholera) and measles (an index of the spread of respiratory infections). The method used is cross-correlation (CCF) analysis, already encountered in sections 4.7.1 and 4.7.2 to establish phase characteristics in the global time series of the marker diseases.

The methodology is a logical extension of that discussed in section 4.7.1. The global time series of reported deaths per 100,000 are now replaced by the regional time series for the two diseases. For each disease, with ten world regions, there are forty-five cross-correlation functions to compute. By analogy with section 4.7.1, we define the short-term lead or lag of one region with respect to another as the value of k at which the correlation is a maximum. Again, for reasons given in section 4.7.2, detrended and deseasonalised regional time series were used. Embedded missing values which would have fragmented the series were replaced with series averages after pre-whitening.

5.7.2 Results for world regions

Figure 5.21 uses vectors to map the leads and lags among the regions. The vectors link each region to those regions with which it had the largest and

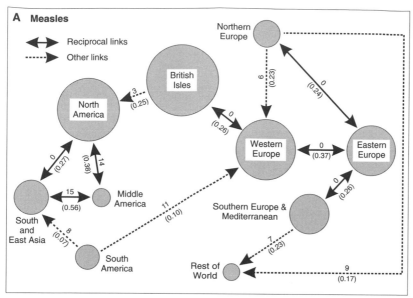

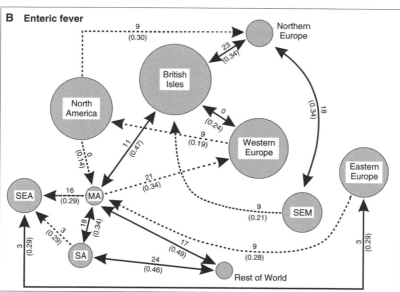

Figure 5.21. Inter-regional spread of disease. Vectors mark corridors of potential spread by linking each region to those regions with which it had the largest and second largest CCF values. Figures give the correlations and the lag in months at which they occurred. Reciprocal links are marked with solid lines, and unidirectional links with pecked lines. Regional circles have been drawn proportional to their 1900 populations. (A) Measles. (B) Enteric fever.

second largest CCF values. Assuming that the leads and lags mark possible diffusion corridors, the arrows point in the direction of spread. Reciprocal links are marked with solid lines, and unidirectional links with pecked lines. The correlation values and the lags at which they occurred are recorded on the vectors.

Measles (map 5.21A): There are two distinct circulation cells, one encompassing the European regions, and the second enclosing the Americas and South and East Asia. The European region is more tightly bonded than the American, with a preponderance of in-phase (lag 0) reciprocal links. In contrast, the lead–lag relationships in the Americas are, with one exception, longer even when reciprocal. The most significant transatlantic link is from the British Isles to North America. The circulation cells identified correspond closely with those isolated by MDS for all diseases, which suggests that the time series of mortality are regionally distinctive either side of the Atlantic. Bearing in mind that the data have been pre-whitened, correlations are modest and, with the exception of the bonds from South America, are statistically significant at the $\alpha = 0.05$ level (two-tailed test) given sample sizes of 300 months.

Enteric fever (map B): There are some major contrasts with the measles map. First, although the reciprocal bonds pick out the core European and American regions as before, leads and lags are much longer almost everywhere (average twelve months compared with five for measles). If we are dealing with a diffusion process, then spread is clearly much slower than for measles. The correlations are also generally somewhat larger (average 0.32 compared with 0.26 for measles). Outside the core regions, there are many more long-distance links than with measles, resulting in a substantially more complex geographical pattern of vectors. The overall impression is of a much more open system than for measles.

5.8 Conclusions

This chapter has focused upon patterns of mortality from our six marker diseases and all causes at the scale of ten major world regions. It is often the case that findings at one geographical level either do not hold at another or else, alternatively, permit more subtle variations to be detected as the spatial scale decreases. In the first part of the chapter, the mortality decline model, the crisis hypothesis, and the 'big-city' hypothesis of excess mortality were re-examined at the regional level to provide a scale comparison with the results obtained in chapter 4 using global time series. For all three hypotheses, the regional analyses broadly confirmed our findings at the world level. So far as the mortality decline model is concerned, at the regional level considered in this chapter, deaths from tuberculosis were on a rising trend almost everywhere; the other marker diseases were on a long-term decline in many areas. The finding for tuberculosis is the same at the regional as at the global level. For the other diseases, the regional results supported the mortality decline model more strongly than did the data analysed at the world scale. For the crisis hypothesis, the increasing amplitude of cyclical swings over time in tuberculosis death rates found at the global scale was seen again in nearly all world regions. Also consistent with the global results was evidence for veracity of a crisis model in the ten regions for deaths from diphtheria and enteric fever. The same mixture of findings for the other marker diseases was found at the regional level as at the global scale. For the 'big-city' hypothesis, of the sixty disease/world region combinations arising with six marker diseases and ten regions, only nine (mainly in developed economies) showed evidence of the excess mortality implied by this hypothesis.

The analysis of mortality data for a set of regions has enabled us to investigate geographical variations in the seasonal incidence of the marker diseases. While there are distinct seasonal features to be seen in the death rates, these effects are more complex than the existing literature seems to suggest. The general features are:

(i)   A reasonably consistent switching of the peak month for incidence from one half of the year to another, depending upon whether the city is in the northern or southern hemisphere. The extent to which this reflects 'indoor crowding' in the hemispherical winter is not clear.

(ii) The unexpected finding that seasonal variability is greater in low than high latitudes. The use of different indices of seasonal variability in disease and a number of variables to measure the effect of environment did not change this conclusion. Nor could the results be laid solely at the door of small sample sizes or small city sizes. We are driven to the conclusion that the impact of climatic variables upon the seasonal incidence of these marker diseases, and the death rates arising therefrom, is considerably more subtle than we had expected. Further research is required to establish whether conventional models of seasonal distributions need modification.

With the regionally based time series data used in this chapter, it is possible to assess the relative time–space intensity of mortality arising from the different diseases using biproportionate scores. Application of this technique led to two very general conclusions: (i) all causes and tuberculosis displayed smaller time–space contrasts than did the other marker diseases; (ii) death rates were relatively concentrated in the Old World up to 1900 and in the New World and Asia after 1900.

The extent to which regional similarities exist in rates of mortality was examined further using multidimensional scaling (MDS). Over the whole period from 1888 to 1912, the European regions formed a distinctive cluster of areas with similar time series behaviour for all the diseases considered. By dividing the study period into two halves (1888–99 and 1900–12), MDS analysis suggested that cohesiveness among the European regions increased with time and, additionally, that a distinctive American region had emerged by 1912. Trend and seasonal features of the regional time series tended to mask regional distinctiveness, especially for enteric fever, measles, scarlet fever, and tuberculosis.

The main emphasis in this chapter has been upon the identification of regional patterns of mortality from the marker diseases. But infection spreads from one area to another, and so the possible inter-regional propagation of two of the marker diseases, measles and enteric fever, as indexed through lead–lag relationships in rates of mortality, was examined in the final section. The cross-correlation bonds suggested that there are distinct European and North American circulation cells for these diseases. The identification of these regional subgroupings is consistent with the MDS results. But there are clear contrasts between the respiratory disease, measles, and the intestinal disease, enteric fever. The much shorter inter-regional lags for measles imply more rapid spread than for enteric fever, while the relative absence of long-distance bonds between regions for measles as compared with enteric fever implies that spread is regional for measles and global for enteric fever.

Preventing the geographical spread of disease from one area to another was one of the driving forces behind the decision of the United States Marine Hospital Service to establish the regular city-by-city recording of selected diseases in the *Weekly Abstract* on an international basis in the 1870s. In the next chapter, we therefore turn to the data at the spatial level at which it was originally collected – the city – and use these data to examine the disease diffusion idea in more detail.

6

The individual city record

London. – One thousand five hundred deaths were registered during the week, including measles, 20; scarlet fever, 9; diphtheria, 40; whooping cough, 50; enteric fever 7, and diarrhea and dysentery, 15. The deaths from all causes correspond to an annual rate of 17.5 a thousand.

Statistical Report for week ending 24 April 1897,
Public Health Reports, vol. XII (1897), p. 486

6.1 Introduction

It is in this chapter that the original mortality data published in the *Weekly Abstract* come into their own. There is a substantial epidemiological and public health literature on many of the 100 cities in our sample. Accordingly, in an appendix to this chapter, we have listed the principal sources on a country-by-country basis for each of the cities. We hope that the listing will give a flavour of the scope of the literature that is available.

Given our 100-city sample, there are at least 2,100 potential time series – 100 cities×7 diseases×3 formats of mortality (crude deaths, death rates, and deaths as a proportion of mortality from all causes) – that we could analyse. A blanket examination of all series is not practicable and would anyway almost certainly lead to an inability to see the wood for the trees. Instead, we outflank the problem by selecting cities and a theme. We begin by choosing the ten largest cities in our world sample and look at their time series for all diseases, simply to illustrate the richness of the database that lies behind the global and regional generalisations made in chapters 4 and 5. As before, we concentrate upon death rates per 100,000 population. Next, we take two of the ten regions – North America (in practice, the United States) and the British Isles – to illustrate the ways in which individual cities can be set within a geographical framework. We then show how such geographical analysis can be extended to all ten regions. The chapter is concluded with a consideration of some city series that display little of the order that we have been distilling from our time series at the global and regional levels in chapters 4 and 5, and which we continue to do here at the city level.

The theme we have chosen is that of spatial diffusion, taking mortality as an imperfect index of morbidity. There are a number of quintessentially geographical questions that can be asked of our city series that relate to the spatial diffusion of disease: do large cities suffer mortality upturns before small cities? Do epidemics of infection spread from one city to another? If so, what is the spatial sequencing? And what is the impact of distance between cities upon the rate and direction of spread?

With these ideas in mind, we now turn to the individual city series.

6.2 The leading world cities

As an indication of the scope of our database, we take from the sample the ten largest cities, based upon their January 1900 populations as given in the *Weekly Abstract*. We have already indicated in section 3.3.2 that the definition of the 'population' of a city remains a slippery concept; there is a range of possible populations (based upon various legal definitions of the city, or real urban areas) rather than a single, unambiguous figure. Nonetheless, we are satisfied that the cities chosen bear a reasonable likeness to the ten largest urban aggregations in the 100-city sample.

The cities are, in size order: London, New York, Paris, Berlin, Vienna, St Petersburg, Chicago, Philadelphia, Moscow, and Bombay. Their populations vary in magnitude from the biggest, London, with 6.65 million inhabitants in 1900, down to Bombay with 0.9 million. Six of the cities are European, three are North American, and one is Asian. Together they make up 46 per cent of the total population of the 100 cities.

6.2.1 Standardising disease rates

With a ten-city selection in which the population of the biggest is over seven times that of the smallest, and disease death rates that range from 1,431 down to 0.04 per 100,000, there is a need, prior to plotting, to standardise the time series in some way that allows ready comparisons to be made. There are many data transformations that could be used, but here we have chosen one of the simplest and most robust solutions, namely standard scores.

For a given city mortality time series, let x_t denote the reported death rate per 100,000 population in month t, and $\bar{x}$ and s_x be the mean and standard deviation respectively of the reported rates taken over the period 1888–1912. Each time series was standardised by calculating the transformation,

$$z_t = \frac{(x_t - \bar{x})}{s_x}. \tag{6.1}$$

The $\{z_t\}$ have zero means and unit variances by construction, and it is the $\{z_t\}$ that are plotted on the vertical axes of each graph in figures 6.1–6.10. For each city, these diagrams illustrate the monthly time series of reported deaths per 100,000 population from 1888 to 1912 from each of the six diseases (line traces) against a backcloth of death rates per 100,000 population from all causes (grey histogram). This backcloth permits an assessment to be made of the varying importance over the study period of each marker disease in contributing to deaths from all causes. Because the $\{z_t\}$ are dimensionless, plots may be directly compared across diseases and cities. Again, to aid comparisons, the same vertical plotting scale has been used for all diseases in a given city, although different vertical scales have had to be used between cities to permit the graphs for each city to be accommodated on a single page.

6.2.2 Comparing diseases within individual cities

Two kinds of comparison may be made on the basis of the charts: across diseases for any given city, and for a given disease between cities. We consider each here, beginning with the within-city comparisons for each city in turn.

(a) London (figure 6.1)

Location and climate: London (latitude 51°30′ N, longitude 0°05′ W) is situated in the chalk basin of the River Thames, southeast England. The climatic regime is maritime; average monthly temperatures range between 37 °F (3 °C) in January and 73 °F (23 °C) in July, with an average annual precipitation of 24 in (597 mm).

Growth, 1888–1912: The population of London increased at an average rate of 70,000 per annum, rising from 5.53 million in 1888 to 7.34 million in 1912.

Sanitation and public health: Significant advances in the sanitary status and public health of London were made in the second half of the nineteenth century; see the chapter appendix for a select bibliography. By the 1890s, a large proportion of the city had access to piped water, a gas supply, and a sewerage system, whilst the development of public transport had opened the suburbs to the less affluent. The prevention of infectious diseases had also received considerable attention from the 1850s and mortality from some diseases, such as scarlet fever, typhoid fever, tuberculosis, and whooping cough, fell significantly to the turn of the century. But other infectious diseases, such as measles, were generally viewed as being beyond the scope of preventive services and mortality did not decline in a systematic manner until the early twentieth century (Daunton, 1991; Hardy, 1993a).

Literature mortality and infectious diseases, 1888–1912: Hardy (1993a) provides a detailed overview of deaths due to specific infectious diseases (diphtheria, pp. 80–109; measles, pp. 28–55; scarlet fever, pp. 56–79; tuberculosis, pp. 211–66; typhoid fever, pp. 151–90; whooping cough, pp. 10–27) and general mortality patterns. Further references are given in the appendix to this chapter.

Time series: The time series shown in figure 6.1 reflect many of the features noted under *Sanitation and public health*. Rates for diphtheria, enteric fever, and scarlet fever declined sharply in the second half of our study period, and the amplitudes of the epidemic cycles diminished; there was also a small negative trend for whooping cough. Scarlet fever displayed a long-term five-year cycle, with seasonal effects superimposed (cf. section 6.2.4). All the series for which there are data have marked seasonal elements. That for measles is the most regular and, by way of contrast with the other diseases, has no discernible trend, biennially larger epidemics, and an annual seasonal upturn. For all practical purposes, data on tuberculosis were not reported in the *Weekly Abstract*.

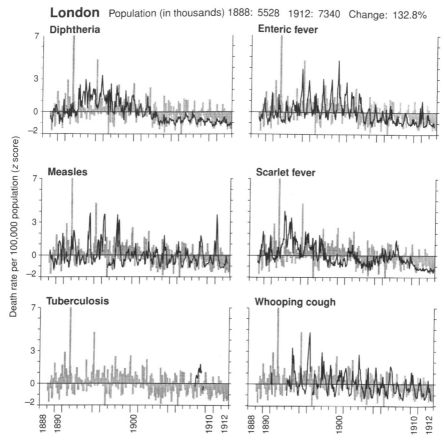

London Population (in thousands) 1888: 5528 1912: 7340 Change: 132.8%

Figure 6.1. London, England. Monthly time series of death rates per 100,000 population, 1888–1912, from six marker diseases (line traces) and all causes (grey stippled histogram). Rates are expressed as standard scores (*z*).

(b) New York (figure 6.2)

Location and climate: New York City (latitude 41°00′ N, longitude 73°55′ W) is situated on the Atlantic coast of the United States at the confluence of the Hudson and East Rivers. The climatic regime is continental; average monthly temperatures range from 28 °F (–2 °C) in February to 73 °F (23 °C) in July, with an average annual precipitation of 42 in (1,060 mm).

Growth, 1888–1912: The period from 1888 to 1912 was one of large-scale urban expansion. Geographically, in 1898 the jurisdiction of the city was extended from Manhattan to include the boroughs of the Bronx, Brooklyn,

Queens, and Richmond. Demographically, the population of the city grew threefold, from 1.53 million (1888) to 4.77 million (1912). Whilst some two-thirds of this population increase was associated with the territorial expansion of the city, it was substantially bolstered by large-scale immigration from Europe.

Sanitation and public health: The squalid and unhealthy state of nineteenth-century New York is described graphically by a number of contemporary authors (see S. Smith, 1972). In 1864, for example, one sanitary inspector described the streets of the city as

composed of house-slops, refuse, vegetables, decayed fruit, store and shop sweepings, ashes, dead animals, and even human excrement. These putrifying organic substances are ground together by constantly passing vehicles. When dried by the summer's heat, they are driven by the wind in every direction in the form of dust. When remaining moist or liquid in the form of a 'slush', they emit deleterious and very offensive exhalations . . . it is a well-recognized cause of diarrheal diseases and fevers. (Cited in S. Smith, 1972, p. 268)

Tenement accommodation, which was home to half a million inhabitants, was of a similarly poor standard:

In very many cases the vaults of privies are situated on the same or higher level, and their contents frequently ooze through the walls into the apartments beside them . . . These are the places that we most frequently meet with typhoid fever and dysentery. (Cited in S. Smith, 1972, p. 269)

Against this background, the second half of the nineteenth century witnessed major advances in the healthiness of the city. Public health measures included improvements in the quality and quantity of the city's water supply, the provision of sewers, street cleansing, and refuse disposal, the regulation of slaughter houses, the establishment of a milk and food inspectorate, and the implementation of an effective building code. But responses to specific infections varied in scope and intensity. Some diseases, such as tuberculosis and diphtheria, became the subject of intense prevention and control campaigns. However, other diseases, such as scarlet fever, measles, and whooping cough, received little attention despite the high fatality rates (Duffy, 1974).

Literature mortality and infectious diseases, 1888–1912: Dwork (1981) provides a comprehensive bibliography of health and disease in New York City, while Duffy (1974) describes the occurrence of major infectious diseases. Further bibliographic details are provided in the appendix to this chapter.

Time series: The public health efforts show up in the time series of the *Weekly Abstract*. There is a sharp discontinuity in the diphtheria series from 1897, with a switch to a lower level and smaller cycles. Tuberculosis rates also fall

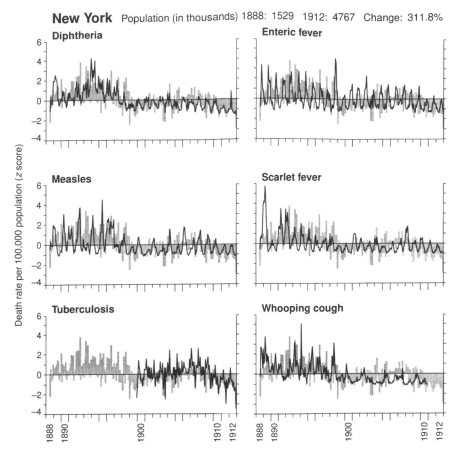

Figure 6.2. New York, USA. Monthly time series of death rates per 100,000 population, 1888–1912, from six marker diseases (line traces) and all causes (grey stippled histogram). Rates are expressed as standard scores (*z*).

sharply after 1909. But, despite the relatively slight attention to scarlet fever, measles, and whooping cough, these series still display sharply lower rates after 1895. Biennial cycles are again evident for measles (note the frequently alternating high/low peaks). Annual seasonal upturns are apparent for diphtheria, enteric fever, measles, and scarlet fever. The series for tuberculosis and whooping cough are altogether more complex; whooping cough appears to have a three-year cycle after 1898.

(c) Paris (figure 6.3)

Location and climate: Paris (latitude 48°50′ N, longitude 2°20′ E) is situated in the Paris Basin of northern France. The climatic regime is maritime; average monthly temperatures range from 36 °F (2 °C) in January to 64 °F (18 °C) in July, with an average annual rainfall of 20 in (508 mm).

Growth, 1888–1912: During the period 1888–1912, the population of Paris increased from 2.3 million to 2.9 million. An estimated 90 per cent of this population increase was attributable to migration with migration peaks apparent in the years 1889 and 1900 (Clout, 1977).

Sanitation and public health: The public health regulations of Paris can be traced to legislation in 1791 and the requirement that prostitutes should be able to present a guarantee of good health. The following sixty years saw a more wide-ranging approach to public health problems, with significant improvements in water distribution, the extension of the sewer system, street cleansing, and waste disposal (La Berge, 1992). But it was Napoleon III who, with the help of Baron Haussmann, transformed Paris in the third quarter of the nineteenth century into a modern city of radiating boulevards and squares, vastly improved water supply, and an immense system of sewers. An outbreak of cholera at mid-century inspired drainage works in the 1860s and 1870s under the planning of Belgrand so that, by 1878, a network of 620 km (385 m) of sewers had been constructed, and the Seine had been substantially freed from organic pollution.

Literature mortality and infectious diseases, 1888–1912: An overview of mortality patterns is provided by Preston and Van de Walle (1978) and Van de Walle and Preston (1974). The appendix to this chapter provides information on the literature relating to specific infectious diseases.

Time series: In view of the improvements in water supply and sanitation, it is worth noting that the time series for enteric fever is, with that for Chicago, the least seasonal and cyclical of the series for this disease among the ten great cities. Apart from two epidemics in 1894 and 1899–1900, it bumps along at an almost constant level. The plots also show that, with the exception of measles, this absence of oscillations is not confined to enteric fever. The frequently well-developed seasonals and cycles present in many of the series for London and New York are often absent or damped. Like London and New York, however, rates were commonly lower in the second half of the period. As with New York, whooping cough shows some evidence of an approximate three-year period of bigger epidemics, and a biennial cycle is evident in the measles series from the turn of the century.

(d) Berlin (figure 6.4)

Location and climate: Berlin (latitude 52°51′ N, longitude 13°24′ E) is situated on the River Spree in northeastern Germany, about 180 km (112 miles) south

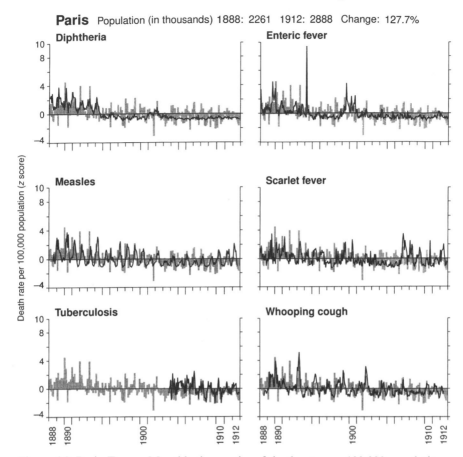

Figure 6.3. Paris, France. Monthly time series of death rates per 100,000 population, 1888–1912, from six marker diseases (line traces) and all causes (grey stippled histogram). Rates are expressed as standard scores (*z*).

of the Baltic Sea. The climatic regime lies on the cusp of continental and maritime influences. Average monthly temperatures range between 30 °F (–1 °C) in January and 66 °F (19 °C) in July, and the average annual rainfall is 23 in (587 mm).

Growth, 1888–1912: Berlin was established as the capital of Germany in 1871. The city experienced rapid population growth from c. 1820, increasing from 1.4 to 2.1 million during the period 1888–1912.

Sanitation and public health: Significant advances in the provision of domestic infrastructure and services were made during the latter decades of the nineteenth century. The mains water supply, initially built in the 1850s for the cleansing of sewage gutters, was extended to over 90 per cent of houses by 1890 whilst, by the same year, almost all properties had been connected to the underground sewage system. In addition, a street cleansing system had been established to deal with the estimated 190,000m³ of rubbish and 100,000 cart-loads of animal dung deposited annually on the city's streets (R. J. Evans, 1987). But the high-level immigration of the 1880s and 1890s created fresh problems in the form of overcrowding, poor housing, and deprivation, especially to the north, east, and south of the administrative and commercial core. *Literature mortality and infectious diseases, 1888–1912*: Mortality patterns in Berlin are discussed in Vögele (1994) and R. J. Evans (1987, in passing).

Time series: The Berlin series are more fragmentary than many of those illustrated so far. Nevertheless, in some, the evidence for cycles rather than secular upturns is clear – two years for measles after 1905, a four-year wave for scarlet fever, and a three-year period for whooping cough.

(e) Vienna (figure 6.5)

Location and climate: Vienna (latitude 48°13′ N, longitude 16°23′ E) is situated on the River Danube in the foothills of the Alps, northeastern Austria. Because of the city's altitude (168 m; 550 ft), the climate is not as continental as its location might suggest. Average monthly temperatures range between 30 °F (–1 °C) in January and 67 °F (19 °C) in July, while the average annual rainfall is 27 in (686 mm).

Growth, 1888–1912: The nineteenth century was a period of rapid urban expansion for Vienna. By mid-century, the population had outstripped the city walls, with an estimated 65,000 residing within the inner walls and a further 440,000 residing between the inner and outer ring. Urban growth during the period 1888–1912 was particularly rapid, with the population of the city increasing from 801,000 in 1888 to 2.1 million in 1912. Much of this growth was associated with high levels of immigration (especially of Czechs and Jews) such that, by 1910, less than half the population was Viennese by birth.

Sanitation and public health: To cope with the growing poverty and poor social conditions in some parts of the city, between 1879 and 1881 the Viennese authorities introduced a series of municipal welfare schemes; by 1888 a system of social security and health insurance had been established (Waissenberger, 1984). But overcrowding and unsanitary conditions remained in many tenement areas. Here, the conditions prevailing in the working-class district of Ottakring are illustrative. In this district, the population increased from 106,000 in 1890 to 178,000 (representing 8 per cent of the city's population) in

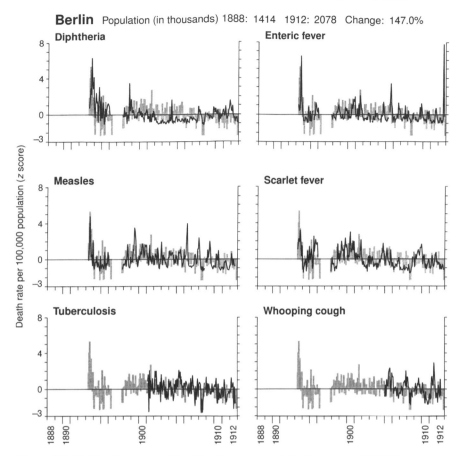

Figure 6.4. Berlin, Germany. Monthly time series of death rates per 100,000 population, 1888–1912, from six marker diseases (line traces) and all causes (grey stippled histogram). Rates are expressed as standard scores (z).

1910. This growth outstripped the provision of domestic services such that, by 1900, 50 per cent of the housing stock lacked running water whilst a single toilet frequently served ten to fourteen families. The overcrowded and unsanitary conditions of this district ensured that death rates from infectious diseases, such as tuberculosis, diphtheria, and measles, were particularly high (Barea, 1992; Boyer, 1981).

Time series: The series for measles and scarlet fever are of particular note. Evidence for a two- to three-year cycle for measles superimposed upon annual seasonal upturns is clearer than in the series so far discussed. For scarlet fever, there is again weak evidence of a longer-term harmonic upon which epidemic outbreaks are stamped.

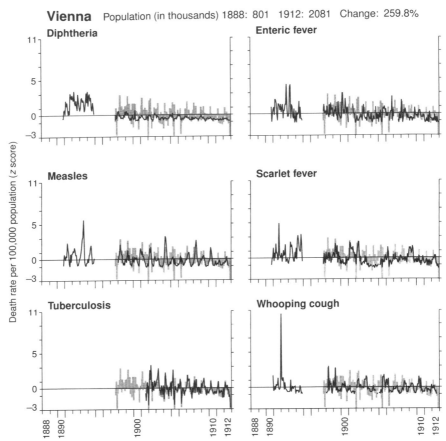

Figure 6.5. Vienna, Austria-Hungary. Monthly time series of death rates per 100,000 population, 1888–1912, from six marker diseases (line traces) and all causes (grey stippled histogram). Rates are expressed as standard scores (z).

(f) St Petersburg (figure 6.6)

Location and climate: The Russian port city of St Petersburg (latitude 60°00′ N, longitude 30°30′ E) is situated on an islet delta where the River Neva empties into the Baltic Sea. The climatic regime is classified as modified continental with maritime influences. Average monthly temperatures range from 18 °F (−8 °C) in February to 64 °F (18 °C) in July. Precipitation is moderate. The average annual rainfall is 23 in (584 mm), and there is snow cover for about one-third of the year.

Growth, 1888–1912: From its foundation in the early eighteenth century, St Petersburg developed as the leading port, commercial and industrial centre, and administrative capital of the Russian Empire. By 1888, the population of the city was rapidly approaching 1 million, and this figure doubled to almost 2 million in the quarter century to 1912. Much of the population increase was attributable to large-scale migration of peasants from the countryside; by 1900, only one-third of the resident population had been born in St Petersburg (Bater, 1986).

Sanitation and public health: St Petersburg is reputed to have been the unhealthiest of all European capitals in the quarter-century to 1912. Overcrowding in the inner city reached exceptionally high levels, with eight city wards recording population densities in excess of 51,000 people/km^2 in 1910; rates of fifteen individuals to each apartment were recorded in some tenements. Indeed, such were the conditions that a British diplomatic report of 1909 noted that 'St Petersburg, compared with large cities of Europe, and even of Russia, has the highest rate of mortality in general and the highest deathrate from infectious diseases' (A. W. Woodhouse, 1909, *British Parliamentary Papers*: Diplomatic and Consular Report, cited in Bater, 1986, p. 59).

Literature mortality and infectious diseases, 1888–1912: Public health and mortality patterns in St Petersburg are described in Bater (1976, 1983, 1986) and Gleason (1990). Further references are given in the appendix to this chapter.

Time series: The measles time series is the only one among the great cities with a rising trend of death rates and oscillations that become increasingly large over the period. One especial feature of many of the St Petersburg series compared with others of the great cities is that they display a longer wavelength cycle with annual upturns superimposed. Scarlet fever shows this most clearly, but there is also a hint that the time series for diphtheria and enteric fever have a similar structure. The peaks in the longer-term wave are also roughly coincident for all three diseases. In view of the comments under *Sanitation and public health*, it is perhaps to be expected that there is little evidence of long-term mortality decline or consistently damping cycles of mortality for any of the six diseases. Mortality decline only begins to be apparent (except for measles) from 1910.

(g) Chicago (figure 6.7)

Location and climate: The city of Chicago (latitude 41°50′ N, longitude 87°35′ W) lies on the southern shore of Lake Michigan, USA, at an altitude of about 76 m (108 ft) above sea level. The climatic regime is continental; average monthly temperatures range between 25 °F (–4 °C) in January and 75 °F (24 °C) in July. The average annual precipitation is 33 in (838mm).

St. Petersburg   Population (in thousands) 1888: 928   1912: 1962   Change: 211.4%

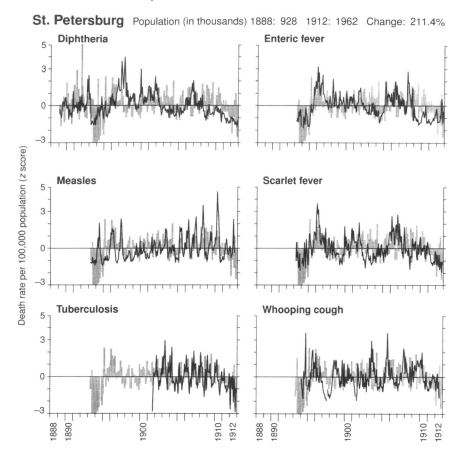

Figure 6.6. St Petersburg, Russia. Monthly time series of death rates per 100,000 population, 1888–1912, from six marker diseases (line traces) and all causes (grey stippled histogram). Rates are expressed as standard scores (*z*).

Growth, 1888–1912: Moderate population growth in the latter years of the nineteenth century was replaced by explosive growth at the beginning of the twentieth century. Between 1888 and 1900, the population grew from 800,000 to 1.1 million, a modest increase but one sufficient to enable Chicago to over-take Philadelphia as the second city of the United States. Between 1900 and 1912, however, the population doubled from 1.1 million to 2.2 million, repre-senting an average annual increase of nearly 85,000 per year. Much of this increase was associated with repeated waves of immigrants, first from Europe, then Mexico and Puerto Rico, and, towards the end of the period, African-Americans from the Deep South.

Sanitation and public health: A permanent board of health was established in Chicago in the immediate aftermath of the 1867 cholera epidemic. The board was responsible for major efforts to improve sanitation and to provide clean public water supplies, an effort that continued right through our study period. The canal schemes associated with the latter were among the great engineering undertakings of their time. Notwithstanding these efforts, one inevitable outcome of the large population influxes of the 1880s and 1890s was poor and overcrowded housing. So, estimates for the early 1890s place the slum population of Chicago at 162,000, or 20 per cent of the total (Duffy, 1990; Pierce, 1970; Spear, 1970).

Literature mortality and infectious diseases, 1888–1912: General mortality patterns are discussed in Higgs (1979). The literature relating to major infectious diseases is outlined in the appendix to this chapter.

Time series: The success of the sanitation and water supply works may be judged from the fact that, despite overcrowding, mortality from the touchstone disease of enteric fever, like that from diphtheria, fell to sharply lower rates after 1900. Further, the epidemic cycles that were an integral component of these series before 1900 effectively disappeared. In the same way, the trend for tuberculosis also remained horizontal. The measles series shows clear evidence of major epidemics every two to three years from 1888–1907 and, from 1903, the oscillations damp in line with the crisis model (see sections 4.4 and 5.3.3). For scarlet fever, major epidemics are about seven years apart; they occur about every three years for whooping cough. Death rates from scarlet fever were also on a gently rising trend over the study period.

(h) Philadelphia (figure 6.8)
Location and climate: Philadelphia (latitude 39°48′ N, longitude 75°22′ W) is situated at the confluence of the Delaware and Schuylkill Rivers in southeast Pennsylvania, about 140 km (87 miles) southwest of New York City. The climatic regime is continental; average monthly temperatures range from 32 °F (0 °C) in January to 75 °F (24 °C) in July, and the mean annual rainfall is 43 in (1079 mm).

Growth, 1888–1912: The population of Philadelphia grew from 1 million in 1888 to 1.5 million in 1912, an average annual increase of 20,000 a year.

Sanitation and public health: Shryock (1966, p. 232) observes that Philadelphia was 'unusual among the larger American towns in that its mortality rate fell somewhat during the second quarter of the nineteenth century'. He attributes this early headway in public health to the high-profile nature of recurrent yellow fever epidemics, particular those of 1798, 1805, and 1820. Two partic-

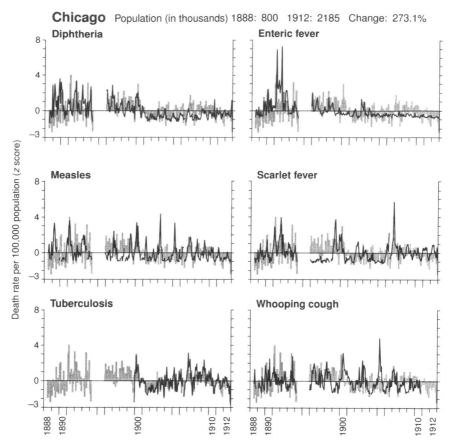

Figure 6.7. Chicago, USA. Monthly time series of death rates per 100,000 population, 1888–1912, from six marker diseases (line traces) and all causes (grey stippled histogram). Rates are expressed as standard scores (z).

ularly notorious killers, typhus fever and malaria, had been brought 'under a considerable degree of control' by the middle of the nineteenth century (Shryock, 1966, p. 232). But, despite these early advances, rapid reductions in mortality awaited the late nineteenth and early twentieth centuries. Thus, between 1870 and 1930 mortality rates for major infectious diseases fell from 600 per 100,000 to 80 per 100,000 (Condran and Cheney, 1982; Condran, Williams, and Cheney, 1985).

Literature mortality and infectious diseases, 1888–1912: General mortality patterns are described in Condran and Cheney (1982), Condran, Williams, and Cheney (1985), and Morman (1984). The appendix to this chapter gives details on the literature relating to major infectious diseases.

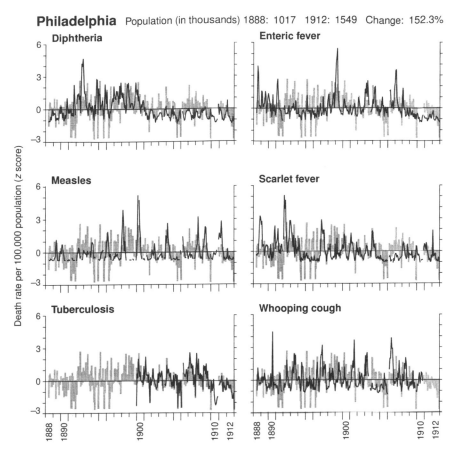

Figure 6.8. Philadelphia, USA. Monthly time series of death rates per 100,000 population, 1888–1912, from six marker diseases (line traces) and all causes (grey stippled histogram). Rates are expressed as standard scores (*z*).

Time series: Philadelphia's diphtheria rates fell sharply after 1900, and epidemic cycles of the disease became strongly damped compared with those in the 1890s. Since diphtheria causes especial levels of mortality among susceptible infants and children, it is noteworthy, in view of the comments under *Sanitation and public health* about declining childhood mortality, that the diphtheria series is the only one of the six plotted in figure 6.8 that displays a downwards shift in trend. So far as the other diseases are concerned, measles shows evidence of major epidemics every two to three years after 1895. The plot in figure 6.8 indicates that the cycles had greater constancy of amplitude after 1900 than before. For scarlet fever, bigger epidemics occurred at roughly five- to seven-year intervals. For tuberculosis, epidemics appeared annually.

Those for whooping cough are spaced at five-year intervals, with lesser epidemics in intervening years.

(i) Moscow (figure 6.9)

Location and climate: The city of Moscow (latitude 55°40′ N, longitude 37°40′ E) lies in the valley of the Moskva River, a tributary of Volga, on the plain of European Russia. The climatic regime is continental, with average monthly temperatures ranging from 14 °F (−10 °C) in January to 64 °F (18 °C) in July. Precipitation is moderate. The annual average is 23 in (581 mm), and there is a prolonged period of snow cover (annual average 146 days).

Growth, 1888–1912: As in many other cities of Europe and North America, the late nineteenth century marked the beginning of a period of rapid industrialisation and urban growth. Between 1888 and 1912, the population expanded by more than 1 million, from 611,000 to 1.62 million, with the average annual growth rate approaching 4 per cent in the later years. This growth was fuelled by the influx of a large and transient population of peasant migrants. At the turn of the century, little over one-quarter of the population was native to Moscow while, of the remainder, almost half had resided in the city for less than six years (Bater, 1983; J. Bradley, 1986).

Sanitation and public health: One result of this rapid and unplanned population growth was a housing shortage. Overcrowding in the city tenements reached severe levels (1912 estimate, 8.7 persons per apartment), and basic domestic services and sanitary facilities were generally lacking. Under these circumstances, and despite increased expenditure on public health and sanitation from the 1890s, mortality rates from infectious diseases remained high throughout the observation period (Bater, 1983; Gleason, 1990).

Literature mortality and infectious diseases, 1888–1912: General mortality patterns are described in Bater (1983), J. Bradley (1986), and Gleason (1990).

Time series: The time series of deaths from enteric fever, measles, and whooping cough display a familiar mixture of regular small upswings in mortality separating major epidemics. These principal epidemics appeared at two- to five-year intervals for enteric fever, two- to four-year intervals for measles, and four- to five-year intervals for whooping cough. Diphtheria rates were especially high at the beginning and end of our period, while the discontinuity in death rates from tuberculosis to a higher level in 1906 must be a recording artefact. Consistent with the high mortality rates noted under *Sanitation and public health*, there is no evidence of a long-run mortality decline in any of the time series; in fact, measles, scarlet fever, tuberculosis, and whooping cough showed slightly rising trends.

Moscow   Population (in thousands) 1888: 611   1912: 1621   Change: 265.3%

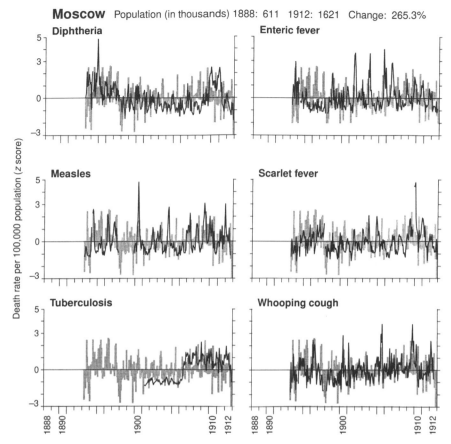

Figure 6.9. Moscow, Russia. Monthly time series of death rates per 100,000 population, 1888–1912, from six marker diseases (line traces) and all causes (grey stippled histogram). Rates are expressed as standard scores (*z*).

(j) Bombay (figure 6.10)

Location and climate: Bombay (latitude 18°52′ N, longitude 72°35′ E) occupies a group of islands lying off the Konkan coast of West India. Bombay Island (comprising seven joined volcanic islets) occupies an area of 65 km² and it consists of a low-lying plain, one-quarter of which lies below sea-level. The climate is subtropical, with a complex regime characterised by four distinct seasons: a cold season, extending from December to February; a hot season from March to May; a rainy (monsoon) season from June to September; a second hot season during October and November. Mean monthly temperatures range from 66 °F (19 °C) in January to 91 °F (33 °C) in May, with a seasonally concentrated precipitation regime giving an average annual rainfall of 71 in (1800 mm).

Growth, 1888–1912: The population of Bombay registered a modest increase between 1888 and 1912, rising from 783,000 to 979,000.

Sanitation and public health: Bombay is the sole Asiatic representative in our sample of ten great cities. In the seventeenth century, it was one of the most unhealthy places in the East, when it was a common proverb that 'Two monsoons were the age of a man' (Karve, 1955, p. 830). The islands were manured with rotting fish and, at low tide, the intervening creeks became putrid swamps. Although improvements were made, nevertheless, at the beginning of our period, Bombay remained squalid and overcrowded. The first waterworks replaced unsanitary wells in the 1870s, and a drainage system was installed in 1879. To cope with the conditions, a City Improvement Trust was set up to make new streets, clear slums, reclaim more land from the sea, and build more sanitary dwellings. But little progress was made until after the Great War, and the city continued to be troubled by the great 'quarantine diseases' throughout our observation period (see, for example, Catanach, 1988). The social and commercial implications of an outbreak of bubonic plague were summarised by the US consul to Bombay in 1897 thus:

The [population] exodus still continues in, if possible, increasing numbers. The general opinion of residents is that fully one-half the population has left the city. Great inconvenience is experienced by all classes in consequence of loss of clerks, servants, and laborers, who have nearly all run away . . . [B]usiness in many branches is completely paralyzed. (S. Comfort (1897), reproduced in *Public Health Reports*, vol. XII (1898), p. 189)

Literature mortality and infectious diseases, 1888–1912: Mortality patterns are described in Klein (1973, 1986).

Time series: Only the time series for enteric fever and measles have a sufficiently complete record to permit comment. Against the public health background sketched above, it is perhaps unsurprising that, alone among the ten great cities, the time series for enteric fever displayed a rising trend over the period of recording. For measles, major epidemics occurred every two to four years with little activity between these peaks.

6.2.3 Comparing diseases across cities

A second method of comparison is to take a single disease and to look at its behaviour measured across all ten cities. On the basis of figures 6.1–6.10, two generalisations stand out.

First, with very few exceptions, the trend in death rates is either horizontal or negative (that is, mean death rates were roughly constant or falling over the study period). This observation is consistent with the mortality decline

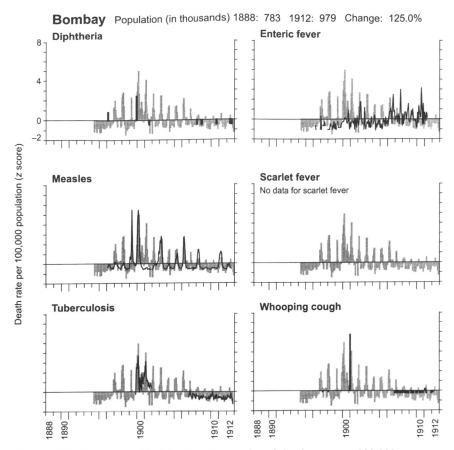

Figure 6.10. Bombay, India. Monthly time series of death rates per 100,000 population, 1888–1912, from six marker diseases (line traces) and all causes (grey stippled histogram). Rates are expressed as standard scores (*z*).

hypothesis examined in the two previous chapters at the global and regional levels.

Second, many of the series, notably those for diphtheria, measles, and scarlet fever, display epidemic behaviour. This is made up of two elements: (i) small-scale upturns in rates on an annual basis (secular events); and (ii) much larger bursts of mortality at intervals of two to five years (cycles). The time series behaviour of the amplitudes of these bursts is, of course, an integral element of the crisis hypothesis discussed at the global and regional levels in sections 4.3 and 5.3.3. Casual inspection of figures 6.1–6.10 indicates that the amplitudes vary in a complex manner both from disease to disease and from city to city. Some – for example, London diphtheria (figure 6.1) and New York whooping cough (figure 6.2) – seem straightforwardly to confirm the crisis model, with smaller-amplitude cycles in the second half of the series than in the first. But for others, like measles in St Petersburg (figure 6.6), the amplitude of cycles increases rather than decreases with time. And finally, in some cities, the amplitudes appear to change very little between 1888 and 1912 (whooping cough in Philadelphia in figure 6.8, for example).

Just as amplitudes change in complex ways, so the spacing of the epidemic cycles is equally heterogeneous, varying between diseases and over the duration of the study period. It is to an examination of the recurrence intervals of these cycles and seasonal swings that we now turn.

6.2.4 Cycles in city disease patterns

To analyse the annual upswings and longer cycles in the city series, we employ the time series decomposition technique of *spectral analysis*. This is described in Jenkins and Watts (1968) and Chatfield (1980).

The basis of spectral analysis is a recognition that a stationary time series, x_t, with zero mean, finite variance, and sampling interval Δt can be accurately approximated by a truncated Fourier series

$$x_t \approx \sum_{j=1}^{J} [A_j \cos(2\pi f_j t) + B_j \sin(2\pi f_j t)], \tag{6.2}$$

where A_j and B_j are random Fourier series coefficients, the $\{f_j\}$ are well-chosen frequencies, and J is sufficiently large. The exact form of the approximation 6.2 used in spectral analysis is called the *spectral representation* of x_t and it results in a plot of the amount of the total variability in the time series (vertical axis) that is accounted for by sine/cosine waves of different wavelengths (horizontal axis). The variance explained is referred to as the *power*, and wavelength is usually expressed as the proportion of one complete wave (peak to peak) per unit time; the reciprocal then gives the wavelength.

Power spectra of all the series illustrated in figures 6.1–6.10 were computed. The method assumes that the series analysed are time-stationary, and so the series were detrended prior to carrying out the spectral decomposition. Figure 6.11 illustrates a sample of the plots based upon death rates per 100,000 population. The peaks at which the seasonal and cyclical components occur have been marked, along with the $\alpha = 0.05$ significance level.

Many writers have commented upon the nature of the seasonal and cyclical features of the diseases studied in this book. Here, we draw upon a selection of recent sources whose work sheds some light on the return intervals for the peaks that appear in the graphs of figure 6.11. The reader should also refer to the corresponding time series plots in figures 6.1–6.10 and to the discussion in section 6.2.2.

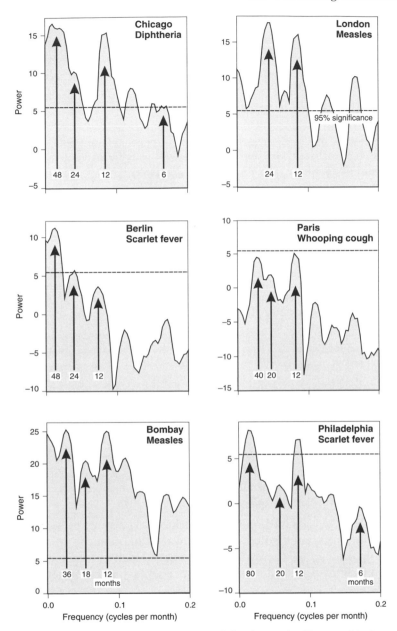

Figure 6.11. City cycles: power spectra of the time series illustrated in figures 6.1–6.10 for selected cities and diseases. The vertical axis gives a measure of the percentage of the variance in the time series that is accounted for by cosine waves of different wavelengths (horizontal axis). Seasonal and cyclical peaks are marked, along with the $\alpha = 0.05$ significance level.

(a) Cyclical features

Noah (1989, p. 178) remarks that: 'Many infections undergo cycles [*sic*] lasting 1, 2, 3 or even four years. Those that occur every year tend to exhibit the most marked seasonal variation.' The 'every year' event is the twelve-month seasonal upswing clearly seen in all the graphs of figure 6.11.

Diphtheria: In New York, 1866–1896,

While the incidence of diphtheria generally increased throughout these years, the morbidity and mortality statistics show four epidemic waves, with the high points coming in the years 1873–76, 1880–82, 1885–89, and 1893–96. (Duffy, 1974, p. 155)

These observations imply an epidemic cycle of three to four years for diphtheria in New York, and the latter two epidemic events are apparent in figure 6.2. The spectrum for Chicago in figure 6.11 also shows evidence of a four-year harmonic.

Measles: In London and other large cities,

measles had a double cycle, of roughly biennial epidemics within a longer cycle of about ten years, during which mortality was higher or lower than in the decades on either side. (Hardy, 1993a, p. 29)

Some of the virus infections . . . have regular patterns of recurrence. [In the UK] measles had a marked biennial cycle until 1968. (Noah, 1989, p. 181)

In figure 6.11, the biennial cycle for measles is the statistically most significant wavelength of the London measles series.

Scarlet fever: In London,

the 1890s marked a turning point in the behaviour of the disease. Previously it had run in epidemic cycles of five years, judging by the mortality peaks. After the epidemic of 1896, however, a seven-year cycle manifested itself, with epidemics occurring in 1901, 1907, 1914, 1921. (Hardy, 1993a, p. 65)

The long wavelength cycles for London referred to by Hardy are to be seen in figure 6.1. In the spectrum for Berlin, the equivalent harmonic is four years, and there is no evidence of this cycle pulling out to seven years. Conversely, the spectrum for Philadelphia does show Hardy's seven-year harmonic.

Whooping cough: In Scotland,

the periodicity of epidemics in Aberdeen was 'somewhat ill-defined' before 1890, but clearly substantially biennial thereafter. In Edinburgh and Perth epidemics occurred generally every three years; in Glasgow every three to four; in Dundee every four. (J. S. Laing, *Public Health*, 13 [1901–2], pp. 586–7; cited in Hardy, 1993a, p. 10)

In London there was some variation in periodicity, with the pattern becoming more unstable as mortality began to fall in the early 1880s. (Hardy, 1993a, p. 10)

Whooping cough and . . . are examples of infections that exhibit cycles of 4 years. (Noah, 1989, p. 181)

The spectrum for Paris shows the complexity that the above quotations would lead us to expect, with peaks at twenty and forty months. The time series plot of figure 6.3 shows why. Up to 1903, comparatively major mortality peaks occurred every two to four years; after the turn of the century, the marked peaks disappeared with the general fall in mortality.

Much of our knowledge of long-term cycles in infectious diseases is based upon European and North American evidence, and there is enormous variability in all parts of the world around the figures for cycle wavelengths quoted above. For example, the power spectrum of the Bombay measles series plotted in figure 6.11 reveals a three-year cycle. Later in this chapter, in section 6.6, we reinforce this caveat by illustrating some highly irregular time series from our 100-city sample.

6.3 Cities in the North American region

A second approach which illustrates the richness of the individual city records is to take one of the regions defined in chapter 5 and then look at all the cities which it comprises. We do this here for two regions, North America (section 6.3) and the British Isles (section 6.4).

6.3.1 The geographical framework

As illustrated in figure 2.9, the number of United States cities for which mortality data were recorded in the *Weekly Abstract* varied enormously over the period from 1888 to 1912. About thirty cities appeared between 1888 and 1894; the number then rose steadily to about 150 by 1912. Given our need for lengthy and complete time series, the list of potential cities for study was fixed by those (twenty-three in all) which appeared regularly in the early editions of the *Weekly Abstract*. From the set of twenty-three, three (Atlanta, Panama, and San Juan) were eventually dropped on the grounds of scant coverage in terms of months in their time series with reports, leaving the set of twenty shown in table 6.1 for analysis in this section.

Table 6.1 gives, on a disease-by-disease basis, the percentage of months over the period for which data are available, along with summary statistics for the time series distribution of reported deaths and death rates. The average annual rates per 100,000 population, 1888–1912, for the pooled data from the twenty cities were: all causes 1,735; diphtheria 48; enteric fever 29; measles 13; scarlet fever 17; tuberculosis 198; whooping cough 13. Thus measles, scarlet fever, and whooping cough carried very similar risks of mortality. Tuberculosis was in a league of its own. Diphtheria and enteric fever were in the middle of the distribution of risks.

Table 6.1. *United States cities: data record by city and disease for persistent cities, 1888–1912, in the Weekly Abstract*

City	1912 population	Disease	Number of months with reports	% of record	Reported deaths, 1888–1912						Average annual rate per 100,000
					Total	Minimum	First quartile	Median	Third quartile	Maximum	
Baltimore	558,485	All causes	297	95.2	224,869	163	681	796	925	1,597	1,851.4
		Diphtheria	288	92.3	4,007	1	6	11	19	64	34.7
		Enteric fever	288	92.3	4,103	1	7	12	20	46	34.0
		Measles	181	58.0	1,022	1	1	3	7	83	8.4
		Scarlet fever	250	80.1	1,371	1	2	4	6.75	57	11.6
		Tuberculosis	165	52.9	17,591	12	96	113	128	194	243.7
		Whooping cough	244	78.2	1,426	1	2	4	9	34	13.0
Boston	670,585	All causes	300	96.2	253,664	182	785.5	892	1004.25	1,576	2,003.4
		Diphtheria	291	93.3	7,285	3	12	19	33.5	116	61.2
		Enteric fever	288	92.3	3,032	1	5	8.5	14	52	24.8
		Measles	235	75.3	1,218	1	2	4	8	34	9.4
		Scarlet fever	270	86.5	2,308	1	3	6	13	34	18.9
		Tuberculosis	165	52.9	15,619	17	84	99	113	170	197.2
		Whooping cough	259	83.0	1,450	1	3	5	7	33	12.7
Chicago	2,185,283	All causes	286	91.7	515,964	231	1,512.75	1,911	2,350.25	3,564	1,504.4
		Diphtheria	279	89.4	14,655	5	33	49	71	171	46.1
		Enteric fever	279	89.4	11,066	2	18.5	29	46.5	334	36.7
		Measles	266	85.3	3,206	1	4	9	17.75	79	9.7
		Scarlet fever	278	89.1	6,308	1	8.25	19	34	154	17.9
		Tuberculosis	164	52.6	38,947	41	198.5	247	309	479	159.1
		Whooping cough	250	80.1	3,427	1	7	12.5	19	75	11.5

City	Population	Cause									
Cincinnati	364,463	All causes	296	94.9	129,760	13	398.5	463	541.25	1,053	1,639.2
		Diphtheria	293	93.9	2,864	1	3	7	13	64	37.0
		Enteric fever	293	93.9	3,110	1	5	9	16	58	39.9
		Measles	157	50.3	788	1	1	3	6	32	10.9
		Scarlet fever	213	68.3	631	1	1	2	4	17	7.9
		Tuberculosis	163	52.2	9,715	11	48.5	62	74	120	208.6
		Whooping cough	176	56.4	537	1	1	2	4	23	8.0
Cleveland	560,663	All causes	308	98.7	136,588	100	369	456	557.5	908	1,651.9
		Diphtheria	297	95.2	3,232	1	6	10	15	44	41.4
		Enteric fever	299	95.8	3,094	1	5	8	13	59	39.8
		Measles	179	57.4	786	1	1	2	5	28	9.3
		Scarlet fever	258	82.7	1,518	1	2	3	7	76	18.0
		Tuberculosis	165	52.9	7,193	2	34	47	60	96	123.3
		Whooping cough	206	66.0	640	1	1	2	4	17	9.0
Denver	213,381	All causes	137	43.9	19,199	27	118	148	197	323	1,108.4
		Diphtheria	113	36.2	452	1	2	3	6	24	25.8
		Enteric fever	104	33.3	683	1	2	4	8	48	43.6
		Measles	44	14.1	93	1	1	1.5	3.25	9	6.0
		Scarlet fever	85	27.2	234	1	1	2	3	21	14.4
		Tuberculosis	53	17.0	2,045	8	33	44	56	187	277.8
		Whooping cough	49	15.7	65	1	1	1	2	4	4.8
Detroit	465,766	All causes	280	89.7	103,216	63	282.5	390	500	881	1,530.9
		Diphtheria	265	84.9	2,772	1	4	7	14	51	47.5
		Enteric fever	124	39.7	515	1	2	3	6	24	13.8
		Measles	45	14.4	121	1	1	2	3	24	4.6
		Scarlet fever	227	72.8	1,031	1	1	3	6	36	16.4
		Tuberculosis	44	14.1	744	1	12.75	23	28.25	45	35.3
		Whooping cough	52	16.7	124	1	1	1.5	3	18	4.9

Table 6.1. (*cont.*)

City	1912 population	Disease	Number of months with reports	% of record	Total	Reported deaths, 1888–1912					Average annual rate per 100,000 population
						Minimum	First quartile	Median	Third quartile	Maximum	
Kansas City, KS	82,331	All causes	75	24.0	5,798	4	80.5	100	118	235	1,609.1
		Diphtheria	38	12.2	93	1	1	2	3	18	29.7
		Enteric fever	56	17.9	200	1	2	3.5	6	11	67.5
		Measles	17	5.4	34	1	1	3	6	9	20.9
		Scarlet fever	21	6.7	21	2	1	2	2	2	8.3
		Tuberculosis	65	20.8	572	2	6	10	13	21	161.2
		Whooping cough	21	6.7	30	1	1	2	2	6	19.4
Kansas City, MO	248,381	All causes	113	36.2	16,036	13	110	152	206	412	792.2
		Diphtheria	75	24.0	186	1	1	2	3.5	10	9.4
		Enteric fever	95	30.4	458	1	2	4	6	26	22.6
		Measles	32	10.3	69	1	1	1	4	12	4.8
		Scarlet fever	67	21.5	139	1	1	1	3	11	7.3
		Tuberculosis	54	17.3	1,063	3	15.25	23.5	28.75	49	91.4
		Whooping cough	55	17.6	89	1	1	1	2.5	6	5.8
Milwaukee	373,857	All causes	304	97.4	96,498	9	286.5	328	390.25	587	1,553.5
		Diphtheria	289	92.6	3,010	1	4	8	13	58	52.3
		Enteric fever	268	85.9	1,426	1	3	5	7	27	23.5
		Measles	157	50.3	580	1	1	3	5	18	10.2
		Scarlet fever	209	67.0	1,009	1	1	3	7	30	16.3
		Tuberculosis	164	52.6	5,205	5	25.75	33	39	108	127.9
		Whooping cough	190	60.9	655	1	1	3	5	19	12.8

City	Population	Cause									
Nashville	110,364	All causes	304	97.4	39,960	11	114.75	136.5	164	254	1,980.4
		Diphtheria	120	38.5	228	1	1	1	2	12	11.5
		Enteric fever	264	84.6	1,026	1	2	3	5	18	51.3
		Measles	67	21.5	215	1	1	2	3	23	13.8
		Scarlet fever	92	29.5	151	1	1	1	2	9	10.1
		Tuberculosis	165	52.9	2,942	2	14	19	23	35	248.1
		Whooping cough	131	42.0	339	1	1	2	3	17	19.8
New Orleans	339,075	All causes	309	99.0	162,476	126	486	543	625	909	2,435.5
		Diphtheria	266	85.3	1,346	1	2	4	6	55	21.1
		Enteric fever	298	95.5	2,349	1	4	7	11	32	34.9
		Measles	105	33.7	456	1	1	2	7	28	8.0
		Scarlet fever	112	35.9	280	1	1	1.5	3	18	4.0
		Tuberculosis	164	52.6	12,287	19	69	78	87	118	299.7
		Whooping cough	181	58.0	467	1	1	2	3	14	7.8
New York	4,766,883	All causes	310	99.4	1,392,454	1,002	3,311.5	4,810.5	6,034.25	8,973	2,115.9
		Diphtheria	302	96.8	40,358	19	94.5	128.5	177	402	67.7
		Enteric fever	302	96.8	12,428	7	24	35.5	56	147	19.0
		Measles	302	96.8	16,957	2	24	45	86.5	209	28.3
		Scarlet fever	302	96.8	17,911	6	25	49.5	82	266	30.1
		Tuberculosis	165	52.9	106,227	166	600	689	751	1,016	206.0
		Whooping cough	278	89.1	9,204	5	19	30.5	45	136	18.5
Newark	347,469	All causes	225	72.1	73,140	43	277	356	427	658	1,546.8
		Diphtheria	214	68.6	1,880	1	5	7	12	48	43.2
		Enteric fever	204	65.4	810	1	2	3	6	26	18.3
		Measles	115	36.9	393	1	1	2	5	18	10.0
		Scarlet fever	181	58.0	1,011	1	2	4	8	38	23.2
		Tuberculosis	164	52.6	8,800	12	45.75	56	67.25	97	265.0
		Whooping cough	158	50.6	529	1	2	3	4	12	12.9

Table 6.1. (cont.)

City	1912 population	Disease	Number of months with reports	% of record	Total	Reported deaths, 1888–1912					Average annual rate per 100,000 population
						Minimum	First quartile	Median	Third quartile	Maximum	
Philadelphia	1,549,008	All causes	294	94.2	506,738	360	1,563.5	1,815.5	2,146.25	3,238	1,726.1
		Diphtheria	297	95.2	15,047	4	29	46	65	203	53.1
		Enteric fever	297	95.2	12,428	2	24	35	51	195	42.8
		Measles	257	82.4	2,971	1	2	6	14	96	9.9
		Scarlet fever	292	93.6	3,975	1	6	10	19	70	13.8
		Tuberculosis	159	51.0	35,860	51	199.5	243	274	417	195.1
		Whooping cough	270	86.5	3,674	1	7	11	18.75	58	13.7
Providence	224,321	All causes	299	95.8	74,881	61	216	257	305.5	427	1,983.9
		Diphtheria	278	89.1	1,426	1	3	5	7	18	38.6
		Enteric fever	253	81.1	870	1	2	3	5	15	24.3
		Measles	155	49.7	768	1	1	3	7	36	19.8
		Scarlet fever	211	67.6	748	1	1	2	4.5	24	20.3
		Tuberculosis	134	42.9	3,558	1	22.25	29	35	55	138.7
		Whooping cough	201	64.4	676	1	1	2	4	43	20.8
San Diego	39,578	All causes	178	57.1	2,775	3	10.25	14	18	84	859.5
		Diphtheria	13	4.2	10	1	1	2	2	4	10.8
		Enteric fever	32	10.3	36	1	1	1	2	5	16.9
		Measles	10	3.2	2	1	1	1	1	1	2.5
		Scarlet fever	14	4.5	6	1	1	1	1	1	5.2
		Tuberculosis	51	16.3	266	1	2	4	10	21	160.4
		Whooping cough	11	3.5	3	1	1	1	1	1	6.2

City										
San Francisco	416,912	All causes	260	83.3	117,512	90	407.5	493	576	850	1,471.3
		Diphtheria	235	75.3	1,545	1	3	5	8.5	45	19.9
		Enteric fever	247	79.2	1,683	1	4	6	9	46	21.5
		Measles	123	39.4	396	1	1	2	4	19	5.4
		Scarlet fever	129	41.3	288	1	1	1	3	21	4.1
		Tuberculosis	149	47.8	9,143	7	49	64	80	131	201.1
		Whooping cough	138	44.2	440	1	1	3	4	18	6.7
Toledo	168,497	All causes	223	71.5	29,326	35	104	138	174.5	310	1,263.2
		Diphtheria	190	60.9	953	1	2	4	7	27	46.3
		Enteric fever	189	60.6	709	1	2	4	5	16	29.8
		Measles	75	24.0	150	1	1	1	3	8	7.5
		Scarlet fever	90	28.8	119	1	1	1	2	5	5.4
		Tuberculosis	146	46.8	2,369	2	13	17	21	36	139.3
		Whooping cough	72	23.1	102	1	1	1	2	7	6.6
Washington, DC	331,069	All causes	304	97.4	126,802	89	369	442	526	934	1,999.4
		Diphtheria	268	85.9	1,853	1	2	5	10	31	30.9
		Enteric fever	295	94.6	3,381	1	5	9	16	56	54.6
		Measles	129	41.3	412	1	1	2	4	22	6.9
		Scarlet fever	143	45.8	256	1	1	1	2	10	4.2
		Tuberculosis	163	52.2	8,310	10	41.5	55	66	104	214.6
		Whooping cough	241	77.2	1,155	1	2	3	6	24	20.4

The geographical locations of the cities are shown in figure 6.12. The cities range in size from the largest, New York (population 4.8 million in 1912), down to the smallest, San Diego (population 39,578 in 1912). The graphs in the lower left of figure 6.12 plot the rank–size distributions of the cities at the beginning and end of the study period. The opportunity is also taken to illustrate both the regional and some of the city series for diphtheria, one of the diseases analysed in some detail in this section. The North American series is plotted as crude mortality. It has been detrended and cropped to define epidemic starts (shown by the ticks on the x-axis); these starts are used in section 6.3.3. The city time series are shown as death rates per 100,000 population, plotted in standard score form (see section 6.2.1).

6.3.2 Spatial autocorrelation and US city epidemics

(a) Disease spread in a set of settlements

For the marker diseases examined in this book, the transmission process is easily specified in general terms: individuals infected with a particular disease mix with those at risk and pass on the infection, thus generating new cases. Most will recover, but some will die to yield the data record studied here. Numbers of reported deaths and death rates are therefore an index, albeit imperfect, of population mixing.

The simplest model of the spread of disease from place to place in a country which reflects this mixing envisages a contagious diffusion process. Propagation occurs from the initial point of introduction to geographically contiguous centres. These, in their turn, transmit the disease to their geographically nearest neighbours and so on. The disease progresses from place to place at the leading edge of a ripple wave, and spatially divorced outbreaks ahead of the wave front do not occur.

Such a geographically highly ordered process is, however, rarely found in practice. One of the commonest circumstances under which a contagious diffusion model is inappropriate is when transmission takes place through a system of cities. The varying population sizes of the settlements result in spread being directed through the urban hierarchy from larger places to smaller. Typically, the initial point of introduction of a disease in a region is its largest city. Then urban centres next in size follow, and so on. In these circumstances, transmission is spatially discrete and fragmented rather than continuous because settlements at high levels of the population size hierarchy are generally some distance apart.

Diffusion processes often display both hierarchical and contagious elements. Simultaneous with the downwards percolation of disease from large settlements to small, spread also frequently takes place from each centre to its geographically nearest neighbours.

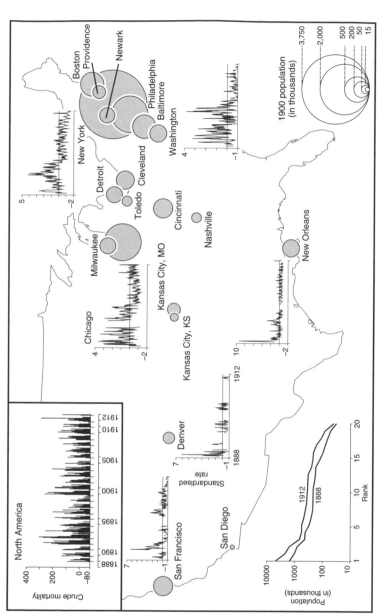

Figure 6.12. United States cities. Location of the twenty study cities, their rank–size population distributions in 1888 and 1912 (lower left), and representative time series of deaths from diphtheria per 100,000 population (z-score format). Circle sizes are proportional to city populations in 1900. The inset graph shows crude mortality (detrended) for the North American region. Ticks show starts of epidemics used in section 6.3.3.

(b) Contagious and hierarchic spread compared

In a classic study of the spread of cholera in the United States for the epidemics of 1832, 1849, and 1866, Pyle (1969) analysed the relative importance of hierarchical and contagious elements in the disease diffusion process. By graphing the date of first report of cholera in cities of the United States against (1) distance from the point of introduction in North America and (2) city population size in each of these epidemics, he was able to construct figure 6.13. In 1832, spread followed a spatial sequence through the main waterway systems of the continent, with outbreaks in towns distant from the points of origin occurring later than outbreaks nearer the sources (figure 6.13A). By 1849, while such spatial effects were still apparent, evidence was also emerging of hierarchical spread, with larger cities reporting outbreaks earlier than smaller cities (figure 6.13B). By 1866, distance effects had disappeared, and spread was in an ordered hierarchical sequence from larger cities to smaller (figure 6.13C).

In the remainder of this section, we use a variety of analytical techniques to examine the relative strengths of the contagious and hierarchical diffusion models in accounting for the spread (as indexed through the city time series of rates of mortality) of each of our six marker diseases in North America. In this subsection, we begin by using the method of autocorrelation on graphs (Haggett, 1976; Cliff, Haggett, Ord, and Versey, 1981, pp. 99–102). To illustrate the approach, full results are first given for diphtheria, and then a summary of findings is presented for the other benchmark diseases.

(c) The results for North America, 1888–1912

The autocorrelation on graphs approach requires us to construct graphs consisting of nodes that represent the cities, and lines or edges connecting the nodes. The connections are made so that the pattern of edges mimics the possible corridors of disease spread corresponding with the diffusion model we wish to test. Accordingly, to check for the existence of distance and hierarchical effects in the spread of each of our six diseases, two graphs were specified:

(1) A nearest neighbour graph defined by setting each element, w_{ij}, in a matrix **W** equal to 1 if cities i and j were nearest neighbours as judged by the straight-line distance in miles between them, and $w_{ij}=0$ otherwise.

(2) A hierarchical graph in which $w_{ij}=1$ if city j was the next larger or the next smaller city in population size to city i and $w_{ij}=0$ otherwise. City populations in 1900 were used.

To determine the goodness-of-fit between each of these graphs and mortality from a given disease, the spatial autocorrelation coefficient, I, was computed for each month of the time series of death rates per 100,000 population. Following Cliff and Ord (1981, pp. 17–21), we define I as

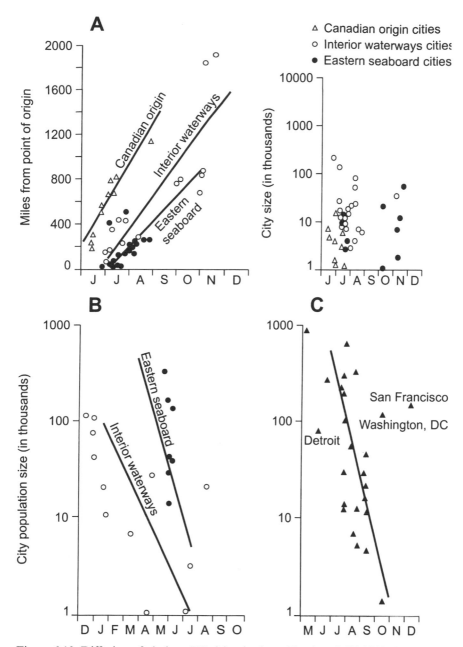

Figure 6.13. Diffusion of cholera, US cities, in the epidemics of (A) 1832, (B) 1849, and (C) 1866. Graphs plot the date of first report in cities in relation to their distance from points of disease introduction and population sizes. Source: based on illustrations in Pyle (1969), figs. 1a, 2a, and 3a, pp. 66, 70, and 73. Figs. 1a, 2a, and 3a from 'Diffusion of cholera in the United States,' by G. F. Pyle, *Geographical Analysis*, vol. 1, no. 1 (January 1969), are reprinted by permission. © Ohio State University Press. All rights reserved.

$$I = \left(\frac{n}{S_0}\right) \frac{\displaystyle\sum_{i=1}^{n}\sum_{j=1}^{n} w_{ij}\, z_i z_j}{\displaystyle\sum_{i=1}^{n} z_i^2} \tag{6.3}$$

where n is the number of cities, x_i is the death rate per 100,000 population in city i in a given month of the time series, and $z_i = x_i - \overline{x}$. The $\{w_{ij}\}$ are drawn from graphs 1 and 2 above. In addition, $S_0 = \displaystyle\sum_{i=1}^{n}\sum_{j=1}^{n} w_{ij}$, $\overline{x} = \dfrac{1}{n}\displaystyle\sum_{i=1}^{n} x_i$, and we adopt the convention that $w_{ii} = 0$. I may be tested for significance as a standard Normal deviate, and the expectation and variance under the null hypothesis of no spatial autocorrelation are given in Cliff and Ord (1981, p. 21). Here, we have evaluated the moments of I under randomisation.

The greater the degree of correspondence between a given graph and the death rate from a disease, the larger will be the spatial autocorrelation coefficient.

Diphtheria   Figure 6.14 plots, as standard scores, the monthly time series of reported deaths per 100,000 population for North America as a backcloth for a plot of the standard Normal deviate for I, computed on a month-by-month basis for the two diffusion graphs defined above. It is evident that the level of spatial autocorrelation has a cyclical behaviour that partially tracks the variations in reported death rates. When mortality peaks occur, levels of spatial autocorrelation on both graphs also tend pick up in a ragged and slightly offset (later) manner; they are lower in inter-epidemic phases. The visual correlation appears stronger for the hierarchy than for the nearest neighbour graph. The implication is that both hierarchical transmission and spatial spread wax and wane in sympathy with many of the epidemics. From 1888 to 1903, there also appears to be a marked two-year cycle in the values of I on the nearest neighbour graph.

These visual associations are explored more formally in figures 6.15 and 6.16. In figure 6.15, the monthly values of the spatial autocorrelation coefficient, I, for each graph have been treated as a time series, from which the autocorrelation and partial autocorrelation functions have been calculated in the manner of section 4.7.1. The ACFs show the cyclical nature of the time series for I on both the nearest neighbour and hierarchy graphs. In addition to high correlations at short lags, the nearest neighbour graph has an approximate four-year cycle. The hierarchy graph has significant peaks at short lags and at twelve (an annual seasonal peak), twenty-four, and thirty-six months. The PACFs confirm the importance of the autocorrelation peaks at short lags on both graphs, as well as the 12-, 24-, and 36-month elements on the hierarchy

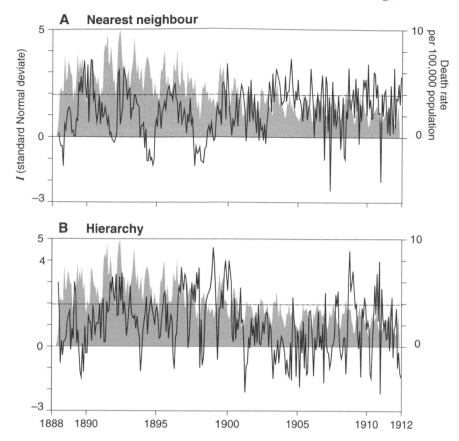

Figure 6.14. Diphtheria, North America, 1888–1912. Monthly reported death rates per 100,000 population (stipple) and corresponding monthly values of spatial autocorrelation coefficient, *I*, as standard Normal deviate (solid line) for different diffusion graphs. (A) Nearest neighbour graph. (B) Population size hierarchy graph. Horizontal pecked lines give 95 per cent significance level for *I* (one-tailed test).

graph. The four-year cycle in the nearest neighbour graph is not in evidence in the PACF.

The features of the ACFs and PACFs in figure 6.15 suggest a process with two main components: (i) the normal rhythm of diphtheria spread, including seasonal effects, takes place principally through the urban size hierarchy; (ii) when there is a major epidemic (every two to four years on the basis of the cycles in *I* plotted in figure 6.14A and the nearest neighbour ACF of figure 6.15), geographical structure also becomes significant, and spatially contagious as well as hierarchical spread takes place.

Figure 6.16 plots the scattergraphs of the ACF and PACF values for *I*

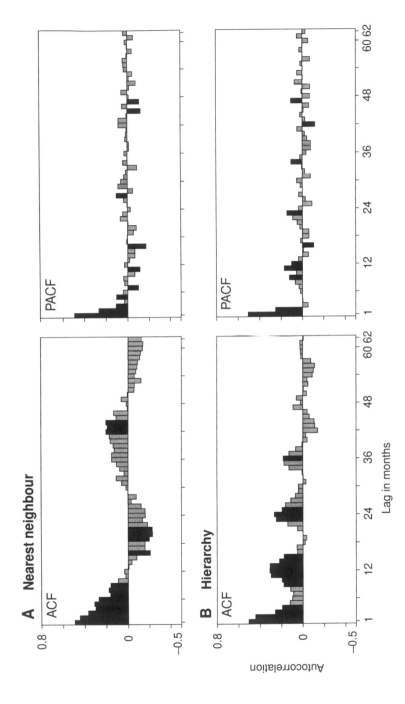

Figure 6.15. Diphtheria, North America, 1888–1912: autocorrelation (ACF) and partial autocorrelation functions (PACF) for spatial autocorrelation coefficients of figure 6.14 when treated as time series. (A) Nearest neighbour graph. (B) Population size hierarchy graph. Significant values at the α=0.05 level (one-tailed test) are black.

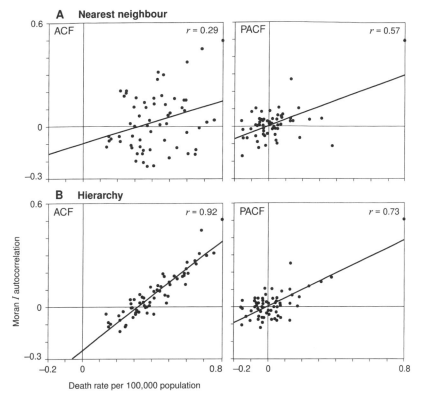

Figure 6.16. Diphtheria, North America, 1888–1912: relationship between corresponding ACF and PACF values for the autocorrelation coefficient, *I* (vertical axis), and monthly death rates per 100,000 population (original data in standard score format, horizontal axis). OLS regression lines are marked, along with the value of the correlation coefficient. (A) Nearest neighbour graph. (B) Population size hierarchy graph.

against the corresponding ACF and PACF values calculated from the time series of reported diphtheria deaths per 100,000 (standard score format). Ordinary least squares regression lines have been fitted. The positive associations on all scattergraphs confirm that both *I* and death rates move broadly in phase, and that epidemic periods, with their higher death rates, enhance spatial and hierarchical transmission. The stronger correlations in 6.16B confirm the generally greater importance of hierarchical diffusion over the study period.

Although the statistical significance of both the nearest neighbour and hierarchical diffusion graphs waxes and wanes in response to the epidemic curve, graphs may vary in their importance by stages of the epidemic cycle. This can be checked by computing the cross-correlation function (see section 4.7.1) between the time series for *I* and the time series of reported death rates. Figure

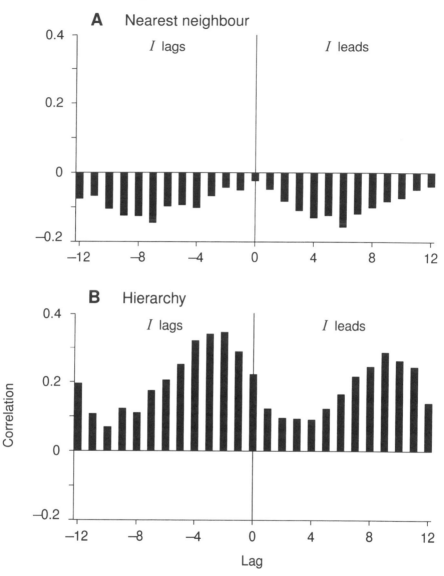

Figure 6.17. Diphtheria, North America, 1888–1912: cross-correlation charts between spatial autocorrelation values, *I*, and reported death rates per 100,000 population. (A) Nearest neighbour graph. (B) Population size hierarchy graph.

6.17 plots these CCFs for each diffusion graph. For the nearest neighbour graph (A), there is a consistent inverse relationship between *I* and death rates, confirming the restricted importance of contagious transmission. This disassociation is at its weakest at lag zero, suggesting that limited propagation among

Table 6.2. *North America: marker diseases,*
1888–1912

Correlations between the ACF and PACF values for the
spatial autocorrelation coefficient *I* (dependent variable)
against the corresponding ACF and PACF values of the
time series of death rates per 100,000 population
(standard score format).

	Graph	
	Nearest neighbour	Hierarchy
ACF		
Diphtheria	0.29	0.92*
Enteric fever	0.66*	0.74*
Measles	0.18	0.34*
Scarlet fever	0.47*	0.63*
Tuberculosis	0.39*	0.28*
Whooping cough	0.20	0.39*
PACF		
Diphtheria	0.57*	0.73*
Enteric fever	0.64*	0.61*
Measles	0.51*	0.47*
Scarlet fever	0.48*	0.58*
Tuberculosis	0.37*	0.31*
Whooping cough	0.33*	0.42*

Note:
* Significant at the $\alpha=0.01$ level (one-tailed test).

nearest neighbours may occur at time of peak mortality. In contrast the hierarchy graph is positively associated with death rates at all lags tested. The largest
CCF value occurs at lag –2, implying hierarchical spread is at its maximum on
average two months after peak mortality rates occur. The gentle reduction in
CCF values as lags increase negatively from this maximum indicates that the
significance of the hierarchy graph diminishes only slowly as diphtheria epidemics wane. Conversely, the shape of the CCF for positive lags testifies that
the hierarchy graph is relatively unimportant in the build-up to peak mortality,
switching rapidly to play a central diffusion role after the peak has passed.

Other diseases   The analysis described above was repeated for the other five
marker diseases (enteric fever, measles, scarlet fever, tuberculosis, and whooping cough). Table 6.2 summarises the findings by giving the correlations

between the (P)ACF values for *I* and the corresponding (P)ACF values for death rates from figure 6.16, along with the equivalent results for the other diseases. The associations are all positive and, given a sample size of sixty-two (the lag to which the ACFs and PACFs were computed), are, with the exception of two nearest neighbour graphs, statistically significant at the $\alpha = 0.01$ level (one-tailed test). As with diphtheria, this implies that the importance of both the nearest neighbour and hierarchical graphs as vehicles for diffusion waxes and wanes in sympathy with the rises and falls in death rates. With the exception of tuberculosis (ACF, PACF), and enteric fever and measles (PACF), the correlations are larger for the hierarchical than for the nearest neighbour graph, confirming the generally greater importance of hierarchical diffusion.

Changes over time   To study changes in the importance of the nearest neighbour and hierarchical graphs over time, figure 6.18 was drawn. The study period was first divided into two equal and non-overlapping halves (1888–1900 and 1900–12), each of 12 1/2 years. For each benchmark disease and diffusion graph, the steps in preparing figure 6.18 were: (1) for the period 1888–1900, calculate the ACF for the time series of standard Normal deviates for *I*, along with the ACF of the monthly reported death rates (in standard score format); (2) compute the correlation coefficient between the two ACFs; (3) repeat steps 1 and 2 for the period, 1900–12; (4) use the correlation coefficients to define the positions of the disease graphs in figure 6.18. If there is no change over time, points will lie on the 45° line. If the time series of *I* echoes more closely the time series of deaths in the second period than in the first, points will lie northwest of the 45° line; if the series for *I* became less like the series for deaths, points will lie southeast of the 45° line.

For each disease, vectors have been added running from the nearest neighbour to the hierarchy graph. Note that tuberculosis had to be omitted from this time-based analysis because recording for this disease only commenced in most cities in the second half of the period.

In figure 6.18, the *x*-axis component of all the vectors is left to right, implying that the hierarchical graph is more closely related to disease patterns (bigger correlation coefficients) than is the corresponding nearest neighbour graph. Only three of the ten points lie northwest of the 45° line, and the split is disease-specific. For enteric fever, scarlet fever, and measles, both graphs fell in the southeast triangle, while for diphtheria they fell in the northwest triangle. Thus, over the study period, the two diffusion graphs became less important correlates of the time series behaviour of enteric fever, scarlet fever, and measles, but they increased in importance for diphtheria.

It is only for whooping cough that the diffusion graphs straddle the 45° line. The nearest neighbour graph (northwest triangle) became more highly correlated with the time series behaviour of this disease, and the hierarchy graph

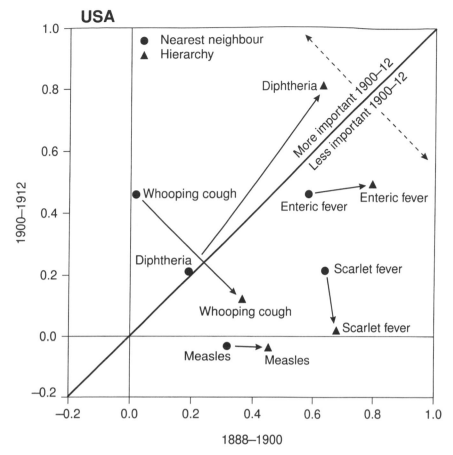

Figure 6.18. North America, 1888–1912: time changes in the importance of nearest neighbour and population hierarchy graphs for disease diffusion. The 45° line corresponds to no change. Axes are correlation coefficients whose calculation is defined in the text. Vectors have been drawn between graph types for each disease.

(southeast triangle) less highly correlated. So, in contrast to Pyle's work on cholera described earlier, there is no evidence from our marker diseases of time-switching from the nearest neighbour to the hierarchy graph as the main mechanism shaping disease diffusion.

6.3.3 US cities as a time-lag surface

An alternative way of isolating any contagious diffusion element that may be present in the propagation of a disease is to look at the expected or *average time-lag* to infection. Given the time series of mortality (or morbidity) for a set of cities, it is possible to determine which cities are generally attacked first in an epidemic, as measured by the early peaking of mortality rates, and those which are relatively unaffected until a later stage of the epidemic. We call this delay the expected or average time-lag to infection. The time sequence for the expected time to infection on a city-by-city basis will provide valuable information about the way in which a disease moves from place to place.

The average time to infection also provides insights into the elusive concept of epidemic velocity. Relatively short average time-lags over a system of cities imply rapidly moving epidemic waves and vice versa. The concept of epidemic velocity has attracted theoretical attention because of its importance for possible preventive measures; the spread of slow-moving waves may be simpler to check than that of rapidly moving waves. Basic references are Mollison (1991) and van den Bosch, Metz, and Diekmann (1990).

(a) Calculation of average time-lags
For each marker disease, time to infection for the twenty North American cities was calculated with reference to the start of epidemics in the regional series generated by pooling the data for the individual cities. For epidemic ℓ, code the first month of the epidemic in the regional series as month 1 and, for city i, note the month in which the disease was first reported in that city as month 2, or 3, or 4, etc. Denote this month as $t_{i\ell}$. The desired quantities are then

$$\bar{t}_i = \left(\frac{1}{m}\right) \sum_{\ell} t_{i\ell} \quad \ell = 1,2,\ldots,m, \qquad (6.4)$$

where i is subscripted over the n cities in the region and there are m epidemics.

Throughout our study period, the populations of most of the North American cities were sufficiently large for each disease to be continuously present, so that a persistent record of mortality occurred in the regional series. Epidemic starts in the regional series were therefore defined by fixing a threshold of reported deaths to be crossed. The thresholds were chosen so as marginally to exceed the general level of deaths reported between the visually evident epidemic spikes. Time trends were removed where necessary before fixing the thresholds. The inset graph in figure 6.12 illustrates the procedure. This shows the time series of crude mortality from diphtheria in North America after removal of the time trend using a linear regression. The residual detrended series has been cropped at −80 to separate the epidemic spikes of mortality from the background mortality, and the dates from which the epidemic starts in individual cities have been measured are marked with ticks on the x-axis of the graph.

For each of the six marker diseases, the average time-lag to infection was computed using equation 6.4 and the procedure described. We then calculated for each city its average time-lag to infection as the mean of the time-lags for the six separate diseases, and these are plotted in figure 6.19. Circles are

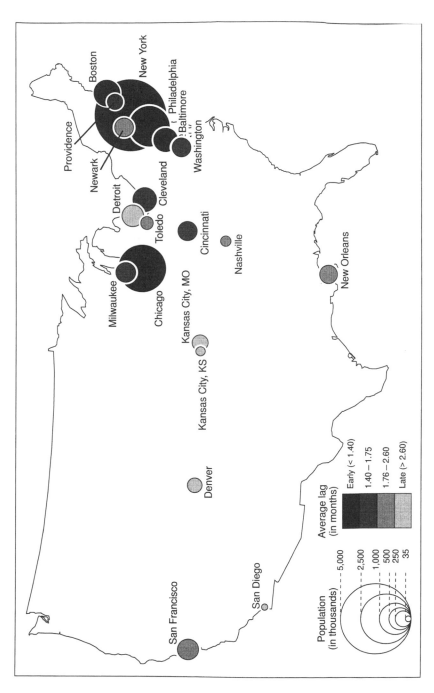

Figure 6.19. US cities: mean time-lags to infection calculated over the six marker diseases.

proportional to city populations and have been shaded dark (early) to light (late) on the basis of time-lags. The first start city for all of the six diseases was New York, so that the annular pattern of shading illustrates the distance effect; the average time-lag to mortality upturns is positively correlated with distance from New York. But the complicating factor is that city size also generally decreases with distance from New York, and we discuss ways of disentangling the size and distance effects further in section 6.5.

(b) Generalisation of average time-lags to surfaces
Maps like that in figure 6.19 can be generalised into time-lag surfaces in a number of ways. We used the procedure discussed in section 5.4.3. Figure 6.20A shows the average time-lags for one of our marker diseases, measles, in the US cities, 1888–1912, as a three-dimensional surface. The viewing position is from northeast to southwest. The block rises away from New York showing that time-lags are longer in smaller cities and cities distant from New York (measles was endemic in New York for the duration of the study period). Thus figure 6.20 indicates that the average result shown in figure 6.19 also holds for a specific disease.

6.3.4 Disease centroids in the United States

An implication of figure 6.20A is that the centres of activity for the transmissible diseases studied in this book may be found in different parts of the United States at different times of the year. This may be tested by computing the month-by-month centroid location of each disease and superimposing these positions upon the time-lag surfaces.

One way of calculating the centroid is described in Kuhn and Kuenne (1962). Assume that the location of the ith city whose disease incidence is to be measured is given a horizontal cartesian coordinate u_i and a vertical map coordinate v_i. Let the reported death rate for i be R_i. The centroid is computed by choosing an initial location at a map coordinate position $\hat{U}, \hat{V}$. This might be, for example, the spatial mean. The centroid of the distribution is now located by an iterative search procedure based upon repeated solution of the equations

$$\hat{U}_{k+1} = \sum_{i=1}^{n} R_i u_i d_{i(k)} \Big/ \sum_{i=1}^{n} R_i d_{i(k)}, \text{ and } \hat{V}_{k+1} = \sum_{i=1}^{n} R_i v_i d_{i(k)} \Big/ \sum_{i=1}^{n} R_i d_{i(k)}. \tag{6.5}$$

until $\hat{U}_{(k+1)} - \hat{U}_{(k)} < \varepsilon$ and $\hat{V}_{(k+1)} - \hat{V}_{(k)} < \varepsilon$ where ε is a pre-specified convergence error level. In these equations, d_i is the distance between the latest centroid and the ith area. The new centroid is denoted by the subscript $(k+1)$. By plotting centroids for successive periods and linking them in sequence, the general direction of movement can be captured.

Figures 6.20B and C plot the centroid trajectories for each disease on a

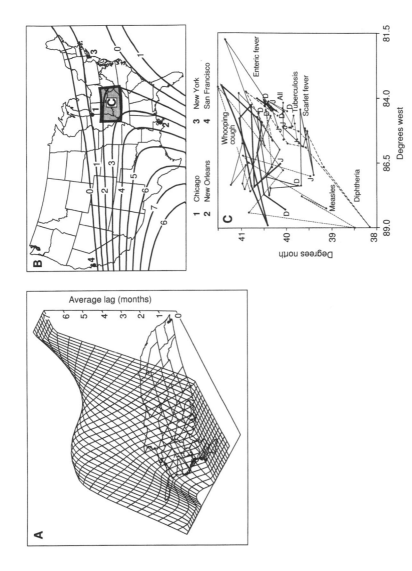

Figure 6.20. United States: average time-lags to infection in months, 1888–1912. (A) Representation of time-lags for measles as a three-dimensional surface, viewed from the northeast. (B) Contour map of average time-lags across all diseases as a context for monthly variations in the geographical location of the Kuhn–Kuenne centroid for each disease and all causes plotted in (C). In C, J = January, D = December. The position of C is marked on B.

month-by-month basis in relation to a contour representation of the map of average time-lags to infection illustrated in figure 6.19. The input data to the centroid calculations consisted of a 20 (cities)×12 (months) matrix of death rates, $\{R_{ij}\}$, where

$$R_{ij} = \frac{1}{T} \sum_{k=1}^{T} r_{ijk}, \quad i=1,\ldots,20\text{(cities)}; \; j=1,\ldots,12\text{(months)}; \; k=1,2,\ldots,25\text{(years)}. \quad (6.6)$$

$T=25$, the number of years in our time series, while r_{ijk} is the reported death rate per 100,000 for city i in month j of year k. The centroid was then calculated for each column of the matrix.

The diagrams show that, depending upon the disease, the monthly centroid trajectories may range over the course of the year from 83° W–91° W and from 38° N–42° N. All causes have the least monthly variation; the centroid remains rooted in one area of the Midwest. This is unsurprising. There is no obvious reason why the geographical centre of deaths from all causes should vary greatly from month to month, except in so far as the six benchmark diseases whose centroids do vary are a component of deaths from all causes; as we have seen in section 5.4, there are complex seasonal variations in the marker diseases.

For the six benchmark diseases, graph 6.20C indicates that there are important geographical variations in the monthly location of the mean centre although, of course, it always remains in the main population locus of the Northeast–Midwest. While variations in location certainly exist, generalisations are harder to come by. However, for diphtheria, measles, and scarlet fever, the centroid in the summer half of the year tends to be located southwest of its position in the winter half. Along with whooping cough, these diseases have similar centroid trajectories, although that for whooping cough is somewhat more variable. The epidemiology of tuberculosis is fundamentally different from the epidemiologies of the other diseases with their short incubation periods (section 3.2), and it has a centroid trajectory that mirrors all causes.

A working hypothesis to account for a southwesterly drift of the disease centroid as between the winter and the summer parts of the year is that infection is moving from the relatively larger east coast cities where endemicity is more likely to the somewhat smaller Midwest cities. Again we see the complex interplay of urban size and distance components in accounting for the geographical distribution of these diseases.

6.3.5 Interaction models and response surfaces

In 1970, A. G. Wilson's pathbreaking monograph, *Entropy in Urban and Regional Modelling*, showed how a wide range of geographical phenomena whose spatial dynamics are driven by population and distance components can be modelled rather than sifted statistically for empirical regularities. We now show how Wilson's style of analysis may be applied to disease distributions.

(a) The entropy-maximising gravity model
To determine the number of deaths attributable to city size and spatial interaction, two steps are involved. First, the gravity model is used to estimate the probabilities of interaction both between and within cities on the basis of their population sizes and distances apart. Second, these probabilities are multiplied by the total number of reported deaths for the set of cities as a whole at some time, t, to generate expected deaths in each of the cities. Rates per unit of population are easily calculated by dividing by city populations.

For each time period, t, the following notational definitions are made: P_i is the population of city i; c_{ij} is the cost of movement between cities i and j. We may estimate the number of interactions between cities i and j, I_{ij}, as

$$I_{ij} = P_i A_i P_j B_j \exp(\beta c_{ij}) \tag{6.7}$$

where

$$A_i = \left[\sum_j P_j B_j \exp(\beta c_{ij}) \right]^{-1} \tag{6.8}$$

$$B_j = \left[\sum_j P_i A_i \exp(\beta c_{ij}) \right]^{-1} \tag{6.9}$$

subject to the constraints

$$\text{(i)} \sum_j I_{ij} = P_i, \text{ (ii)} \sum_i I_{ij} = P_j, \text{ and (iii)} \sum_i \sum_j P_{ij} c_{ij} = C. \tag{6.10}$$

Constraints (i) and (ii) prevent the estimated interactions from exceeding the population totals of the cities, while constraint (iii) ensures that the costs of the interactions taken over all cities cannot exceed some total cost constraint. Algorithms for solving the set of relations (6.7)–(6.10) are given in Baxter (1976, pp. 309–31). Critically from the viewpoint of the analysis described here, provided that the $\{P_i\}$ are scaled to sum to unity (and are therefore empirical probabilities), the estimated interactions, $\{\hat{I}_{ij}\}$, will be probabilities; that is,

$$\sum_i \sum_j \hat{I}_{ij} = 1.$$ Multiplying these probabilities by the observed total of reported deaths in any time period distributes these deaths among the cities according to the interaction model.

(b) Interpretation of model parameters
The coefficient β is the so-called friction of distance parameter, while the $\{A_i\}$ and $\{B_j\}$ are Normalisation values associated with the population sizes of the

origin and destination cities respectively. In the following subsections, the model is applied to data on reported deaths from the six marker diseases in the US cities. The procedure is developed in full for tuberculosis, and summary results are presented for the other diseases.

Obviously, a full matrix of interactions will be generated by the model. There will be flows estimated between $i{\rightarrow}j$ and $j{\rightarrow}i$. Also, when $i{=}j$, we handle within-city mixing.

(c) US cities as a response surface

Inter-city distances (in miles) have been used as a surrogate for costs of movement, so that larger distances imply greater cost and, *ceteris paribus*, less interaction. Figure 6.21A plots the total reported deaths from tuberculosis, 1888–1912, per 100,000 population as a three-dimensional surface. As in figure 6.20, surface values have been estimated by fitting local quadratic polynomials to the city rates using distance weighted least squares. Diagram A shows that rates fell steadily from northeast to southwest across the United States, with the highest rates in the then heavy industrial areas of the Northeast.

As long ago as 1954, Geary argued that the aim of spatial modelling is to account for any systematic geographical pattern present in the data and, accordingly, that such modelling should follow certain well-defined steps: (a) establish, using a test of spatial autocorrelation, that there is systematic spatial pattern in the data that can be accounted for by the proposed model; (b) fit the model and test the residuals from the model for spatial autocorrelation. If there is no spatial autocorrelation in the residuals, the proposed model is successful in that it has accounted for all the systematic spatial variation in the data. If residual spatial autocorrelation is found, the model should be revised until the residuals are found to be autocorrelation-free.

Applying this strategy to the tuberculosis data, the standard Normal score for the spatial autocorrelation coefficient, I, given in equation (6.3), is $z{=}3.38$ when evaluated under Normality so that, in Geary's (1954) terms, there is systematic spatial variation in the death rates of figure 6.21A to model. Following Cliff and Ord (1981, p. 168), the pattern of spatial weights, $\{w_{ij}\}$, in (6.3) should be chosen to represent the spatial autocorrelation pattern hypothesised under the alternative hypothesis, H_1. Since we are attempting to model both within- and between-city interactions generating tuberculosis, we set $w_{ij}{=}1$ in three instances: (i) if $i{=}j$ (the within-city effect); (ii) city i was either the next larger or smaller city than j in population size (hierarchical effects); or (iii) cities i and j were nearest neighbours using straight-line distances (contagious diffusion effects); $w_{ij}{=}0$ elsewhere.

Figure 6.21B plots as a contour map the death rates per 100,000 population arising from within-city mixing estimated from the maximum entropy model – that is, the rates obtained for $i{=}j$ in equation (6.7). In fitting (6.7), we set

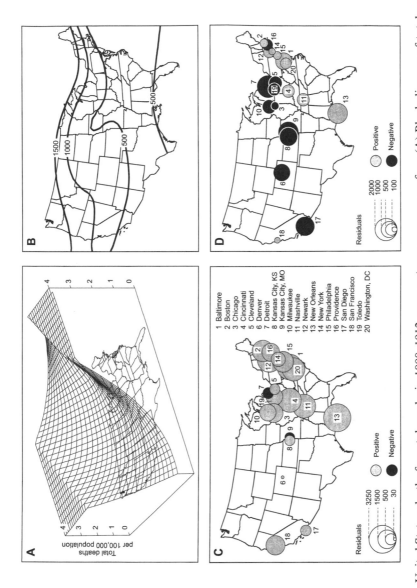

Figure 6.21. United States: deaths from tuberculosis, 1888–1912, as an entropy-response surface. (A) Block diagram of total reported deaths, 1888–1912, per 100,000. (B) Deaths per 100,000 population from within-city mixing estimated by entropy model. (C) Residuals from B. (D) Residuals from estimates of deaths by the entropy model after allowing for within and between city mixing. z-scores on A, C, and D are tests for spatial autocorrelation.

$c_{ij}=1$ if $i=j$ and, to parallel the test for spatial autocorrelation above, if city i was either the next larger or smaller city than j in population size, or if cities i and j were nearest neighbours using straight-line distances; $c_{ij}=999$ otherwise, an arbitrarily large 'cost' to force non-zero estimates of deaths on to terms with $c_{ij}=1$. The configuration of the resulting surface shown in diagram 6.21B has some similarities with that for the raw data in A. Rates are highest in the northeast and fall towards the south.

Figure 6.21C uses proportional circles to map the residuals from the within-city surface. Positive residuals (model underestimates death rates) have been left white; negative residuals (model overestimates deaths) are black. The residuals were tested for spatial autocorrelation using a weights matrix for H_1 that set $w_{ij}=1$ for situations (ii) and (iii) described above, so that we are testing only for between-city hierarchical and neighbourhood effects. The standard Normal score for I was $z=0.87$, so that no significant spatial autocorrelation remained to be accounted for after allowing for within-city mixing. Given the constrained estimation, only two cities – Detroit and Kansas City (Missouri) – have negative residuals. As map 6.21C shows, the largest residuals are found on the northeastern seaboard and on a southwards line down to New Orleans.

To show how the analysis would have proceeded from this point if the residuals had been significantly autocorrelated, figure 6.21D uses proportional circles to map the residuals from both the within- and between-city elements together. These residuals were again tested for spatial autocorrelation, and a standard Normal score of $z=1.63$ was obtained. This is not significant at conventional significance levels, so we conclude that the proposed entropy model has accounted for all the systematic spatial variation in tuberculosis death rates at this period. For this spatial autocorrelation test, the weights matrix for H_1 was a fully connected graph except for situations (i)–(iii) described earlier, where we set $w_{ij}=0$. As a result, we tested for all possible patterns of spatial autocorrelation in the residuals except those already allowed for by fitting the entropy model.

As map 6.21D (which has been plotted using the same scale of circles as C) shows, residuals are uniformly smaller once the deaths generated by spatial interaction terms are included. There is also geographical banding of positive and negative residuals but, as noted above, this is not statistically significant. Given that the autocorrelation in map 6.21A is removed by the within-city mixing component rather than the between-city element, it appears that the latter is relatively unimportant compared with within-city mixing in accounting for tuberculosis deaths. This is consistent with our findings earlier in this section.

The modelling procedure described above was repeated for the other diseases. Table 6.3 gives the spatial autocorrelation values at each stage; those for tuberculosis are included for completeness. This table shows that, for all diseases, there is significant positive spatial autocorrelation in the raw data.

Table 6.3. *Spatial autocorrelation among United States cities*

Standard Normal deviates for tests of spatial autocorrelation in raw data and residuals from the entropy interaction model fitted to deaths from all causes and each of the marker diseases.

Disease	Raw data	Residuals from within-city component	Residuals from within- and between-city components
All causes	3.92*	1.48	−2.23*
Diphtheria	4.89*	2.35*	−3.34*
Enteric fever	2.87*	0.66	−1.04
Measles	2.32*	−0.36	−0.45
Scarlet fever	4.49*	2.25*	−2.90*
Tuberculosis	3.38*	0.87	−1.63
Whooping cough	2.21*	−0.13	−0.32

* Significant at the $\alpha=0.05$ level (two-tailed test).

Except for diphtheria and scarlet fever, the autocorrelation in the raw data appears to be eliminated by the within-city component of the entropy model, and to yield random residuals. However, a slightly more complex picture emerges when the residuals from the within- and between-city components of the entropy model are tested for autocorrelation. As described above, the weights matrix used at this stage tested for all remaining patterns of spatial autocorrelation. Negative autocorrelation was systematically detected in all residuals, and all causes were added to diphtheria and scarlet fever in being statistically significant. Notwithstanding these complexities, however, the main conclusion is that within- rather than between-city effects are more important in determining death rates.

6.4 Cities in the British Isles region

The various analyses described in the previous section may be repeated for any of the other world regions. In this section, we check the North American results in the British Isles region before applying one of the techniques described – average time-lag maps – to all ten regions.

6.4.1 The geographical framework

Once regular reporting commenced, the number of cities in the British Isles region for which mortality data were recorded in the *Weekly Abstract* did not vary greatly over the study period, and this stands in marked contrast to North

America. Between two and five cities appeared in 1887–8; this number rose to around twenty from 1893, at which level it remained until 1912. The maximum number of British cities reported in any one week was twenty-three.

In choosing our cities for inclusion, we again focused upon those which appeared regularly in the *Weekly Abstract* over the period from 1888, and this led to the identification of nineteen for which data were repeatedly recorded. Three of these (Plymouth, South Shields, and Sunderland) were eventually dropped because of missing data, leaving the sixteen shown in table 6.4 to form the basis of the analysis described in this section. A select bibliography of the epidemiological and public health literature for these sixteen cities is given in the appendix to this chapter.

Table 6.4 gives, on a disease-by-disease basis, the percentage of months over the period for which data are available for these sixteen cities, along with summary statistics for the time series distribution of reported deaths and death rates. The average annual rates per 100,000 population, 1888–1912, for the pooled data from the sixteen cities were: all causes 1,500; diphtheria 22; enteric fever 11; measles 38; scarlet fever 12; tuberculosis 45; whooping cough 29. In terms of orders of magnitude, the rate for all causes is very comparable with that for the United States, but the figure for tuberculosis is only a quarter of the North American value. The rates for diphtheria and enteric fever are under half the US values; measles is about three times larger, whooping cough twice, and scarlet fever the same.

The geographical distribution of the British cities is shown in figure 6.22. Circles have been drawn proportional to their mid-term populations. The graph in the upper left of the diagram illustrates the rank–size distributions of the cities in 1888 and 1912. The size distribution is much more primate than that for the United States (figure 6.12). London is approximately ten times larger than the next biggest British city (Glasgow); in the United States, New York was somewhat more than three times larger than the next biggest American city, Chicago. It is this primacy that produces the marked 'elbow' in the rank–size curves for the British Isles. The geographical distribution of the British cities provides reasonable spatial coverage of the British Isles region. There are two cities from Ireland, four from Scotland, one from Wales, and nine from England. Of the English cities, four are clustered in the industrial heartland of Yorkshire–Lancashire.

Figure 6.22 also shows the time series of deaths from measles per 100,000 population for selected cities. For ease of plotting, these have been graphed in standard score format (see section 6.2.1). The charts again illustrate the variety to be seen at the individual city level. Repeating biennial cycles (cf. section 6.2.4) are evident in the series for Belfast, Dublin, London, and Sheffield, but with marked contrasts in their amplitudes – those for Sheffield increasing with time; those for Dublin declining, for example. The London series displays annual seasonal peaks interwoven with the biennial cycle.

Table 6.4. *British Isles cities: data record by city and disease for persistent cities, 1888–1912, in the Weekly Abstract*

City	1912 population	Disease	Number of months with reports	% of record	Reported deaths, 1888–1912							Average annual rate per 100,000 population
					Total	Minimum	First quartile	Median	Third quartile	Maximum		
Belfast	391,051	All causes	295	94.6	153,861	87	421.5	523	644.5	996		1,927.6
		Diphtheria	267	85.6	963	1	2	3	5.0	16		12.3
		Enteric fever	275	88.1	3,575	1	5	9	16.0	133		47.1
		Measles	198	63.5	3,140	1	3	7	19.5	161		47.5
		Scarlet fever	225	72.1	754	1	1	2	4.0	19		10.1
		Tuberculosis	82	26.3	7,691	16	79	92	108.8	159		252.6
		Whooping cough	228	73.1	3,111	1	6	10	17.3	65		46.2
Birmingham	842,517	All causes	235	75.3	183,232	181	661.5	760	876.0	1,551		1,682.1
		Diphtheria	232	74.4	2,067	1	5	7	12.0	34		19.1
		Enteric fever	220	70.5	1,394	1	3	5	9.0	32		13.3
		Measles	210	67.3	4,167	1	6	13	24.0	163		39.1
		Scarlet fever	232	74.4	1,930	1	4	6	10.0	36		17.7
		Tuberculosis	26	8.3	779	6	11.25	17.5	38.0	99		11.3
		Whooping cough	230	73.7	4,276	1	8	14	24.8	102		39.4
Bristol	359,400	All causes	289	92.6	105,360	46	289	364	446.0	1,021		1,400.2
		Diphtheria	263	84.3	1,357	1	2	4	7.0	25		17.1
		Enteric fever	201	64.4	546	1	1	2	3.0	24		7.7
		Measles	185	59.3	2,118	1	2	5	13.0	115		32.8
		Scarlet fever	230	73.7	669	1	1	2	4.0	17		9.4
		Tuberculosis	49	15.7	1,274	5	18	28	33.0	43		70.2
		Whooping cough	214	68.6	1,781	1	3	6	10.8	48		28.9

Table 6.4. (*cont.*)

City	1912 population	Disease	Number of months with reports	% of record	Total	Minimum	First quartile	Median	Third quartile	Maximum	Average annual rate per 100,000 population
Cardiff	184,633	All causes	198	63.5	36,909	39	154	189.5	226.0	393	1,105.5
		Diphtheria	159	51.0	647	1	2	3	6.0	16	19.6
		Enteric fever	108	34.6	179	1	1	1	2.0	6	5.6
		Measles	93	29.8	669	1	1	3	8.0	76	22.8
		Scarlet fever	116	37.2	325	1	1	2	3.0	31	10.9
		Tuberculosis	91	29.2	1,568	3	13.5	17	21.0	31	85.4
		Whooping cough	165	52.9	831	1	2	4	6.0	24	27.0
Dublin	406,536	All causes	234	75.0	172,840	168	622	730	833.0	1,458	2,329.5
		Diphtheria	184	59.0	928	1	3	4	7.0	20	13.6
		Enteric fever	231	74.0	1,634	1	3	6	9.0	36	22.3
		Measles	165	52.9	2,708	1	3	7	19.0	172	38.3
		Scarlet fever	202	64.7	853	1	2	3	6.0	27	11.6
		Tuberculosis	143	45.8	18,014	19	107.5	130	146.0	208	358.0
		Whooping cough	183	58.7	2,270	1	5	9	15.0	96	35.6
Dundee	171,006	All causes	215	68.9	52,961	46	208.5	243	285.0	464	1,692.5
		Diphtheria	171	54.8	488	1	1	2	4.0	11	15.5
		Enteric fever	106	34.0	241	1	1	2	3.0	10	7.8
		Measles	112	35.9	1,113	1	2	4	10.3	126	35.3
		Scarlet fever	128	41.0	267	1	1	1.5	3.0	9	9.0
		Tuberculosis	45	14.4	799	2	14	19	23.0	32	47.0
		Whooping cough	194	62.2	1,291	1	3	5	8.0	34	41.4

Reported deaths, 1888–1912

City	Population	Cause								
Edinburgh	321,200	All causes	299	95.8	124,936	70	355	421	488.0	951	1,647.3
		Diphtheria	281	90.1	1,242	1	2	4	6.0	16	16.7
		Enteric fever	207	66.3	577	1	1	2	4.0	13	8.0
		Measles	219	70.2	2,373	1	2	6	14.0	101	32.4
		Scarlet fever	263	84.3	1,044	1	2	3	5.0	46	14.0
		Tuberculosis	50	16.0	1,802	4	32	36.5	44.8	59	88.3
		Whooping cough	253	81.1	2,594	1	4	8	14.0	56	33.6
Glasgow	785,600	All causes	299	95.8	354,371	270	1,000	1,158	1,370.5	2,501	2,013.4
		Diphtheria	298	95.5	3,482	1	7	11	15.8	38	20.5
		Enteric fever	293	93.9	2,824	1	5	8	13.0	40	16.5
		Measles	249	79.8	9,468	1	10	21	57.0	260	53.4
		Scarlet fever	296	94.9	3,326	1	6	9.5	15.0	55	19.8
		Tuberculosis	3	1.0	20	4	5	6	8.0	10	1.2
		Whooping cough	251	80.4	11,935	1	22	42	62.0	266	65.9
Leeds	445,568	All causes	235	75.3	145,040	316	529.5	604	697.5	1,082	1,673.1
		Diphtheria	226	72.4	1,838	1	3	5.5	10.0	49	21.2
		Enteric fever	211	67.6	1,118	1	2	4	6.0	37	16.5
		Measles	221	70.8	3,291	1	5	11	19.0	151	38.1
		Scarlet fever	221	70.8	1,105	1	2	4	7.0	53	12.9
		Tuberculosis	137	43.9	6,173	7	36	45	54.0	127	112.6
		Whooping cough	230	73.7	2,664	1	6	10	15.0	47	30.8
Leith	81,000	All causes	289	92.6	27,706	14	74	96	117.0	258	1,428.8
		Diphtheria	182	58.3	361	1	1	2	3.0	7	18.8
		Enteric fever	112	35.9	147	1	1	1	1.3	3	8.1
		Measles	113	36.2	505	1	1	2	4.0	39	31.1
		Scarlet fever	128	41.0	306	1	1	1	2.3	22	16.1
		Tuberculosis	137	43.9	1,383	1	7	10	13.0	25	140.8
		Whooping cough	160	51.3	597	1	1	2	4.0	26	38.0

Table 6.4. (cont.)

City	1912 population	Disease	Reported deaths, 1888–1912								Average annual rate per 100,000 population
			Number of months with reports	% of record	Total	Minimum	First quartile	Median	Third quartile	Maximum	
Liverpool	752,055	All causes	270	86.5	320,492	629	1,015.25	1,155.5	1,330.8	2,009	2,137.0
		Diphtheria	269	86.2	2,669	1	6	9	13.0	28	17.3
		Enteric fever	262	84.0	2,553	1	4	8	14.0	32	18.0
		Measles	231	74.0	6,964	1	12	21	38.5	149	49.1
		Scarlet fever	270	86.5	4,334	1	9.25	14	19.0	77	29.1
		Tuberculosis	67	21.5	5,861	16	72	91	104.5	148	112.6
		Whooping cough	233	74.7	6,024	3	13	22	33.0	89	42.9
London	7,340,119	All causes	286	91.7	2,298,084	3,333	6,644.75	7,902	9,148.3	20,767	1,475.4
		Diphtheria	286	91.7	41,439	27	80.25	126	195.0	416	27.2
		Enteric fever	283	90.7	13,092	5	21.5	39	62.0	205	8.5
		Measles	281	90.1	61,789	20	108	180	279.0	922	39.9
		Scarlet fever	286	91.7	17,122	7	35	52	78.0	183	11.2
		Tuberculosis	22	7.1	6,590	19	44.25	247.5	502.5	701	17.2
		Whooping cough	236	75.6	40,465	18	102	153.5	224.5	624	26.9
Manchester	714,427	All causes	236	75.6	224,397	240	829.25	928.5	1,065.3	1,594	1,921.6
		Diphtheria	236	75.6	2,070	1	5	9	11.0	27	17.7
		Enteric fever	230	73.7	1,559	1	4	6	9.0	28	13.6
		Measles	233	74.7	7,156	2	13	23	43.0	139	61.8
		Scarlet fever	233	74.7	2,059	1	5	8	12.0	24	17.9
		Tuberculosis	148	47.4	11,955	13	68	83	95.3	147	146.9
		Whooping cough	233	74.7	4,795	2	11	18	25.0	121	41.1

City	Population	Cause								
Newcastle	269,193	All causes	236	75.6	80,027	77	294	329.5	381.3	624	1,617.2
		Diphtheria	210	67.3	688	1	1	3	4.0	21	13.5
		Enteric fever	133	42.6	284	1	1	2	2.0	13	6.1
		Measles	202	64.7	1,675	1	3	6	11.0	42	35.9
		Scarlet fever	170	54.5	485	1	1	2	3.0	29	9.8
		Tuberculosis	63	20.2	1,322	1	11	19	31.0	52	48.6
		Whooping cough	217	69.6	1,591	1	4	6	9.0	29	34.0
Sheffield	454,653	All causes	235	75.3	138,437	233	491	569	672.0	1,271	1,738.1
		Diphtheria	227	72.8	2,106	1	3	5	8.0	80	27.5
		Enteric fever	217	69.6	1,402	1	2	4	7.0	41	18.5
		Measles	219	70.2	4,438	1	3	9	23.0	304	54.7
		Scarlet fever	228	73.1	1,409	1	3	5	8.0	26	17.7
		Tuberculosis	139	44.6	7,035	12	35	51	63.5	100	135.3
		Whooping cough	224	71.8	2,698	1	5	9	15.0	74	34.1
Southampton	120,896	All causes	236	75.6	28,163	17	93	117	141.0	243	1,487.2
		Diphtheria	159	51.0	378	1	1	2	3.0	22	20.1
		Enteric fever	104	33.3	189	1	1	1	2.0	9	10.9
		Measles	90	28.8	488	1	1	3	6.0	64	30.5
		Scarlet fever	67	21.5	115	1	1	1	2.0	10	7.8
		Tuberculosis	141	45.2	1,517	1	8	10	14.0	25	100.7
		Whooping cough	150	48.1	427	1	1	2	3.8	16	21.9

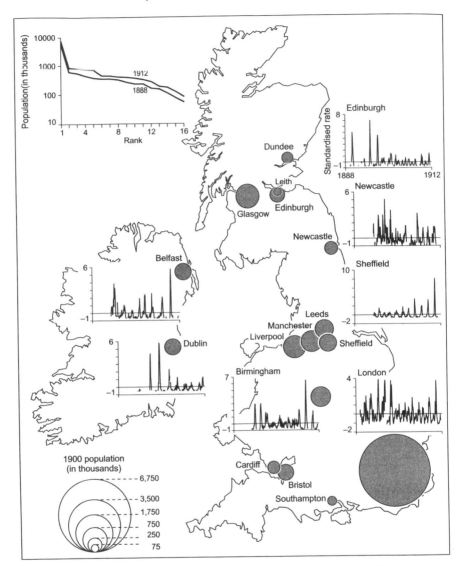

Figure 6.22. Cities in the British Isles. Locations of the sixteen study cities, their rank–size population distributions in 1888 and 1912 (upper left), and representative time series of deaths from measles per 100,000 population (*z*-score format). Circle sizes are proportional to city populations in 1900.

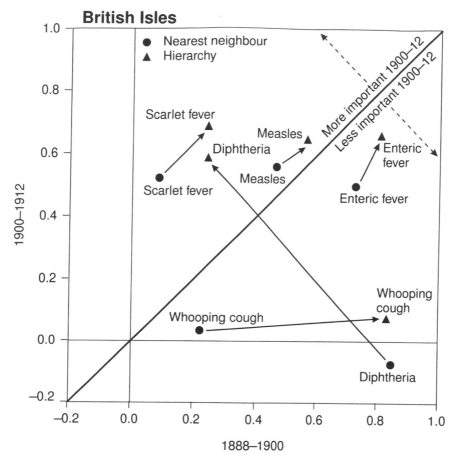

Figure 6.23. British Isles, 1888–1912: time changes in the importance of nearest neighbour and population size hierarchy graphs for disease diffusion. The 45° line corresponds to no change. Axes are correlation coefficients whose calculation is defined in the text. Vectors have been drawn between graph types for each disease.

Compared with these cities, others (Birmingham, Edinburgh, and Newcastle) have much more irregular cyclical components.

6.4.2 Results: comparative analysis

(a) Autocorrelation on graphs

Figure 6.23 repeats the methodology of figure 6.18 for the British cities and, in three respects, the results are similar. First, the diagram shows that, except for diphtheria, the *x*-axis component of the vectors is left to right implying, as in the United States, that the hierarchical graph is generally more closely related to disease patterns (bigger correlation coefficients) than is the corresponding nearest neighbour graph. Second, there is no bias in the number of nearest neighbour (circles) and hierarchy (triangles) graphs lying each side of the 45° line, so that again there is no evidence of a systematic time switch from one graph to the other as a vehicle for diffusion. Third, the graphs for only one disease – in the British region, diphtheria – fell either side of the 45° line.

There are two main differences as compared with the US cities. In contrast to the 3:7 split in the United States, in the British Isles region there is a 5:5 split in the number of points lying either side of the 45° line. Thus there is less evidence in the British Isles of a diminution over the study period in the importance of these graphs as diffusion corridors. Second, the diseases for which both graphs occur either in the northwest triangle or else in the southeast triangle differ. In the British region, scarlet fever and measles are plotted in the northwest, while whooping cough and enteric fever are plotted in the southeast. Only enteric fever occurred in the same triangle in both world regions.

In summary, the principal similarity between the North American and British Isles regions is that, in both, hierarchical diffusion is more important than contagious diffusion for the marker diseases.

(b) British city epidemics as a time-lag surface
The analysis described in sections 6.3.3 and 6.3.4 was repeated in the sixteen British cities. The surfaces and centroid locations are plotted in figure 6.24. There are strong parallels with the findings for the United States. For measles, the block diagram in figure 6.24A shows that, as with measles in the United States, average time-lags to infection are shortest in the main population belt (here, the London–Manchester axis), and that they rise in all directions from this central valley of short lag times.

So far as disease centroids are concerned, comparison of figures 6.20B and 6.24B shows that deaths from all causes again display the least monthly variation. The trajectories for enteric fever, scarlet fever, tuberculosis, and whooping cough are aligned along the southeast–northwest trough of short average time-lags; those for diphtheria and measles remain in the southern part of this trough. A picture equally complex as that for the United States emerges when attempts are made to generalise about the monthly locations of disease centroids. For enteric fever and whooping cough, centroids in the winter half of the year lie southeast of those in the summer half. For scarlet fever and tuberculosis, this is less obviously so.

Taken together, figures 6.24A and B imply that, as in the United States, the time sequence of diffusion for the marker diseases is dictated partly by hierarchical spread and partly as a function of distance between cities.

(c) British cities as a response surface
The analysis carried out for the US cities in section 6.3.5 was also repeated for the British cities. Table 6.5 summarises the spatial autocorrelation results. As

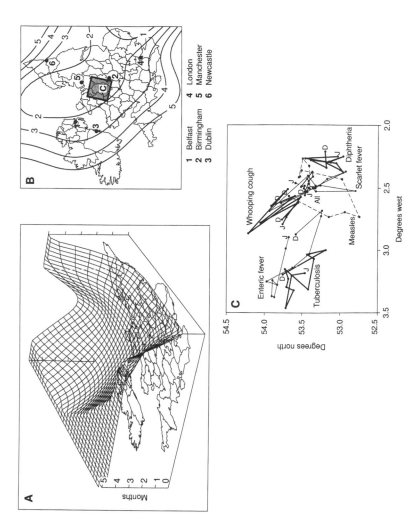

Figure 6.24. British Isles: average time-lags to infection in months, 1888–1912. (A) Representation of time-lags for measles as a three-dimensional surface, *viewed from the southeast*. (B) Contour map of average time-lags across all diseases as a context for monthly variations in the geographical location of the Kuhn–Kuenne centroid for each disease and all causes plotted in (C). In C, J=January, D=December. The position of C is marked on B.

Table 6.5. *Spatial autocorrelation among British cities*

Standard Normal deviates for tests of spatial autocorrelation in raw data and residuals from the entropy interaction model fitted to deaths from all causes and to each of the marker diseases.

Disease	Raw data	Residuals from within-city component	Residuals from within- and between-city components
All causes	2.26*	−1.39	−0.20
Diphtheria	2.18*	−2.29*	−0.05
Enteric fever	3.18*	0.50	−1.21
Measles	2.73*	−1.46	−0.72
Scarlet fever	3.21*	−0.16	−1.26
Tuberculosis	2.86*	0.81	−0.81
Whooping cough	3.14*	−0.25	−1.04

* Significant at the $\alpha = 0.05$ level (two-tailed test).

in the United States, all the original death rates displayed significant positive spatial autocorrelation. Except for diphtheria, the within-city element of the entropy-maximising model accounted for the significant spatial pattern in the disease distributions, leaving spatially random residuals. It is noteworthy that diphtheria was one of the two diseases in the North American region for which this component of the entropy model failed to remove all the significant spatial autocorrelation. Addition of the between-city diffusion element succeeded in eliminating the remaining spatial autocorrelation. As with the United States, we conclude that within-city mixing was the main engine generating the patterns of death rates witnessed at the turn of the century.

6.5 Cities in all regions

6.5.1 Average time-lag maps

Our analysis of the data in the *Weekly Abstract* for the North American and British Isles regions has suggested that the spatial diffusion of all the marker diseases occurs partly through a 'drain-down' mechanism from larger to smaller cities, and partly by contagious spread among geographically proximate cities. In this section, we take one of the methods used previously, that of time-lag mapping, to check whether these components of diffusion are to be found in all ten world regions.

To calculate average time-lags, each disease was first studied separately, and the procedure described in section 6.3.3 was followed. For a given disease, the average time-lag to infection for the cities comprising each of the ten world regions was calculated from equation 6.4 with reference to the start of epidemics in the regional series of which the cities were a part.

6.5.2 *Results: ten-region comparisons*

Figure 6.25 graphs the $\{\bar{t}_{ij}\}$ (in months, vertical axis) generated from equation 6.4 against city population sizes (log scale) for each of the six diseases separately and (top) for an average graph formed by calculating the mean lag across all six diseases. The OLS regression lines fitted to the lag-time/population size relationship for the cities of each world region are also plotted. These have been produced beyond the point clusters to facilitate labelling. Although variability is to be seen from region to region and from disease to disease, the overriding feature is the generally inverse correlation between city size and time to infection. That is, the larger the city, the shorter the time to infection.

To check whether the average time-lag to infection is a function of the distance of cities within a region from the city of first flare-up, stepwise multiple regressions were fitted to time-lags against log of population size and log of the straight-line distance between each city and city of first flare-up in its world region. To illustrate the style of the analysis, table 6.6 gives the full results applied to the time-lag for each city, averaged across all six diseases (dependent variable).

Three features of the table deserve comment:

(1) Sample sizes are too small for many regions for much significance to be attached to the findings for these areas; they are quoted here for completeness.

(2) Notwithstanding this caveat, both for the pool of 100 cities and all regions except Middle America, there is an inverse relationship between population size and average time-lag – that is, larger cities entered epidemic phases, as judged by mortality upturns, earlier than smaller cities. This result confirms the simple regressions graphed in figure 6.25. In addition, the population variable is entered before the distance variable in eight of the eleven regressions.

(3) Where the distance variable is statistically significant (all 100 cities and the 20 cities of North America), there is a positive relationship between average time-lag and distance implying, *ceteris paribus*, that the further a city is from the origin of an epidemic in a given region, the later the epidemic will start in that city (see figure 6.19).

Taken together, these results suggest that city size effects dominate epidemic start times. It remains an open question as to whether this simply reflects greater disease endemicity in larger cities or whether, for the lower levels of the population hierarchy at least, there is cascade transmission of infection from larger cities to smaller to initiate epidemics. Indeed, both effects may jointly

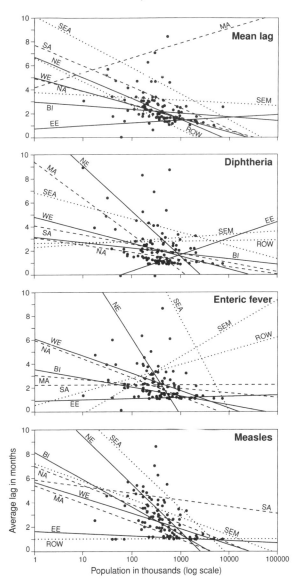

Figure 6.25. Average time-lags, ten world regions. Regression relationships between
average time to epidemic flare-up and city population size by disease and world
region. OLS linear trend lines have been fitted to the regional subsets of points
shown as scattergraphs. Lines have been produced beyond the point clouds for
identification purposes only. The mean lag graph is the average relationship over the
six individual diseases. Solid lines have been used for the European regions, pecked
lines for the Americas, and dotted lines for the remainder. BI=British Isles;
EE=Eastern Europe; MA=Middle America; NA=North America; NE=Northern
Europe; SA=South America; SEA=South East Asia; SEM=Southern Europe and
Mediterranean; ROW=Rest of World; WE=Western Europe.

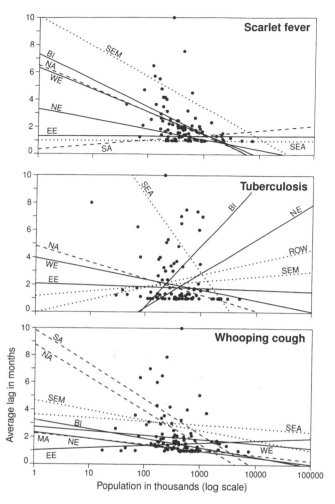

Figure 6.25. (*cont.*)

determine epidemic start times in any particular city, and this seems to be the implication of finding 3 above.

Table 6.7 follows the format of 6.6, but gives only the statistically significant regression results (not stepwise) with reasonable sample sizes for each of the six diseases separately. For the population variable, this table reinforces our previous conclusions. An inverse relationship between time-lag and population size was found except for tuberculosis in the British Isles. For the distance variable, the interpretation is more complex. The significant values split equally between inverse and positive relationships with time-lag, implying that spread may occur both upwards and downwards through the city systems.

It is tempting to argue, on the basis of table 6.7, that the structured patterns

Table 6.6. *Average time-lags by cities in ten world regions*

Stepwise multiple regression results for average time-lag to epidemic starts in cities as a function of population size and distance from start city in each world region. The average is calculated as the mean of the time lags for each city on the individual marker diseases.

				Coefficients				
Disease	Region	n	Constant	Population (log)	Distance (log)	R^2	$r(P,D)$	Process
Average, all six	All	100	16.87	−2.48* (−4.07)		0.16*		Hierarchy and
			9.84	−1.99* (−3.22)	1.63* (2.61)	0.22*	−0.31*	distance
	British Isles	16	3.59	−0.25 (−0.73)		0.04		
			2.95	−0.23 (−0.63)	0.24 (0.36)	0.05	−0.18	
	Eastern Europe	7	2.54		−0.40 (−0.84)	0.15		
			3.37	−0.13 (−0.17)	−0.41 (−0.74)	0.16	−0.06	
	Northern Europe	5	10.39	−1.43 (−2.34)		0.73		
			11.34	−1.48 (−1.61)	−0.30 (−0.14)	0.74	−0.35	
	Southern Europe and Mediterranean	11	2.05		0.46 (0.48)	0.03		
			5.61	−0.80 (−0.58)	0.71 (0.65)	0.07	0.39	
	Western Europe	16	8.35	−1.12* (−1.83)		0.21		
			7.87	−1.45* (−1.94)	1.00 (0.79)	0.24	−0.56	Hierarchy
	Middle America	8	−8.02	4.30 (1.00)		0.25		
			71.80	4.50 (0.90)	−27.0 (−0.44)	0.32	−0.03	
	North America	20	11.91	−1.76* (−4.09)		0.50		
			7.29	−1.37* (−2.96)	0.90* (1.75)	0.58	−0.48	Hierarchy and distance
	South America	5	7.27		−1.10 (−0.24)	0.03		

Table 6.6. (*cont.*)

Disease	Region	n	Constant	Coefficients		R^2	$r(P,D)$	Process
				Population (log)	Distance (log)			
			18.02	−1.00 (−0.08)	−2.50 (−0.14)	0.04	−0.94	
	South and East Asia	7	27.25	−3.80 (−0.64)		0.09		
			38.44	−4.50 (−0.63)	−2.20 (−0.31)	0.12	−0.35	
	Rest of World	5	9.42	−1.09 (−1.97)		0.80		

* Significant at the $\alpha=0.05$ level (one-tailed test); *t*-values in parentheses.

are to be found exclusively in the developed world, but other world regions are ruled out on the grounds of sample size.

6.6 Some atypical series

This chapter has been concerned with a search for order in the time series of our six marker diseases at the city level. We complete our analysis at this spatial scale by illustrating in figure 6.26 five series that display atypical features of one kind or another and a sixth, whooping cough in Leeds (England), that is remarkable in its typical characteristics.

Sheffield, England (diphtheria): Except for a four-year window from 1899–1903, the monthly death rate averaged almost exactly 1 per 100,000 population. During that four-year period, death rates spiralled without warning to a sustained and higher level that reached a maximum of twenty-two in December 1899. After 1903, the normal time series run recommenced.

Colombo, Ceylon (enteric fever): This series is the exact opposite of what would be expected from the mortality decline and crisis hypotheses described in sections 4.3 and 4.4. From 1894, when records began, until 1905, the long-term trend in monthly rates was horizontal at around 5 per 100,000 population. In 1905, a strongly rising trend in rates set in, and this was accompanied by substantially increased amplitudes in the cycles of mortality.

Madras, India (measles): This time series is made exceptional by the three spires of mortality in 1898, 1900, and 1906. In March 1898, 147 deaths were reported, a rate of 30 per 100,000 population. In section 7.2.3, we discuss the

Table 6.7. *Average time-lags by disease in ten world regions*

Significant regression results by disease for average time to epidemic starts as a
function of population size and distance from start city in each region.

Disease	Region	n	Constant	Population (log)	Distance (log)	R^2	Process
Diphtheria	All	100	9.59	−1.40* (−3.61)	0.24 (−0.54)	0.16	Hierarchy
Enteric fever	British Isles	16	8.89	−1.09 (−3.29)	−0.54 (−1.23)	0.49	Hierarchy
	North America	20	4.34	−1.20 (−1.60)	1.56* (−1.87)	0.42	Distance
Measles	All	100	15.4	−2.94* (−3.34)	1.64* (1.96)	0.20	Hierarchy and distance
	British Isles	16	22.8	−3.77* (−5.45)	0.15 (0.16)	0.72	Hierarchy
Scarlet fever	All	100	15.9	−2.66* (−4.33)	0.54 (1.04)	0.22	Hierarchy
	British Isles	16	25.4	−3.24* (−3.38)	−2.24 (−1.76)	0.53	Hierarchy
	North America	20	10.22	−1.77* (−5.40)	0.62 (1.70)	0.77	Hierarchy
Tuberculosis	British Isles	16	−25.0	4.46* (3.77)	1.43 (0.33)	0.55	Hierarchy
	Eastern Europe	7	−12.3	5.12 (2.44)	−6.16* (−3.39)	0.80	Upwards spread
	Western Europe	16	2.62	−2.69 (−1.89)	5.89* (2.54)	0.38	Distance
Whooping cough	British Isles	16	9.21	−1.06* (−2.25)	−0.80 (−1.27)	0.34	Hierarchy
	North America	20	13.92	−2.65* (−2.25)	1.21 (1.01)	0.36	Hierarchy
	Western Europe	16	10.9	0.40 (0.33)	−4.79* (−3.06)	0.44	Upwards spread

* Significant at the $\alpha=0.05$ level (one-tailed test); *t*-values in parentheses.

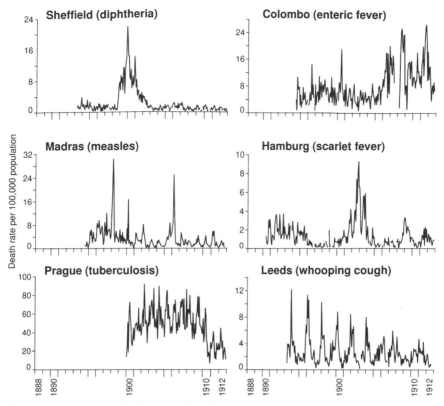

Figure 6.26. Some atypical time series. Six exceptional city time series of monthly death rates per 100,000 from the marker diseases.

changing United States experience of mortality from measles, and show that, over a thirty-year period from 1960–90, the average annual rate was 1.09 deaths per 1,000 reported cases. The implication of this gearing is that c. 150,000 cases might have occurred in Madras around April 1898 in a population of nearly half a million. This yields an attack rate of around 30 per cent, on a par with the great measles epidemics of history such as that in Fiji in 1875 (see Cliff, Haggett, and Smallman-Raynor, 1993, pp. 130–7). The epidemics of 1900 and 1906 were not much smaller.

Hamburg, Germany (scarlet fever): There are two distinctive features of this time series. First, from 1901–3, the city suffered three successive springs of exceptionally high mortality from the disease, with rates two to three times greater than those experienced over the remainder of the period. Second, there appears to be a long wavelength cycle of six to seven years in mortality underlying the annual seasonal swings.

Prague, Austria–Hungary (tuberculosis): On an annual basis, this is a well-behaved time series with the seasonal swings that are characteristic of many of the city, regional, and global time series of our marker diseases. But, beneath the annual cycle of mortality, there is a quadratic trend peaking around 1905 and falling thereafter. In addition, the seasonal highs and lows are damped in the last two years of the series. These features contrast with our findings at the global and regional scales (sections 4.3, 4.4, and 5.3) where tuberculosis was shown to be a disease of increasing significance as a cause of death almost everywhere. Yet despite the apparent decline in mortality from tuberculosis after 1905, Prague had the fourth highest median death rate over the period among our 100 cities.

Leeds, England (whooping cough): By way of an antidote to the series discussed so far in this section, the Leeds series is exceptional as a model of good behaviour. The evidence presented in sections 4.4 and 5.3 on the crisis hypothesis was at best equivocal in its support. In the Leeds series, the trend is level throughout (no mortality decline) but, as predicted by the crisis model, the mortality peaks decline so evenly from 1893, when the data record begins, that it is almost possible to put a ruler across the tops. Moreover, the peaks of mortality are stamped out at three-year intervals (cf. Noah (1989) in section 6.2.4), although they are increasingly complex after 1905.

The graphs shown in figure 6.26 underline the danger of studies which generalise from the results for a single city. In effect, a researcher could find examples of mortality trends to suit (or refute) any one of the wide range of models of mortality change in the historical demography literature.

6.7 Conclusions

In this chapter, we have illustrated the richness of the database upon which our analysis of mortality patterns at global and regional levels was based. We have also continued our search for order in mortality rates at a further and lower spatial scale, that of the city – the level for which the data reported in the *Weekly Abstract* were originally collected.

For the ten largest (in terms of mid-term populations) cities in our world sample, we showed that the long-term trend in death rates was roughly horizontal or falling for nearly all city/disease combinations suggesting that, in these great cities, the mortality decline model is a reasonable approximation to behaviour. So far as seasonal and cyclical events were concerned, much greater variability was found and, although no formal analysis of the crisis hypothesis was attempted, visual inspection of the plots in figures 6.1–6.10 readily illustrates the variety to be found. Certainly evidence for ubiquitous time-damping in the amplitudes of cycles expected under the crisis model was not apparent.

The return time for peaks in mortality rates was examined using spectral decomposition. This technique readily identified both the seasonal and cyclical returns in the mortality rates in our ten cities. But, while cycles in mortality for some of the marker diseases conformed with conventional wisdom, the technique showed that, even in the ten biggest cities in the global sample, there were considerable fluctuations around the 'norms'. Indeed, the city series plotted in figures 6.12 and 6.22 reinforce the point; although there are a number of repeating empirical themes to be found in these time series, equally there are many that do not seem to fit conventional models of the demographic/mortality transition.

The six marker diseases considered in this book are all either wholly or partly transmissible from person to person by the respiratory or intestinal routes. For such diseases, the ways in which they are propagated from city to city is an important question, and one that we have attempted to answer using a number of techniques of geographical analysis. For two of the ten world regions, North America and the British Isles, testing for spatial auto-correlation in rates of mortality on different diffusion graphs and entropy surface modelling were used to identify patterns of spread. Although diffusion occurred from city to city, it appeared that, once infection was present in a city, the main engine causing recurrent peaks of mortality was within-city transmission rather than repeated reinfection from outside. Since most of the US and British cities in our sample were large enough over the period from 1888 to 1912 to maintain indigenous reservoirs of infection for these diseases, our findings present a consistent story: the amplitude and spacing of cyclical recurrences probably reflects the rate of build-up of local susceptible populations through births. See Bartlett (1957, 1960), Black (1966) and Cliff, Haggett, and Smallman-Raynor (1993, pp. 10–12) for a review of the models proposed to link recurrence intervals, endemicity, and population growth.

In cities that are too small to maintain permanent local reservoirs of infection, then the spread of disease from large cities is the only mechanism by which a new epidemic can recommence (see section 7.5.1). Using the concept of average time-lag to infection, the relationship between times of peak mortality and city size was examined for all the cities in each of the ten world regions. It was shown that city size and timing of mortality peaks are positively correlated – the larger the city, the earlier the peak, implying possible passage of disease from larger to smaller cities. Taken with the findings described in the previous paragraph, we may tentatively suggest the following qualitative model to account for the mortality patterns witnessed in these regional systems of cities:
(i)   Some very large cities act as permanent reservoirs of infection.
(ii) In any epidemic, these peak earlier than smaller cities because infection is already present.

(iii) In smaller cities, epidemics are restarted by infection carried to them from the reservoir cities. This spread is driven mainly through the urban size hierarchy, from larger to smaller cities (cf. Pyle's (1969) work on cholera discussed in section 6.3.2).

(iv) Once infection is introduced, the disease is maintained by spread among the local susceptible population which is ultimately exhausted and the epidemic wave passes.

(v) The process restarts once local susceptible populations build up to a threshold size that will sustain infection arriving from a reservoir city.

The analyses described in chapters 4–6 are distinctive in the global nature of our sample of cities, the fine temporal resolution (potentially weekly) of the data, the emphasis upon different geographical scales, and a dominantly cross-sectional treatment. But, as compared with many studies in historical demography and epidemiology, the time span of our series, from 1888 to 1912, is brief indeed. In the next chapter, we address this problem by enlarging our temporal span to look at patterns of mortality from the marker diseases over the course of the twentieth century. We conclude by examining the marker diseases in the context of global mortality from all diseases, old, new, and emerging.

Appendix to chapter 6

For the 100-city sample studied in this book, this appendix lists some of the principal references relating to their public health, mortality, and morbidity, 1888–1912, from all causes and our six marker diseases of diphtheria, enteric (typhoid and paratyphoid) fever, measles, scarlet fever, tuberculosis, and whooping cough. Cities are listed alphabetically by their country at the time according to the distribution given in table 3.3. The full reference for each source appears in the list of references at the end of the book.

AUSTRALIA. **Melbourne:** diphtheria, state of Victoria (Cumpston, 1989, pp. 292–9); measles, state of Victoria (Cumpston, 1989, pp. 305–9); scarlet fever, state of Victoria (Cumpston, 1989, pp. 300–4); tuberculosis, state of Victoria (Cumpston, 1989, pp. 276–91); typhoid fever (Jamieson, 1903; Springthorpe, 1909), state of Victoria (Cumpston, 1989, pp. 230–8); whooping cough (Cumpston, 1989, pp. 310–12).

AUSTRIA-HUNGARY. **Prague:** typhoid fever (Skalicka, 1903), 1910 (Keltner, 1911).

BELGIUM. **Brussels:** typhoid fever, 1893–1906 ('Tableau de la mortalité', 1907).

BRAZIL. **Bahia:** tuberculosis (de Meirelles, 1897–8). **Pernambuco:** public health (Levine, 1978). **Rio de Janeiro:** historical urban development (Rios, 1972).

BURMA. **Rangoon:** typhoid fever (Fitz Gerald, 1897).

CUBA. **Havana:** scarlet fever (Lebredo, 1904).

DENMARK. **Copenhagen:** historical urban development (Holm, 1972); diphtheria (Carlsen & Heiberg, 1897; Heiberg, 1895), 1895–1901 (Carlsen & Heiberg, 1903); scarlet fever (Heiberg, 1907), 1885–1900 (Heiberg, 1907–8); tuberculosis (Hansen, 1904).

EGYPT. **Alexandria:** typhoid fever (Phillips, 1910); **Cairo:** historical urban development (Tawab, 1972); typhoid fever (Phillips, 1910).

ENGLAND. **Birmingham:** historical urban development (Swaisland, 1972); mortality patterns, nineteenth century (R. Woods, 1978, 1984), 1881–90 (Welton, 1897); diphtheria (A. Hill, 1895–6); scarlet fever, early twentieth century (H. M. Woods, 1933); tuberculosis (F. B. Smith, 1988, in passing). **Bristol:** mortality patterns, 1881–90 (Welton, 1897); tuberculosis (F. B. Smith, 1988, in passing). **Leeds:** mortality patterns, 1881–90 (Welton, 1897); tuberculosis (F. B. Smith, 1988, in passing). **Liverpool:** mortality patterns, 1881–90 (Welton, 1897); diphtheria (Hope, 1931, pp. 69–71); measles (Hope, 1931, pp. 69–71); scarlet fever (Hope, 1931, pp. 69–71), early twentieth century (H. M. Woods, 1933); tuberculosis (Hope, 1931, pp. 71–6); typhoid fever (Hope, 1931, pp. 69–71; Stallybrass, 1911–12); whooping cough (Hope, 1931, pp. 69–71). **London:** public health, 1881–1906 (Jephson, 1907, pp. 288–433); mortality patterns, 1881–90 (Welton, 1897); historical urban development (Regan, 1972); diphtheria (Hardy, 1993a, pp. 80–109; W. R. Smith, 1896; Sykes, 1893–4, 1894), 1890–7 (Parkes, 1898–9), 1895–1914 (Goodall, Greenwood, & Russell, 1929), 1896–8 (Dixey, 1898), early twentieth century (Forbes, 1927); measles (Hardy, 1993a, pp. 28–55); scarlet fever (Hardy, 1993a, pp. 56–79), 1895–1914 (Goodall, Greenwood, & Russell, 1929), early twentieth century (H. M. Woods, 1933); tuberculosis (Hardy, 1993a, pp. 211–66; F. B. Smith, 1988, in passing), 1850–1910 (UK, Medical Research Committee, 1918); typhoid fever (Grattan, 1910; Hardy, 1993a, pp. 151–190; Hodgetts & Amyot, 1905), 1851–1900 (B. Luckin, 1984), 1895–1914 (Goodall, Greenwood, & Russell, 1929); whooping cough (Hardy, 1993a, pp. 10–27); general discussion of health (Daunton, 1991); early modern period discussion of health (Landers, 1993). **Manchester:** mortality patterns, nineteenth century (Pooley & Pooley, 1984), 1881–90 (Welton, 1897); childhood mortality, nineteenth century (Cruickshank, 1981); scarlet fever, early twentieth century (H. M. Woods, 1933); tuberculosis (F. B. Smith, 1988, in passing); typhoid fever (Niven, 1897). **Newcastle:** mortality patterns, 1881–90 (Welton, 1897); tuberculosis (F. B. Smith, 1988, in passing). **Sheffield:** mortality patterns, 1881–90 (Welton, 1897); tuberculosis (F. B. Smith, 1988, in passing). **Southampton:** mortality patterns, 1881–90 (Welton, 1897).

FRANCE. **Le Havre:** typhoid (Brouardel, 1894; Gilbert, 1896), 1894 ('Typhoid fever at Havre', 1894), 1902 (Frottier, 1903), 1911 (Vigne & Loir, 1911). **Lyon:** mortality patterns (Preston & Van de Walle, 1978); diphtheria, 1886–1910 (Séchan, 1911), 1901–5 (Musy, 1906); typhoid fever (Pic, 1906; Wolff, 1911); whooping cough (Sarda, 1907). **Paris:** historical urban development (Delouvrier, 1972); mortality patterns (Preston & Van de Walle, 1978; Van de Walle & Preston, 1974); measles (Debré & Joannon, 1926; Gagnière, 1907); scarlet fever (Gagnière, 1907); tuberculosis (Marié-Davy, 1905; A. Mitchell, 1990); typhoid fever (Bucquoy, 1894a, 1894b; Chabal, 1904; Rochard, 1894), 1876–94 (Lancreaux, 1894), 1884–93 (de Pietra Santa, 1894), 1894 (Bucquoy, 1894a, 1984b; Thoinot & Dubief, 1896; Vallin, 1894), 1904 (Lemoine, 1904).

GERMANY. **Berlin:** mortality patterns (Vögele, 1994). **Cologne:** infant mortality from infectious diseases (Vögele, 1994). **Frankfurt:** infant mortality from infectious diseases (Vögele, 1994); diphtheria, 1903 (Henius, 1904). **Hamburg:** infant mortality from infectious diseases (Vögele, 1994); diphtheria (R. J. Evans, 1987, pp. 195–6); measles (R. J. Evans, 1987, p. 195); scarlet fever (R. J. Evans, 1987, pp. 195–6); tuberculosis (R. J. Evans, 1987, pp. 183–9); typhoid fever (R. J. Evans, 1987, pp. 189–194); whooping cough (R. J. Evans, 1987, p. 195). **Munich:** infant mortality from infectious diseases

(Vögele, 1994); tuberculosis (Goldschmidt & Luxenburger, 1896); typhoid fever (Childs, 1898). **Nuremberg:** diphtheria, 1896 (Cnopf, 1898).

HOLLAND. **Amsterdam:** historical urban development (Leemans, 1972).

INDIA. **Bombay:** public health (Harrison, 1994); social structure (Kosambi, 1986); mortality patterns, 1870–1914 (Klein, 1973, 1986). **Calcutta:** public health (Harrison, 1994); historical urban development (Ashraf & Green, 1972); mortality patterns (Klein, 1973); typhoid fever (Rogers, 1907). **Madras:** public health (Harrison, 1994).

IRELAND. **Belfast:** tuberculosis (F. B. Smith, 1988, in passing); typhoid fever (Lindsay, 1898; Mair, 1909), 1898 (J. L. Smith & Tennant, 1898). **Dublin:** tuberculosis (F. B. Smith, 1988, in passing); typhoid fever (D. E. Flinn, 1909).

ITALY. **Catania:** diphtheria, 1877–96 (Giaquinta, 1898); typhoid fever, 1887–92 (Di Mattei, 1894), 1893–9 (Basile, 1903). **Naples:** diphtheria (Montefusco, 1914); typhoid fever (Caro, 1898).

JAPAN. **Osaka:** historical urban development (Royama, 1972).

MALAYA. **Singapore:** public health (Tan, 1991).

MEXICO. **Mexico City:** historical urban development (Fried, 1972); diphtheria (Fabela, 1907); tuberculosis (Terrés, 1903); typhoid fever (Troconis Alcalá, 1906).

NORWAY. **Christiania:** typhoid fever, 1896 (Harbitz, 1897).

RUSSIA. **Moscow:** historical urban development (Khromov, Preobrazhensky, Promyslov, Roganov, & Sinitsyn, 1981); public health (Bater, 1983, pp. 312–15; J. Bradley, 1986; Gleason, 1990). **Odessa:** historical urban development (Subtelny, 1988); public health and mortality (Skinner, 1986), nineteenth century (Herlihy, 1978). **St Petersburg:** public health and mortality patterns (Bater, 1976, 1983, 1986; Frieden, 1981; Gleason, 1990; Hutchinson, 1990), 1890–1914 (Bater, 1985); whooping cough (Kozlova, 1973). **Warsaw:** historical urban development (Zawadzki, 1972); public health (Corrsin, 1986).

SCOTLAND. **Dundee:** public health and mortality (Jackson, 1979, pp. 386–426); diphtheria (Jackson, 1979, pp. 393–5); measles (Jackson, 1979, pp. 395–6); tuberculosis (Jackson, 1979, pp. 389–90); typhoid fever (Jackson, 1979, 391–2); whooping cough (Jackson, 1979, p. 395). **Edinburgh:** public health and mortality (Keir, 1966, pp. 320–68); diphtheria (Tait, 1974, pp. 43–4); measles (Tait, 1974, pp. 48–50); scarlet fever (Tait, 1974, pp. 43–4); tuberculosis (Tait, 1974, pp. 57–60); typhoid fever (Tait, 1974, pp. 46–8); whooping cough (Tait, 1974, p. 53). **Glasgow:** public health (Chalmers, 1905, 1930; Checkland & Lamb, 1982; Cunnison & Gilfillan, 1958, pp. 475–515), 1905–46 (MacGregor, 1967); discussion of diphtheria, measles, scarlet fever, typhoid, tuberculosis, and whooping cough, 1855–1911 (Pennington, 1979), 1905–46 (MacGregor, 1967); diphtheria (J. B. Russel, 1895–6; Chalmers, 1930, pp. 311–36; Cunnison & Gilfillan, 1958, p. 494); measles (Chalmers, 1930, pp. 337–50; Cunnison & Gilfillan, 1958, p. 496); scarlet fever (Chalmers, 1930, pp. 311–20; Cunnison & Gilfillan, 1958, pp. 495–6); tuberculosis (Chalmers, 1930, pp. 91–142; Cunnison & Gilfillan, 1958, pp. 486–90; Pennington, 1982; F. B. Smith, 1988, in passing); typhoid fever (Chalmers, 1930, pp. 300–10; Cunnison & Gilfillan, 1958, p. 492); whooping cough (Cunnison & Gilfillan, 1958, p. 496).

SOUTH AFRICA. **Cape Town:** public health (Laidler & Gelfand, 1971); typhoid fever (J. A. Mitchell, 1907). **Durban:** public health (Laidler & Gelfand, 1971).

SWEDEN. **Stockholm:** historical urban development (Mehr, 1972); diphtheria, 1903–4 (I. Anderson, 1904).

SWITZERLAND. **Zurich:** typhoid, 1901–9 (Goldberg, 1911).

TURKEY. **Constantinople:** demographic structure (Duben & Behar, 1991; Karpat, 1985, pp. 86–106).

UNITED STATES OF AMERICA. **Baltimore:** mortality patterns, 1850–1915 (Meeker, 1971–2), 1871–1900 (Higgs, 1979); public health (Howard, 1924); diphtheria (Howard, 1924, pp. 350–63); measles (Howard, 1924, pp. 314–22); scarlet fever (Howard, 1924, pp. 299–314), 1912 (White, 1929); tuberculosis (Howard, 1924, pp. 380–417); typhoid fever (Ford & Watson, 1911; Howard, 1924, pp. 256–68; Janney, 1903–4; Osler, 1894–5; Stokes, 1908); whooping cough (Howard, 1924, pp. 337–50). **Boston:** mortality patterns, 1871–1900 (Higgs, 1979); diphtheria, early twentieth century (Forbes, 1927); scarlet fever (Donally, 1915); tuberculosis, 1885–1903 (Stone & Wilson, 1905); typhoid fever (Brough, 1904). **Chicago:** historical urban development (Rakove, 1972); mortality patterns, 1871–1900 (Higgs, 1979); diphtheria (Rawlings, 1910), early twentieth century (Forbes, 1927); measles (Young, 1912); scarlet fever (Rawlings, 1910), 1911–12 (Capps & Miller, 1912); tuberculosis (Sachs, 1904); typhoid fever, 1902 (N. W. Jones, 1906). **Cincinnati:** mortality patterns, 1871–1900 (Higgs, 1979); typhoid fever, 1850–1915 (Meeker, 1971–2). **Cleveland:** tuberculosis (Howard, 1903), 1895–1901 (Welty, 1903); typhoid fever (Perkins, 1911), 1890–1902 (Moorehouse, 1903), 1903–4 (Whipple, 1906), 1904 (Moorehouse, 1905). **Denver:** typhoid fever (McLauthlin, 1896). **Detroit:** typhoid fever (Clark, 1910; Strong, 1910). **Milwaukee:** mortality patterns, 1871–1900 (Higgs, 1979); typhoid fever ('Typhoid fever in Milwaukee', 1910). **Nashville:** public health (Doyle, 1985, pp. 82–6). **New Orleans:** mortality patterns, 1871–1900 (Higgs, 1979); diphtheria (J. Jones, 1894–5a), 1886–94 (J. Jones 1894–5b); typhoid fever, 1850–1915 (Meeker, 1971–2). **New York City:** historical urban development (Sayre, 1972); comprehensive bibliography of health and disease (Dwork, 1981); mortality patterns, 1871–1900 (Higgs, 1979); diphtheria (Duffy, 1974, pp. 154–7; Kleinman, 1992), late nineteenth century (Quiroga, 1990), early twentieth century (Forbes, 1927; W. T. Russell, 1943); measles (Duffy, 1974, p. 158); scarlet fever (Donally, 1915; Duffy, 1974, p. 158; Seibert, 1904); tuberculosis (Billings, 1912; Duffy, 1974, pp. 159–61; Miller, 1904; Shively, 1903; L. G. Wilson, 1990), 1889–1900 (Fox, 1975), early twentieth century (Drolet & Lowell, 1952); typhoid fever (Bolduan, 1912; Clerc, 1910; Duffy, 1974, pp. 161–5), 1905 (Billings, 1906a, 1906b); whooping cough (Duffy, 1974, p. 158). **Newark:** mortality patterns, 1871–1900 (Higgs, 1979); public health and disease, 1832–95 (Galishoff, 1988), 1895–1918 (Galishoff, 1975, pp. 120–34); tuberculosis, 1895–1918 (Galishoff, 1975, pp. 120–34). **Philadelphia:** public health (Alewitz, 1989; Fissell, 1992); mortality patterns (Condran & Cheney, 1982; Condran, Williams, & Cheney, 1985; Morman, 1984), 1871–1900 (Higgs, 1979); measles (Phillips, 1910; Ostheimer, 1910); scarlet fever, 1912 (White, 1929); tuberculosis (Deacon, 1911); typhoid fever (Dixon & Royer, 1910–11; Faries, 1904–5; Neff, 1912; McCarthy, 1987), 1850–1915 (Meeker, 1971–2). **Providence:** mortality patterns, 1871–1900 (Higgs, 1979); typhoid fever, 1850–1915 (Meeker, 1971–2). **San Francisco:** mortality patterns, 1871–1900 (Higgs, 1979); typhoid fever (Ryfkogel, 1907). **Toledo:** mortality patterns, 1871–1900 (Higgs, 1979). **Washington, DC:** typhoid fever (Kober, 1897; Sedgwick, 1911), 1850–1915 (Meeker, 1971–2), 1908 (Rosenau, Lumsden, & Kastle, 1909).

URUGUAY. **Montevideo**: typhoid (Consejo Nacional de Higiene, 1912).

WALES. **Cardiff:** mortality patterns, 1881–90 (Welton, 1897); diphtheria (Walford, 1898–9); tuberculosis (F. B. Smith, 1988, in passing).

7

Epidemics: looking forwards

There has been a gratifying progressive decrease in contagious diseases . . .
Tuberculosis, however, is an exception . . . [T]he provisional governor has
recently appropriated the sum of $60,000 for the construction of the necessary
machinery and equipment for the establishment of a free tuberculosis
sanitarium for the poor of both sexes.

Minister Morgan, Report on Tuberculosis in Cuba
Public Health Reports, vol. XXII (1907), p. 805

7.1 Introduction

With the decision by Surgeon General Robert Blue (plate 2.6) in 1912 to discontinue the overseas city tables, the world coverage of the *Weekly Abstract* came to an end. The weekly reports were, of course, to continue and flourish to this day as the Centers for Disease Control and Prevention's *Morbidity and Mortality Weekly Report*, but the city data were restricted to the United States and its territories. Other international bodies such as the League of Nations Health Bureau and the World Health Organization were to progressively take on the global recording role.

But, although the global monitoring provided by the *Weekly Abstract* ceased, the global scourges it described did not. Accordingly, in this chapter, we use other evidence to sketch the pattern of mortality attributable to epidemic diseases from the first decades of this century through to the present day. We first look at each of our six marker diseases on a disease-by-disease basis and reconstruct the principal trends for each (section 7.2). We then turn to the broad picture of mortality decline during the present century and try to identify the factors behind it (section 7.3). Since this covers a massive arena of demographic debate, we can only summarise the main positions of the protagonists and propose a way in which the debate might be clarified.

Because this book is being written in the last decade of the twentieth century, at a time when epidemiological change is very fluid, we spend the second half of the chapter looking forwards. In section 7.4, we examine those changes in global environments – both natural and manmade – which are shaping the pattern of future epidemic diseases. In section 7.5, we outline the different disease control strategies now open to governments and provide examples of the ways in which major interventions have shaped, and will continue to shape, the pattern of epidemic diseases. Finally, in section 7.6, we bring together some of the major strands developed in this book and show how, in the process of looking forward, we become ever more dependent upon the accurate reconstruction and decipherment of our epidemic past. It is in this reconstruction and decipherment that the purpose of our research lies.

7.2 Post-1900 changes in disease mortality

In this section, we look at the historical record of disease mortality in this century for each of the six diseases that formed the cornerstone of our study of the period from 1888 to 1912. For each disease, we look first at the statistical evidence of change and then at some of the putative explanations that have been put forward to account for the changes observed. To give a measure of uniformity to our discussion, for each disease we have used the mortality data assembled by Alderson (1981) in his *International Mortality Statistics*.

These cover thirty-one countries, mainly in Europe, for each of the fifteen quinquennial periods from 1901–5 to 1971–5 inclusive.

To allow for the variable demographic composition of each of the countries, Alderson employed mortality and age-structure data for each country at each period to compute a standardised mortality ratio (SMR) by the indirect method for 180 causes of death in both males and females and for all persons (except, of course, for gender-specific diseases like breast and testicular cancer where only the data relevant to the appropriate gender are given). The various ways in which SMRs may be calculated are summarised in Benjamin (1968, ch. 6). The basic idea behind SMRs is, however, straightforward. If a country has a relatively 'old' population (as, for example, in Western economies) there may be an excess of deaths from diseases of age simply because the country concerned has an undue proportion of older people. In these circumstances, the conventional mortality rate will not reflect the true risk of death from such causes. By the same token, countries with high birth rates and young populations may have excess deaths from certain diseases that especially afflict the young.

Thus mortality from many diseases is not independent of either the geographical environment or the age–sex composition of the population at any moment in time. Without standardising for this effect, inter-area comparisons of the impact of different diseases over long time periods are restricted, especially if the demographic composition of the population changes very much. SMRs allow for these effects by referencing each country's mortality to the mortality expected in a 'standard' population, generating a ratio with the standard population in the denominator. Thus a ratio greater than 1 (or some multiple of this) denotes an excess of deaths from a given cause as compared with the standard population.

To establish the main trends of mortality for our six marker diseases and all causes over the course of this century, we have used Alderson's data on these diseases for twelve of his countries which have particularly continuous demographic and mortality records: Australia, Belgium, Denmark, England and Wales, Italy, Japan, the Netherlands, Norway, Portugal, Sweden, Switzerland, and the United States of America. Median SMRs based on these twelve countries were used to establish world trends in mortality.

7.2.1 Diphtheria

(a) The nature of diphtheria decline

For diphtheria, figure 7.1 illustrates the trend for the fifteen quinquennial periods from 1901–5 to 1971–5. The heavy line plots the median SMR value for the twelve countries (see discussion above), while the shaded area forms an envelope delimiting the range of values from the highest to the lowest SMR in each five-year time period.

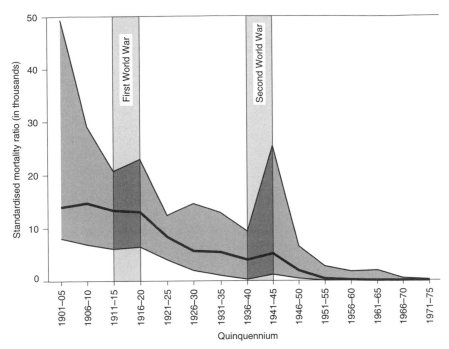

Figure 7.1. Trends in diphtheria mortality in the developed world, 1901–1975.
Median value (heavy line) of standardised mortality ratios (SMRs) for males in
twelve countries (Australia, Belgium, Denmark, England and Wales, Italy, Japan,
Netherlands, Norway, Portugal, Sweden, Switzerland, United States of America).
The shaded area forms an envelope which delimits the range of values from the
highest to lowest SMR in each five-year time period. Source: based on data in
Alderson (1981), tab. 24, p. 161.

Compared with the median SMR of 13,969 for the initial quinquennium
(1901–5) at the start of the century, the median for diphtheria had fallen over
a thousand-fold to only 9.5 by the last quinquennium (1971–5). Taking into
account the enclosing envelope, the decline was particularly marked between
1901 and 1915, and in the years immediately after the two world wars. By 1925,
the median SMR value had fallen to one-half of its beginning-of-century
value and, by 1950, it had reached one-tenth of its initial value. The unremit-
ting decline in SMRs was checked during both world wars, and some countries suffered sharp rises as witnessed by the shape of the upper edge of the
envelope.

In comparative terms, the fall in diphtheria SMRs is (together with scarlet
fever and whooping cough) the most striking of the six diseases. This is shown
in figure 7.2 which plots, on a logarithmic scale, the course of all diseases over
the period 1901–75, with the initial SMRs set to 100 for ease of comparison.

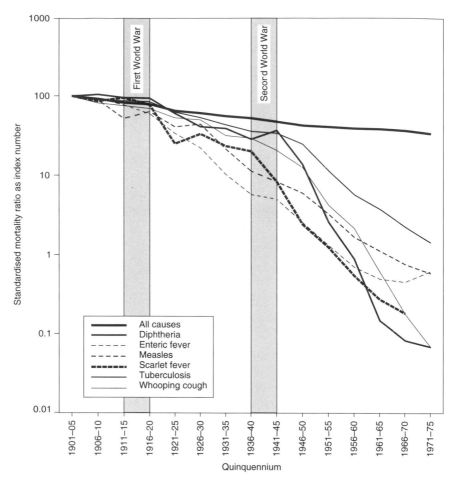

Figure 7.2. Trends in mortality in the developed world for six epidemic diseases, 1901–1975. Median values computed for male SMRs on the same basis as figure 7.1 for six marker diseases and deaths from all causes. For ease of comparison between the diseases, all have been indexed to a value of 100 for the 1901–5 quinquennium and plotted on a logarithmic axis. Source: based on data in Alderson (1981), tabs. 1 (p. 113), 17 (p. 147), 21 (p. 155), 24 (p. 161), 25 (p. 164), 33 (p. 182), 178 (p. 475).

With the continuing decline in diphtheria in the developed world, it is increasingly difficult to track the very few deaths now attributed to this cause outside the developing world.

The international pattern is reinforced by studies at the national level. Thus MacIntyre (1926; cited in Lancaster, 1990, p. 110), who analysed deaths from diphtheria in England and Wales from 1871 to 1924, noted that the peak years (with over 8,000 deaths per year) occurred in the 1890s but that, over the fifty-year period, there was little reduction in the absolute number of deaths per year (from 2,900 in the 1870s to 2,500 in 1921). This contrasts with scarlet fever and typhoid fever which both showed reductions of around 95 per cent over the same time span. If we link MacIntyre's findings with Alderson's data, the implication seems to be that the especially rapid decline in diphtheria mortality is a feature of the twentieth century.

(b) The causes of diphtheria decline
Despite a picture of long-term decline since 1900, detailed study of records for individual countries shows that incidence of the disease oscillates irregularly from year to year. It may be that the relative frequencies of the three types of diphtheria (see section 3.2.3) have also varied, and this proposition has been used by Lancaster (1990) to explain some of the irregularities in mortality. The data of Goodall, Greenwood, and Russell (1929) on patients admitted to the Eastern Fever Hospital, Homerton, London, may be taken as typical of the experience before the introduction of widespread active immunisation campaigns. Admissions were running at over 1,000 per annum for the first five years of the century but, by the Great War, had more than halved. For young children (ages zero to five years) the case–fatality rates were 17, 15, and 12 per cent in the quinquennia 1900–4, 1905–9, and 1910–14, respectively. Thus there were declines in both case incidence and case–fatality rates over these years.

Madsen and Madsen (1956) have also called attention to the relationship between different death rates recorded in Denmark and the different types of diphtheria bacteria prevalent there at particular times. Low rates in the 1930s were followed by peak years during the Second World War (see figure 7.1) since when diphtheria has largely disappeared as a cause of mortality. Of the three types of *Cornyebacterium diphtheriae* (*gravis*, *intermedius*, and *mitis*) McLeod (1943) in studies of Australian, British, and Central European records found that *gravis* and *mitis* were associated with higher mortality rates.

As discussed later (see table 7.3), immunisation against diphtheria became possible after 1923, and this preventive measure has hastened the decline of the disease. It is currently one of the diseases targeted by the World Health Organization for global elimination as part of its Expanded Programme on Immunization. By the early 1990s, immunisation levels averaged nearly 70 per cent in all countries of the world, and ranged between a low of 2 per cent (Guinea) and effectively blanket coverage in the major industrialised countries.

7.2.2 Enteric fever

(a) The nature of typhoid and paratyphoid decline
Typhoid and paratyphoid are used here as equivalent to the 'enteric fever' analysed in chapters 4–6. The change in mortality from typhoid and para-

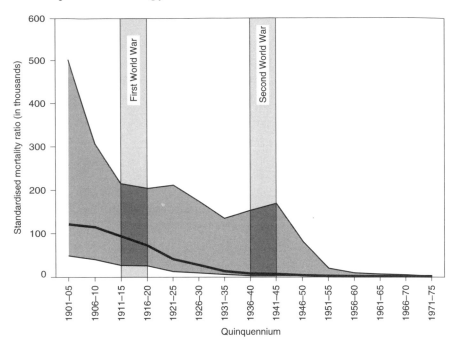

Figure 7.3. Trends in enteric fever (typhoid and paratyphoid) mortality in the developed world, 1901–1975. Median value (heavy line) and range of standardised mortality ratios (SMRs) for males in twelve countries plotted on the same basis as figure 7.1. Source: based on data in Alderson (1981), tab. 17, p. 147.

typhoid is shown in figure 7.3 for the fifteen quinquennial periods from 1901–5 to 1971–5. The heavy line plots the median SMR value for the twelve countries (see discussion above), while the shaded area forms an envelope delimiting the range of values from the highest to the lowest SMR in each five-year time period.

Compared with the SMR of 121,400 for the first quinquennium of the century, values for typhoid and paratyphoid had fallen 160-fold to a value of only 750 by the last quinquennium (1971–5). Taking into account the range of SMR values, the decline was particularly marked in the period up to the Great War and after 1945: by 1920 the SMR value had fallen to one-half of the beginning-of-century value and, by 1933, it had reached one-tenth of its initial value. In contrast to diphtheria, SMRs did not pick up to any marked degree in either of the world wars. Reference back to figure 7.2 shows that, in comparative terms, the fall of enteric fever SMRs is (together with measles) in the middle range of the six diseases. Since 1975, the small numbers of typhoid deaths in the twelve countries have made extension of Alderson's analysis impractical; even in 1975, the World Health Organization recorded only forty-eight deaths from this cause in the twelve and, by 1990, this had fallen to only six deaths.

Regionally based analyses of enteric fever data from the first quarter of the twentieth century enable us to say something about the age distribution and country-by-country variation in fatality at the time. Lancaster (1990, p. 72) has studied the trends in mortality from enteric fever for England and Wales by age group for the six decades between 1870 and 1930. He found that the death rate was consistently highest among young adults between twenty and twenty-four years of age. But, for all age groups, the death rate fell over the period: from 324 per million in the 1870s to 11 per million in the 1920s. Gay (1918) has drawn attention to country-by-country variations in case–fatality rates. At that date, in the United States, typhoid fever ranked fifth among the infectious diseases as a cause of death, where it was exceeded in importance by tuberculosis, pneumonia, infantile diarrhoea, and diphtheria. He estimated the case–fatality rate for typhoid fever at about 1:10 in the United States. Gay also cites Murchison's statistics from the London Fever Hospital which give a case–fatality rate of 17 per cent, and he suggests that this rate was approximately equal to that of 'the best hospitals in France, Germany, and England' (Gay, 1918, p. 15).

(b) The causes of enteric fever decline
In a classic account, Gay (1918) stated that typhoid fever had historically been one of the great causes of death and disability internationally, and that it remained important in 1918. But he also noted that scientific studies had led to a complete conception of the disease process and that this had resulted in practical consequences of great significance: 'No human disease, under varying conditions of life, in war and in peace, has been more rapidly checked, and none gives greater promise of eventual complete suppression' (Gay, 1918, p. 13).

Progressive reduction in urban pollution played a critical role in bringing about the decline of the enteric fevers. The provision of an adequate water supply, when coupled with the proper disposal of excreta and the protection of food and milk from infection, had a sustained impact. The ready availability of clean water was central, and so the decline of the disease as a major cause of death had to wait the spin-off of the public health movements in the second half of the nineteenth century. For example, London did not obtain a water supply of assured quantity and quality until after the Public Health Act of 1875; it was later still in many English provincial towns. Gay (1918) provides confirmation of the importance of clean water supplies for the decline in enteric fever death rates; crude mortality fell in both Vienna and Munich when mountain spring water was brought into each city in 1867 and 1870 respectively. In the United States at the turn of the century, improvements in city water supplies meant that mortality rates in rural areas generally exceeded those in urban areas.

In a historical survey of typhoid fever, Ashcroft (1964) developed a four-level model with the following elements:

Level 1: Hygiene is very bad and *Salmonella typhi* is ubiquitous; infection occurs in infancy or early childhood and is either symptomless or unrecognised.

Level 2: Hygiene is poor and *S. typhi* is common; first infections occur in childhood rather than in infancy and are recognisable, although often mild.

Level 3: Hygiene is not uniformly good; outbreaks may involve all age groups.

Level 4: Hygiene is excellent; *S. typhi* and typhoid are both rare.

Lancaster (1990) notes that, in the First World War, active immunisation of populations was introduced. Mortality rates from enteric fever were kept low (see figure 7.3), but it is by no means clear from the data whether the active immunisation was the effective cause of this; it is possible that its effect was negligible. Improved handling of milk and food, both important potential vehicles of infection, was increased in the inter-war years, as was the disposal of excreta in the great European cities. Lancaster (1990) notes that shellfish have been important in the spread of enteric fever, and were thought to have caused 25,000 deaths in France during the years 1920–34.

By the 1920s in England, the major problems of enteric fever had been solved. Consequently, as noted in Scott (1934) and Greenwood (1935), when outbreaks occurred, it was often the task of medical officers of health merely to determine which link in the chain of hygiene had been broken. As the century progressed, food handlers became less important vectors, partly as a result of better education and partly because of public health action on the safety of food; for example, measures were taken to ensure that uncooked vegetables, shellfish, ice creams, and the like were not contaminated in processing. Nevertheless, despite the precautions, epidemics still appeared from time to time. So Parker (1984) and G. S. Wilson (1984) provide accounts of an epidemiological investigation of a widespread typhoid epidemic that affected southeast England in 1941 and 1942. Phage-typing indicated that all cases were infected from a single source, milk supplied by a farmer who carried the bacillus. Another epidemic could be traced to tinned meat infected in Argentina (Lancaster, 1990, pp. 73–4).

7.2.3 Measles

(a) The nature of the measles decline
The fall in mortality for measles is shown in figure 7.4 for the fifteen quinquennial periods from 1901–5 to 1971–5. The heavy line plots the median SMR value for the twelve countries (see discussion above), while the shaded

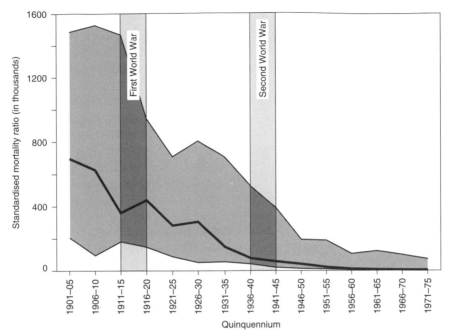

Figure 7.4. Trends in measles mortality in the developed world, 1901–1975. Median value (heavy line) and range of standardised mortality ratios (SMRs) for males in twelve countries plotted on the same basis as figure 7.1. Source: based on data in Alderson (1981), tab. 33, p. 182.

area forms an envelope delimiting the range of values from the highest to the lowest SMR in each five-year time period.

Compared with the median SMR of 696,950 for the quinquennium at the start of the century (1901–5), the median had fallen 170-fold to just 4,050 by the last quinquennium (1971–5). The decline was particularly marked from 1901 to 1935. By 1921, the SMR value had fallen to one-half of its value at the beginning of century and, by 1940, it had reached one-tenth of its initial value. Comparison of the graph with those for diphtheria and enteric fever (figures 7.1 and 7.3) shows that the pattern for measles was fundamentally different from these diseases prior to the Great War; the upper edge of the envelope showed no downwards trend. Reference back to figure 7.2 shows that, in comparative terms, the fall of SMRs for measles is (together with enteric fever) in the middle range of the six diseases. Since 1975, the small numbers of measles deaths in the twelve countries have made extension of Alderson's analysis impractical. By 1975, the World Health Organization recorded only 352 deaths from this cause in the twelve countries and, by 1990, this total had fallen to just sixty-three deaths. The contrast is stark when we turn to the

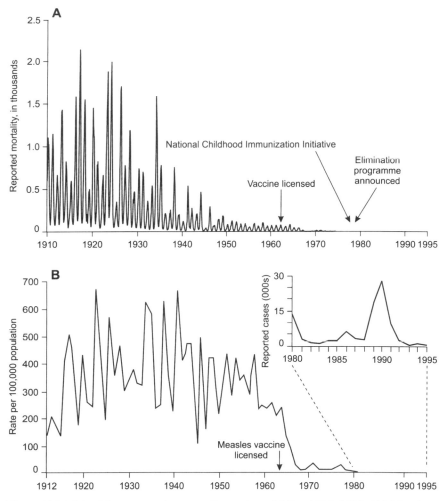

Figure 7.5. United States measles mortality and morbidity, 1910–1995. (A) Measles deaths by month, January 1910–December 1988. (B) (Main graph) Annual measles morbidity 1912–90 plotted as cases per 100,000. (Inset graph) Reported cases in thousands for the years 1980–95. Source: Cliff, Haggett, and Smallman-Raynor (1993), figs. 9.2 and 9.3, pp. 220, 224, and new data.

developing world; in 1990, WHO estimated that over 1.5 million deaths annually were still attributable to this cause.

Measles provides a very good example of the complex relationships between mortality, morbidity, and major clinical intervention through vaccination which, for measles, became available after 1963. We illustrate this for one country, the United States, in figure 7.5. Graph A plots the changes in

Table 7.1. *Measles in the United States, 1960–1990*

Relationship between mortality, morbidity, and population size.

Year	Deaths/1 m population	Deaths/1,000 cases	Cases/100,000 population
1960	2.11	0.86	245.4
1961	2.37	1.02	231.7
1962	2.2	0.85	259.2
1963	1.93	0.96	204.3
1964	2.2	0.92	239.7
1965	1.43	1.05	135.3
1966	1.33	1.28	104.4
1967	0.41	1.29	31.8
1968	0.12	1.08	11.1
1969	0.2	1.59	12.8
1970	0.44	1.88	23.2
1971	0.44	1.20	36.5
1972	0.12	0.74	15.5
1973	0.11	0.86	12.7
1974	0.1	0.91	10.5
1975	0.09	0.82	11.4
1976	0.06	0.29	19.2
1977	0.07	0.26	26.5
1978	0.05	0.41	12.3
1979	0.03	0.44	6.2
1980	0.05	0.81	6.0
1981	0.01	0.64	1.4
1982	0.01	1.17	0.8
1983	0.02	2.67	0.7
1984	0.004	0.39	1.1
1985	0.02	1.42	1.2
1986	0.01	0.32	2.6
1987	0.01	0.55	1.5
1988	0.01	0.88	1.4
1989			7.3
1990			11.2

measles mortality since 1910. The decline has been dramatic: in a single peak month in 1917 over 2,000 measles deaths were recorded; by contrast, in the 1980s, measles-related deaths were negligible. Detailed figures for each year appear in table 7.1 for the period 1960 to 1990. In the 1960s, the number of deaths in all years totalled 2,690, equivalent to an annual death rate of 1.43 deaths per million population and a case–fatality rate of 1.09 deaths per 1,000 measles cases. By the 1970s, deaths were sharply down to about one-ninth: 304

for the whole decade. This is equivalent to an annual death rate of 0.15 per million population. The case–fatality rate showed a less dramatic fall from 1.09 (in 1960–9) to 0.74 deaths per 1,000 measles cases. By the 1980s, measles deaths were down to a total of thirty-one (1980–8), equivalent to an annual rate over the period of 0.01 deaths per million population and a fatality rate of just 0.09 deaths per 1,000 measles cases.

Annual measles morbidity in the United States since 1912 is graphed in figure 7.5B. As with mortality, the record of decline is striking: in four peak years in the pre-vaccination decades, measles incidence was at an annual rate of over 600 per 100,000 population. In the early 1980s, the equivalent annual rates were less than 1 per 100,000 population, a decrease of over 99.8 per cent. In the 1960s, the number of cases in all years totalled 2.77 million, equivalent to an annual morbidity rate of 148 cases per 100,000 population. By the 1970s, measles incidence was sharply down to about one-eighth: 367,000 for the whole decade. This is equivalent to an annual morbidity rate of 17 cases per 100,000 population. By the 1980s, measles cases were down still further to 57,000, equivalent to an annual morbidity rate of 2.4 cases per 100,000 population. The contrast in morbidity rates between the worst year in table 7.1 (1962) and the best (1983) is 370:1; note, however, the case upturn in 1989–90.

(b)   The causes of the measles decline
As we saw earlier in figure 4.1, to account for mortality decline from any of the six infectious diseases examined in this book, a complex mixture of improvements in medical care, standards of living, and the environment might be adduced, as well as intervention by immunisation to prevent sickness in the first place (see section 7.3.2). Figure 7.4 has shown that measles mortality had been falling from the start of the century, and a puzzle continues to be posed as to the precise reasons for these decades of decline. It is the only one of our six marker diseases to be caused by a virus (section 3.2.3), and so the likelihood is that improvements in diet and general nursing care to prevent lethal complications occurring among the sick are the main causes. From 1963, however, vaccination became an option, and measles is the disease among our six markers for which the impact of vaccination is most clearly seen. This disease, like diphtheria, tuberculosis, and whooping cough among the markers, has been targeted by the World Health Organization for global eradication. We follow Fenner (1986) in confining the term *eradication* to the total global removal of the infectious agent (except, as with smallpox, for preserved laboratory samples). *Elimination* is used to refer to the stamping out of the disease in a particular country or region, but it leaves open the possibility of reinfection from another part of the world.

The roots of the world campaign for measles eradication lie in the United States. As we have already seen, in the United States in the early years of the twentieth century, thousands of deaths were caused by measles each year and, at mid-century, an annual average of more than half a million measles cases and nearly 500 deaths were reported in the decade from 1950–9. It was against this background that the Centers for Disease Control, Atlanta, Georgia, evolved in the United States a programme for the elimination of indigenous measles once a safe and effective vaccine was licensed for use in 1963. As we discuss later in this chapter (section 7.5.1), it is estimated that a population of the order of 250,000–300,000 is required to maintain endemic measles. Work in Africa by Macdonald in the early 1960s, reported by Thacker and Millar (1991), led him to suggest that one way of reducing the 'at risk' population in large countries below this endemicity threshold was by mass vaccination, so breaking the chains of measles infection. In the countries studied by Macdonald, he argued that an annual mass vaccination campaign reaching at least 90 per cent of the susceptible children would have the required effect.

In 1966, Sencer (reported in Sencer, Dull, and Langmuir, 1967) announced that the epidemiological basis existed for the eradication of measles from the United States using a programme with four tactical elements: (a) routine immunisation of infants at one year of age; (b) immunisation at school entry of children not previously immunised (catch-up immunisation); (c) surveillance; and (d) epidemic control. The immunisation target aimed for was 90–5 per cent of the childhood population.

Following the announcement of possible measles eradication, considerable effort was put into mass measles immunisation programmes throughout the United States. Federal funds were appropriated and, over the next three years, an estimated 19.5 million doses of vaccine were administered. The discontinuity induced in the time series of reported cases is clear from figure 7.5B.

In 1962, the year before measles vaccine was introduced, there were 481,500 cases of measles reported in the United States. By 1966, this number had been reduced by more than 50 per cent to 204,000 and, by 1968, the reported incidence had plummeted to 22,000, less than 5 per cent of the 1962 level. But, in 1969, a vaccine against rubella (German measles) was licensed and all federal funds were targeted against rubella; no federal funds were allocated to the measles immunisation programme from 1969–71. As a result, public sector vaccination declined. The susceptible population rose and, as figure 7.5B bears witness, the number of reported measles cases rose sharply, reaching 75,000 cases in 1971.

By the mid-1970s, it was evident that the campaign against measles was running out of steam and that steady increases in incidence were occurring. To remedy this situation, a nationwide childhood immunisation initiative was launched in April 1977, followed by the announcement in October 1978 of a programme to eliminate indigenous measles from the United States by 1 October 1982. The immunisation goal aimed for was again Macdonald's 90 per cent of the childhood population.

This second push against the disease caused the contraction of infection

Table 7.2. *Measles in the United States, 1960–1980*

Changes in incidence by age group based on four
reporting areas (New York City; Washington, DC;
Illinois; Massachusetts).

Age group	Incidence		Decline (percent)
	1960–4	1976–80	
Below 5 years	766.0	40.7	−95
5–9 years	1,236.9	29.0	−98
10–14 years	169.1	33.6	−80
15 years and over	10.0	3.3	−67

Source: Frank, Orenstein, Bart, Bart, El-Tantawy,
David, and Hinman (1985), tab. 2, p. 883.

from most of the settled parts of the United States in 1978 to restricted areas
of the Pacific Northwest, California, Florida, the northeastern seaboard, and
parts of the Midwest by 1983. In that year, twelve states and the District of
Columbia reported no measles cases, and twenty-six states and the District of
Columbia reported no indigenous cases. Four states (Indiana, 406; Illinois,
216; California, 181; Florida, 159) accounted for 64 per cent of the 1,497 cases.
Of the 3,139 US counties, only 168 (5 per cent) reported any measles cases. In
contrast, measles was reported from 195 counties in 1982 and from 988 in 1978
when the Measles Elimination Program began. The persistence of indigenous
measles in many of the 1983 regions may be explained by the importation of
cases from Mexico and Canada.

The contribution of vaccination to a reduction in morbidity rates was not
uniform across all age groups. A study of four reporting areas (see table 7.2)
over the early 1960s compared with the late 1970s showed a 95 per cent reduction in measles incidence among children up to five years old, but a reduction
of 80 per cent amongst older children (ten to fourteen years old), and only 67
per cent amongst those aged fifteen years and older. In interpreting all figures
for measles morbidity, it is important to recall that the completeness of
measles registration in the United States is not known with confidence. It is
generally believed that measles reporting is at least 80 per cent of cases actually occurring (Hinman, Brandling-Bennett, Bernier, Kirby, and Evans, 1980),
and that it is more complete in rural than in urban areas, particularly when the
latter experience large outbreaks (Cliff, Haggett, and Smallman-Raynor, 1993,
p. 225).

Unfortunately, total elimination in the United States still has not been
achieved. Vaccination levels have fallen back and the continued importation

of measles cases from overseas resulted in a resurgence of cases to 6,200 in 1986.

The US lead was followed up with varying degrees of vigour in other Western countries and was pressed in developing countries through WHO's Expanded Programme on Immunization. But, by 1995, the position achieved was spatially very patchy. A few countries (for example, Hungary, Israel, and Sweden) claimed vaccination rates of over 95 per cent. In contrast the average coverage for Africa was 51 per cent, Latin America 81 per cent, and South and East Asia 84 per cent. Worldwide, currently 45 million cases of measles occur each year; 1 to 2 million victims die – mostly young children in third-world countries. By 1993, the global coverage of measles vaccination was 78 per cent, well below the 90 per cent target originally set by WHO for 1995.

It has become progressively clear that, no matter how high coverage is, the infectivity of measles is likely to make global eradication a very long-term prospect. Even a vaccine coverage of 100 per cent will leave vaccine recipients susceptible unless the vaccine was more effective than the present 80+ per cent level. The US experience suggests that vigilant efforts to maintain high vaccination levels, strong surveillance, and an aggressive response against imported cases in measles-free zones are required to hold the ground already gained. Any immediate hopes of the global eradication of measles seems remote but, for measles at least, a feasible scenario is that more developed countries will follow the lead of the USA and try to eliminate measles nationally as an endemic disease. For this to be achieved, however, the great divergence of attitudes to, and of programmes against, measles in the developed world will need to be unified. Whether the coalescence of disease-free zones in developed countries would ever allow a sustained attack on measles reservoirs in developing countries will depend as much on politics and economics as on epidemiology.

7.2.4 Scarlet fever

(a) The nature of the scarlet fever decline

The fall in mortality from scarlet fever is shown in figure 7.6 for the fifteen quinquennial periods from 1901–5 to 1966–70. (Note that data for the quinquennium 1971–5 were not available in a standard form.) This chart plots the median SMR value for the twelve index countries (see discussion above) as a heavy line; the shaded area forms an envelope delimiting the range of values from the highest to the lowest SMR in each five-year time period.

Compared with the median SMR of 16,530 in the first quinquennium of the century, the median had fallen 550-fold to only thirty by the last quinquennium (1966–70). This decline was particularly marked in the first two decades: by 1921 the median had slipped to one-half of the beginning-of-century value

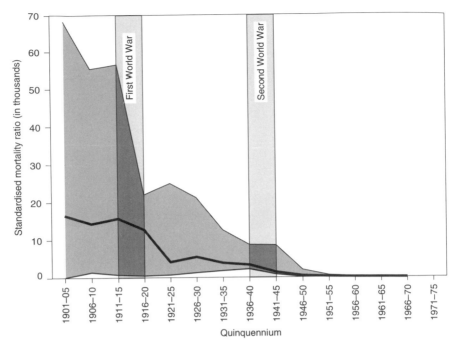

Figure 7.6. Trends in scarlet fever mortality in the developed world, 1901 1975.
Median value (heavy line) and range of standardised mortality ratios (SMRs) for
males in twelve countries plotted on the same basis as figure 7.1. Source: based on
data in Alderson (1981), tab. 21, p. 155.

and, by 1942, it had reached one-tenth of its initial value. Reference back to
figure 7.2 shows that, in comparative terms, the decline in SMRs for scarlet
fever is (together with diphtheria and whooping cough) among the most striking of the six diseases. Since 1975, the small numbers of scarlet fever deaths in
the twelve countries has made extension of Alderson's analysis impractical.

Accounts of the changing significance of scarlet fever as a cause of mortality in individual countries are cameos of the behaviour of the median
values. For example, MacIntyre (1926) has traced the regular fall in scarlet
fever deaths in England and Wales: from an annual average of over 17,000
deaths in the 1870s to around 900 per year by the mid-1920s. In Australia,
Cumpston (1927) has told a similar story. The first cases occurred in Tasmania
in 1833, followed by Victoria and New South Wales in 1841. The disease was
episodically a major cause of mortality until c. 1910. Since then, it has become
a minor and now very rare cause of mortality in that country.

(b) The causes of the scarlet fever decline
The development of penicillin and its derivatives after 1940 was important in
the elimination of scarlet fever as a significance cause of mortality in the last

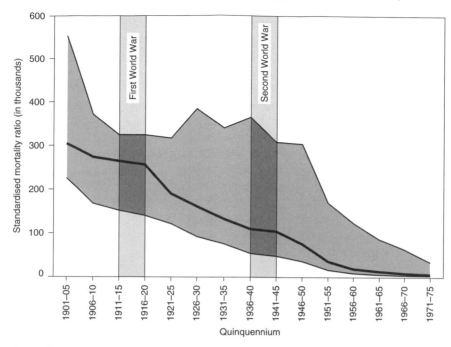

Figure 7.7. Trends in pulmonary tuberculosis mortality in the developed world, 1901–1975. Median value (heavy line) and range of standardised mortality ratios (SMRs) for males in twelve countries plotted on the same basis as figure 7.1. Source: based on data in Alderson (1981), tab. 1, p. 113.

half century – penicillin in its several forms is an accepted and highly effective treatment. Penicillin-resistant strains of streptococcus have not occurred to date. Antibiotic therapy is maintained for ten or more days and helps to ame-liorate the condition, although bacteria may persist in the pharynx of a third of patients. More recently developed antibiotics, such as erythromycin for penicillin-sensitive patients and clindanycin or a cephalosporin where both penicillin and erythromycin are contraindicated, have added to the armoury of clinicians and reduced scarlet fever to negligible proportions.

7.2.5 *Tuberculosis*

(a) The nature of the tuberculosis decline
The fall in mortality from tuberculosis is shown in figure 7.7 for the fifteen quinquennial periods from 1901–5 to 1971–5. This plots as a heavy line the median SMR value for the twelve countries used elsewhere in this section; the shaded area forms an envelope delimiting the range of values from the highest to the lowest SMR in each five-year time period.

Compared with the median SMR of 305,000 for the quinquennium from

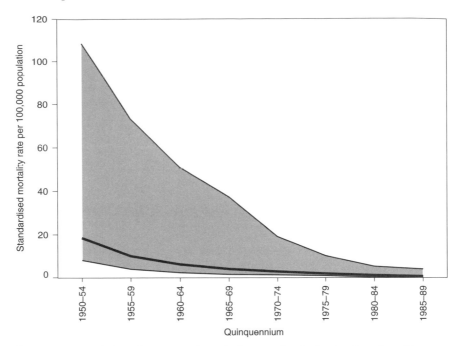

Figure 7.8. Trends in pulmonary tuberculosis mortality in the developed world, 1950–1989. Median value (heavy line) and range envelope for World Health Organization age-standardised death rate per 100,000 population using the same twelve countries as in figure 7.7. The two graphs have been calculated on a slightly different basis so only the generalised forms of the downward trends are comparable.

1901–5, the median had fallen seventy-fold to a value of only 4,350 by the last quinquennium (1971–5). The decline was almost linear over the period: by 1928, it had slipped to one-half of its beginning-of-century value and, by 1954, it had reached one-tenth of its initial value. However, reference back to figure 7.2 shows that, in comparative terms, the decline for tuberculosis is the least striking of the six diseases. Over the period from 1901 to 1975, pulmonary tuberculosis remained a major cause of death in some countries. This is illustrated in figure 7.7 by the upper edge of the envelope that plots the maximum SMR for each quinquennium. The resistance of some countries to the trend in the median is especially marked from 1920 to 1950.

After the Second World War, the general decline in mortality from pulmonary tuberculosis continued as the World Health Organization data plotted in figure 7.8 indicate. This illustrates the age-standardised death rate between 1950 and 1989 by five-year periods for the same twelve countries recorded by Alderson. As before, the heavy line plots the median, while the shaded envelope gives the maximum and minimum values in each quinquennium. For the twelve countries, deaths from pulmonary tuberculosis stood at 145,000 in 1950 and, by 1990, had been reduced by two-thirds to 5,500.

During the 1980s, the picture for tuberculosis mortality began to change again. Both mortality and morbidity have plateaued or increased in areas and population groups with a high prevalence of HIV infection (that is, especially in the developing nations). Disseminated/extrapulmonary/non-cavitary tuberculosis is highly diagnostic of AIDS (Smallman-Raynor, Cliff, and Haggett, 1992, p. 41); it is associated with the generalised immunosuppression that accompanies HIV infection.

The geographical and temporal variability in mortality from tuberculosis illustrated above is also to be found in other studies. Lancaster (1990, pp. 83–6) has analysed the rates for mortality for tuberculosis for the period 1908–80 for a number of countries. Deaths per million per annum ranged from 950 at the start of the period to 2 at the end.

The generally downwards trend in tuberculosis mortality over course of this century appears also to have been accompanied by shifts in the age distribution. Lancaster's analysis of data for England and Wales indicates that, in the epochs before 1920, there was a high death rate in infancy and a minimum in the childhood decade; the rates then rose rapidly to a high level in early adult life and remain high up to the age of seventy-five years. The maximum has tended to shift over the decades so that it now appears at rather later ages. In recent decades, there has been only low mortality in the younger age groups.

There is also some evidence of differential mortality rates by gender. Analysis of English data by Springett (1952) revealed that in females, attack rates, notification rates, and mortality rates were all greatest in young adult life. In contrast, among males, mortality rates were highest in the older age groups. Springett concluded that the deaths in older age groups could be attributed to delayed effects of infections acquired many years earlier. But, in general, mortality rates increase with age and, in old persons, they are higher in males than females (Benenson, 1990, p. 459).

(b) The causes of the tuberculosis decline
There are a number of reasons for the decline in mortality from tuberculosis. First, after 1945, the use of pasteurisation for milk and the development of tuberculosis-free cattle herds increasingly shut off one of the reservoirs of infection of the disease. Second, improvements in public health, especially the reduction of overcrowding in the homes of the urban poor, reduced the opportunity for spread via the respiratory route (see sections 3.2.2 and 3.2.3). Third was the development of a tuberculin test (1908) leading to the earlier isolation of infected patients and improved drugs for treatment after 1952.

The role of TB vaccination: In their study of tuberculosis death rates from 1851 to 1967, Topley and Wilson (1975) noted that the proportionate decrease in the death rates in the decade from 1949 to 1959 was as great as that in the ninety years between 1855 and 1945. The authors attributed this sharp decline in the 1950s to the use of chemotherapy rather than to any age cohort interpretation of the changes (Lancaster, 1990, p. 87).

Preventive inoculation against tuberculosis using live but attenuated tubercle bacilli had been available from 1921 when it was introduced as a vaccine in France by Albert Calmette and Camille Guérin. The strain designated BCG (Bacillus Calmette–Guérin) was widely utilised in France, Central Europe, and the Balkans after its introduction; its use spread to Scandinavia and South America in the 1930s, but was little employed in the USA until after 1940; the United States still remains one of the countries where BCG vaccination is not routinely carried out. The generalised international use of BCG vaccination occurred after the Second World War. Vaccination of uninfected (tuberculin-negative) persons can induce tuberculin sensitivity in over 90 per cent of those vaccinated. The protection conferred has varied markedly in field trails. This may be related to population characteristics, the quality of the vaccine, or the strain of BCG employed. Some controlled trials have provided evidence that protection may last as long as twenty years, while others have shown no protection at all.

For tuberculosis, the treatment was revolutionised after 1952 as the new drug, isoniazid, was shown to be effective in preventing the progression of latent tubercule infection to clinical disease in a high proportion of individuals. It is routinely recommended for infected persons under thirty-five years of age; among older persons, the increased risk of isoniazid-associated hepatitis makes this treatment less appropriate. But this treatment and the subsequent development of drug cocktails led to the virtual disappearance of the disease and its associated sanitoria during the 1950s and 1960s. It is thus particularly disturbing to note the increasingly generalised return of the disease as a complication of HIV infection in many parts of the world.

7.2.6 Whooping cough

(a) The nature of the whooping cough decline
The fall in mortality from whooping cough is shown in figure 7.9 for the fifteen quinquennial periods from 1901–5 to 1971–5. This plots the median SMR for the twelve marker countries as a heavy line; the shaded area forms an envelope delimiting the range of values from the highest to the lowest SMR in each five-year time period.

Compared with the median SMR of 14,760 in the initial quinquennium of the century, values for whooping cough had fallen by nearly 1,500-fold to only

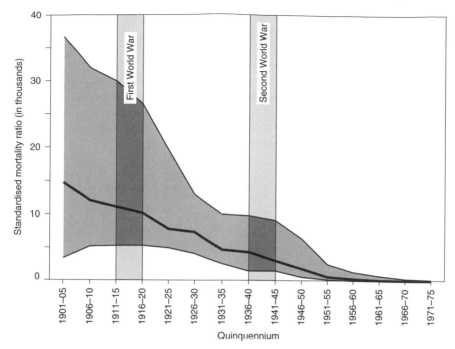

Figure 7.9. Trends in whooping cough mortality in the developed world, 1901–1975. Median value (heavy line) and range of standardised mortality ratios (SMRs) for males in twelve countries plotted on the same basis as figure 7.1. Source: based on data in Alderson (1981), tab. 25, p. 164.

ten by the last quinquennium of data (1971–5). This fall was almost linear over the three-quarters of a century, but the sharpest decline in the worse-affected countries occurred between 1901 and 1930 (upper edge of envelope). By 1928, the median SMR had reached one-half of its beginning-of-century value and, by 1949, it stood at just one-tenth. Reference back to figure 7.2 shows that, in comparative terms, the decline in the median SMR for whooping cough was, along with diphtheria and scarlet fever, among the most striking of the six diseases.

(b) The causes of the whooping cough decline
Accounting for the twentieth-century decline in mortality from whooping cough must be founded upon an understanding of the age distribution of cases and the timing of vaccine development. It is primarily a disease of early childhood and, at the beginning of this century, 3 to 5 of every 1,000 children born died of the disease. These generalisations may be developed using data from Lancaster (1990, pp. 112–13): the *Registrar General's Statistical Review of England and Wales for the Six Years, 1940–1945*, shows that about four out

of five of the notifications were of children under the age of five years. Further, the case–fatality rates were very much higher in infancy than at higher ages. In England and Wales at ages zero, one and two, and three and four, these were, for males (females), 63 (73), 9 (13), and 1 (3) in 1944, with case notification rates of 14 (15), 19 (22), and 21 (24) per 1,000. Pertussis is also remarkable in being one of the few infective diseases to have a significantly lower death rate among males than females; this is also to be seen in Lancaster's figures. The reasons for this are not understood, but it is a persistent feature of the mortality in all countries under a variety of climatic and hygienic conditions (A. B. Hill, 1933).

Vaccine protection against pertussis became available from the mid-1930s. Prior to this date, the decline in mortality seen in figure 7.9 must be principally accounted for by improvements in (i) public health, especially the reduction of overcrowding in the homes of the urban poor, which reduced the opportunity for spread of this respiratory disease (see sections 3.2.2 and 3.2.3), and (ii) standards of nutrition reducing the vulnerability of infants and young children to fatal complications such as broncho-pneumonia. As Sauer (1955, p. 588) comments:

The mildest cases occur, as a rule, in sturdy children . . . During cold weather, the most serious complication is bronchopneumonia, especially in infants of the poor, where poor hygiene and congested living conditions prevail.

Once vaccines offering protection against the disease had been discovered, the potential to hasten its decline was enhanced. The first vaccine trials took place in 1933, and developments of the initial versions were in widespread use by the later 1940s (Hardy, 1993c, p. 1095). The impact of vaccination may seen from a case study of the city of Evanston, Illinois. This city adopted immunisation against whooping cough in 1934, and reported only three cases of the disease in 1944 when the city had a population of 70,000. This was the lowest case total in the history of the city prior to that date. During the ten years prior to immunisation, the average annual number of reported cases was 351. There has not been a single whooping cough death in the city since 1934.

But internationally the picture was different. Although, as we have noted above, vaccination was widespread by mid-century, immunisation was still mainly confined to developed countries, and globally the disease continued to cause more deaths in the first years of life than diphtheria, scarlet fever, and smallpox combined (Sauer, 1955, p. 588). The generalised use of pertussis vaccine had to await the initiation of the World Health Organization's Expanded Programme on Immunization in 1974 (see section 7.5.2). Nevertheless, even in the developed nations, a problem with whooping cough still persists. Public awareness of possibly supposed complications of vaccination has led to periodic falls in rates of vaccination in countries like Japan and Britain where immunisation is voluntary, and this allows the disease to return.

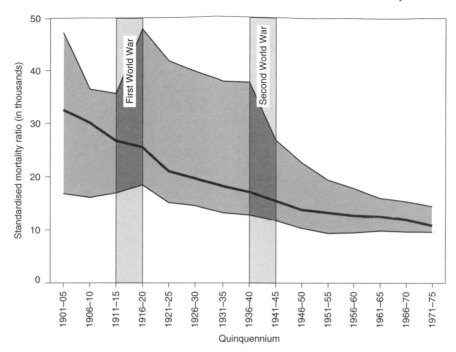

Figure 7.10. Trends in deaths from all causes in the developed world, 1901–1975. Median value (heavy line) and range of standardised mortality ratios (SMRs) for males in twelve countries plotted on the same basis as figure 7.1. Source: based on data in Alderson (1981), tab. 178, p. 475.

7.2.7 Deaths from all causes

For completeness, it is useful to subject deaths from all causes based upon the Alderson SMR data to the same analysis as we have the six individual diseases. The general decline in mortality is shown in figure 7.10 for the fifteen quinquennial periods from 1901–5 to 1971–5. This graph plots the median SMR value for the twelve marker countries (see discussion above) as a heavy line, while the shaded area forms an envelope delimiting the range of values from the highest to the lowest SMR in each five-year time period.

Compared with a median SMR of 32,500 in the first quinquennium of the century (1901–5), the figure had fallen threefold to a value of 10,900 by the last quinquennium (1971–5). For the median, the decline was fairly constant and gentle over the period: by 1941, it had fallen to one-half of its millennium value and, by 1971–5, it had shrunk to one-third of its initial size. For some countries, the experience was different. As the upper edge of the shaded envelope indicates, the effect of the First World War was to push the maximum SMR in each quinquennium to a high level, from which it declined in a parallel

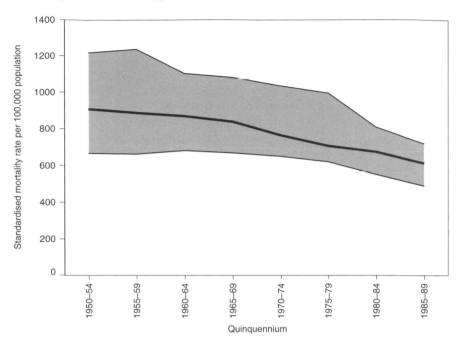

Figure 7.11. Trends in deaths from all causes in the developed world, 1950–1989. Median value and ranges for World Health Organization age-standardised death rate per 100,000 population using the same twelve countries as in figure 7.10. The two graphs have been calculated on a slightly different basis so only the generalised forms of the downward trends are comparable.

fashion to the twelve-country median over the period of the Depression and the Second World War. It was only after 1945 that these outlier SMRs converged rapidly on the twelve-country median.

The post-Second World War decline is illustrated further in figure 7.11 using World Health Organization data. This graph plots the age-standardised death rate between 1950 and 1989 by five-year periods for the same twelve countries recorded by Alderson. As before, the heavy line plots the median, while the shaded envelope delimits the maximum and minimum value in each quinquennium. For the twelve countries, the death rate from all causes stood at 905 per 100,000 population in 1950 and, by 1990, this had been reduced by one-third to 611.

Finally, reference back to figure 7.2 shows that, as we would expect, in comparative terms, the fall in SMRs for deaths from all causes is much less striking than that for any of the six communicable diseases.

A detailed analysis of the geographically disaggregated patterns of decline in deaths from all causes over the course of this century would be a massive undertaking, and take us well outside the scope of this book. For the period to mid-century, the topic has also been discussed in a number of major studies (for example, Erhardt and Berlin, 1974; Preston, 1976; and Wrigley, 1969), and the reader should consult these sources.

7.3 The causes of epidemic disease decline

In the preceding section we have commented upon the downward trend of mortality displayed by each of our six marker diseases. We now draw these points together and set them in the context of the wider debate over the causes of mortality decline in the twentieth century.

7.3.1 Mortality decline: some general issues

Up to this point, the SMR data provided by Alderson has been analysed on a disease-by-disease basis. We now look at the general conclusions which can be drawn by considering the results from all six diseases taken together. We examine this (i) in the time domain by comparing one five-year period with another and (ii) in the spatial domain by comparing the results for one set of countries with those for another.

(a) Changes over time: quinquennial comparisons

One simple but robust way of assessing time changes in Alderson's SMR data is to chart the relative change in the median value for each disease on a period-by-period basis. For any given disease, let M_t denote the median SMR in quinquennium t. Then the relative change, ΔM_t, as a percentage may be expressed as

$$\Delta M_t = 100(M_t - M_{t-1})/M_{t-1}. \tag{7.1}$$

Negative values denote a fall.

Figure 7.12 summarises the results obtained for all six diseases; ΔM_t is plotted on the vertical axis, and time on the horizontal axis. Again we follow the convention of plotting the median of the six diseases on equation 7.1 as a heavy line, while the shaded envelope indicates the range of values. As we would expect, with diminishing disease mortalities, the general pattern of change is negative. But what is more interesting is that progress has not been uniform: in some quinquennia, there was loss of ground and median mortalities actually *increased* albeit for short and temporary intervals. These reversals in the downward trend occurred at four times: (i) around the First World War, (ii) the inter-war Depression years, (iii) the Second World War, and (iv) at the end of the data period in the 1970s. The first three reversals are logical but the fourth, at the end of the period, is counterintuitive. It may well be that, by then, the very small number of deaths meant that insignificant variations

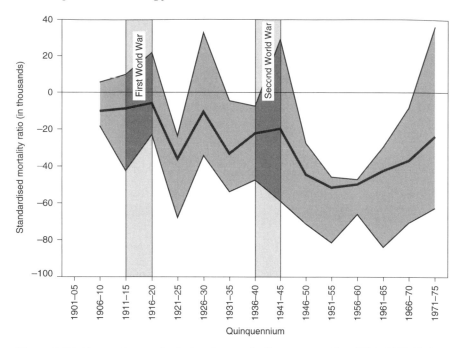

Figure 7.12. Comparisons of relative changes in disease mortality, 1901–1975. Using comparisons for each of the six marker diseases, the median value of changes from one quinquennium to another is shown. The shaded envelope represents the range in values.

in the SMR could have a large impact on equation 7.1 since the measure is relative to prevailing levels.

The graph also shows evidence of cyclicity. There are very strong 'surges' of improvement following the two world wars. The twenty-five year period after the Second World War in which no disease showed evidence of any increase is particularly striking. The factors that lay behind these changes, including the success or otherwise of national and WHO campaigns for disease elimination, are discussed in the next section of this chapter.

(b) Changes over space: variation between countries
A second approach is to look at variations in the SMRs over space as evidenced by the twelve countries included in our survey. If we look back at the individual SMR graphs based on Alderson's data (figures 7.1, 7.3, 7.4, 7.6, 7.7, 7.9, and 7.10), we recall that each median (shown by a heavy line) is surrounded by a shaded area forming an envelope that delimits the range of values from the highest to the lowest SMR country in each five-year time period. To allow comparison of the variability in the SMRs between the seven

envelopes, we computed a dimensionless measure of their variability, the coefficient of variation, CV. CV was defined as

$$CV = 100(s/\overline{x}), \tag{7.2}$$

where, for a given disease, $\overline{x}$ and s are the arithmetic mean and standard deviation respectively of the SMR values of the twelve countries in each quinquennium. The coefficient is large where there is great variation in relation to the mean, and small when the variation is relatively small.

Figure 7.13 plots these coefficients of variation in a standardised format by setting the CV for each disease in the first quinquennium (1901–5) equal to 100, and indexing later values with respect to first values. In contrast to the diagrams for the six diseases given in section 7.2, which showed a monotonous decrease in the median SMRs over time, this diagram suggests that the variability of the SMRs has *increased* over time in a striking way.

An epidemiological interpretation of this graph suggests that the study period can be divided into two phases:

(i)   An early phase from the millennium through to the end of the Second World War, during which variability was comparatively low. Over this interval, SMRs for the six diseases and all causes were high (see the diagrams in section 7.2), and most countries shared a common level of large but declining mortality.

(ii) A later phase since the end of the Second World War when mortality as measured by the SMRs has continued to decline but international variability has gone up. This implies that some countries made much more rapid progress towards disease elimination than others.

The finding is remarkable in that it is based on the experience of twelve countries which form part of the developed world. In terms of the SMR data published in Alderson, only Portugal clearly displayed a mortality pattern (at least over the seventy-five years studied) that suggested a different and less favourable epidemiological history than that of the other eleven countries in our sample. We can only speculate that, if we had been able to include developing countries in our selection of countries (this was precluded by the availability of reliable mortality data for the time period), then the contrasts might have been still greater.

7.3.2 *Explaining mortality change*

The fact we can demonstrate clearly that (i) disease mortality declined for the first three quarters of this century (albeit in a cyclic rather than linear fashion) and that (ii) the variations in decline between countries increased as the century wore on (section 7.3.1) throws little light on why these declines and variations occurred. We look briefly at the debate over the reasons for change and develop a model for testing some of the alternative hypotheses.

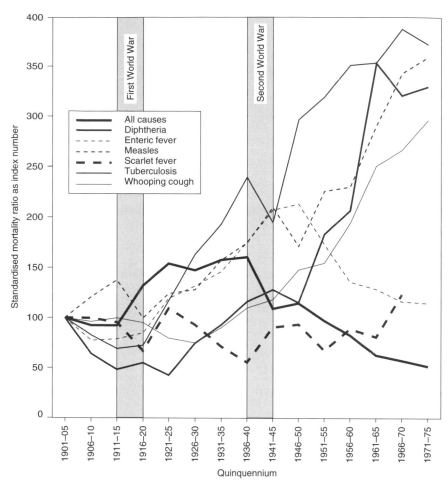

Figure 7.13. Increased variation in the range of SMR values for six marker diseases and all causes, 1901–1975. The coefficient of variation has been used as a measure of the relative dispersion in the SMR values (see explanation in text). Each disease has been standardised on an initial value of 100 in the first quinquennium (1901–5), and subsequent values have been indexed with respect to this initial value.

(a) The continuing debate on mortality decline
The lively debate on the causes of the overall mortality decline did not stop with data at the end of the nineteenth century. As the discussion in section 4.2 indicated, the views over the 'long decline' have drawn on demographic information which spans from the start of the eighteenth century through to the end of the twentieth. So the rumbling battle that followed McKeown's thesis on *The Modern Rise of Population* (1976) on the role of nutrition has seen a

number of studies which have questioned the arguments by using twentieth-century data: Vallin and Meslé's (1988) study, *Les causes de décès en France de 1925 à 1978* is a case in point. Like many recent studies, this eschews a grand central theory and sees mortality decline as the end product of a complex bundle of factors which interact in different time periods and different demographic regions. This continuing shift towards such models of cautious complexity led Schofield and Reher (1991, p. 7) to comment: 'there may have been multiple paths to mortality transition which have yet to be unearthed by scholars'.

But there are two areas in which debates using twentieth-century data (and still more the data of the next century) may have advantages over those from earlier periods. First, more is now known about the changing nature of disease itself. The best example is that of influenza where the recognition that the influenza A virus was subject to both major shifts and minor drifts (Cliff, Haggett, and Ord, 1986) is a major explanation for mortality changes. The 1918–19 pandemic (with its estimated 20 million deaths worldwide) and the lesser pandemics of Asian, Hong Kong, and 'Red' flu in more recent decades each illustrate the direct effect of disease change on mortality, as do the minor 'drift' changes which boost winter mortality on a regular two- or three-year cycle. This contrasts with earlier periods when changes in the virulence of diseases is more speculative. For example, Lancaster (1990, p. 115) conjectures that the decline in mortality from scarlet fever from the nineteenth century may be attributable to the existence of scarlet fever strains operating in earlier centuries which are no longer in circulation 'for no other explanation [of the decline] has ever been given'. In the absence of direct virological or bacteriological knowledge, changes in virulence remains a potentially powerful explanation of last resort in the hypothesis locker.

A second difference in studying the present century is (a) the dramatic increase in medical knowledge and (b) its consequent effect on prevention and treatment. The links between (a) and (b) are shown in table 7.3 which summarises some of the major advances in medical treatment and prevention in so far as they affect our six marker diseases. Figure 7.14 sets these advances in the context of the number of publications annually for each disease, 1879–1990, as recorded in *Index Medicus*. The publication record reflects, *inter alia*, the chief discoveries as well as major downturns of publications, lagged to reflect time between submission and publication, during the world wars. As with figure 7.12, the pattern of publications has cyclical components. We note the following features of figure 7.14:

(i)   For diphtheria, the unexplained spike of publications in the late 1890s, and, compared with the background level, the larger number of publications in the late 1920s and 1930s after the development of diphtheria toxoid for immunisation.

(ii) For the enteric fevers, the high level of publications from 1897 to 1918

Table 7.3. *Some major twentieth-century microbiological advances with implications for the six marker diseases*

The diseases are diphtheria, enteric fever, measles, scarlet fever, tuberculosis, and whooping cough.

Date(s)	Event	Discoverer and/or developer	Disease implications
1906–1921	BCG vaccine	Calmette, Guérin	Method of immunising children against tuberculosis
1907	Scarlet fever serum	Moser Garbritchewsky	Serum from horses immunised with cultures of streptococci for scarlet fever immunisation
1908	Tuberculin test	Mantoux	Diagnostic test for recognising tuberculosis
1914–1918	Anti-typhoid vaccine	Wight and Semple	Successful deployment of anti-typhoid vaccine first developed in 1897
1918	Antibodies in measles convalescents	Nicolle	Sero-prevention and sero-attenuation in measles
1923	Toxoid for immunisation	Glenny and Hopkins	Use of toxoid for human immunisation against diphtheria
1924	Test for scarlet fever	Dick and Dick	Dick test to determine susceptibility of a subject to scarlet fever
1928	Penicillin	Fleming	Treatment of diphtheria and scarlet fever
1933	Whooping cough vaccine	Madsen	Trials in Faeroe Islands of whooping cough vaccine; only slight influence on prevalence but decreased severity of attack
1943	Streptomycin	Waksman	Antibiotic treatment of tuberculosis
1944	Human immune serum globulin	Cohn	Measles
1948	Chloramphenicol		Antibiotic for typhoid fever treatment; resistance strains since early 1970 caused switch to other antibiotics
1952	Isoniazid	Robitzek and Selikoff	Treatment of tuberculosis

Table 7.3. (*cont.*)

Date(s)	Event	Discoverer and/or developer	Disease implications
1954	Measles virus	Enders and Peebles	Isolation of measles virus
1955	Cycloserine		Treatment of tuberculocis
1963	Measles virus licensed	Enders, Katz, and Milanovic	Licensing of attenuated live virus produced by Enders and colleagues in 1958

following the manufacture of anti-typhoid vaccine and during its successful mass deployment in the Great War.

(iii) For measles, the comparatively large output after 1960 coinciding with isolation of the causative virus, vaccine developments, and the US Measles Elimination Program discussed in section 7.2.3.

(iv) For scarlet fever, the steady decline in publications and interest after 1930 as the availability of penicillin and other antibiotics cause this disease to begin its slide into history.

(v) For tuberculosis, the vastly greater number of publications than for any of the other five diseases; the upturns in publications following improvements in prevention and treatment; and the reversal of the falling trend in publications after 1980 consequent upon the re-emergence of tuberculosis as a major global health threat in association with the HIV pandemic, and the emergence of drug-resistant strains of tuberculosis.

(b) Treatment vs prevention
Nature of the hypotheses: The enhanced role of medical technology in the present century allows some light to be thrown on the relative roles of treatment and prevention in disease reduction.

(i) The *treatment hypothesis* states that mortality decline arises from improvements in the treatment of patients who are unfortunate enough to succumb to a particular disease. Thus we should expect, *ceteris paribus*, the improved treatment of a disease to be marked by a reduction in the number of cases which become deaths. This may be assessed by computing a (scaled) case–fatality ratio: here we use the reported number of deaths per 1,000 reported cases. A time series plot of this case–fatality ratio should have a declining trend under the treatment hypothesis.

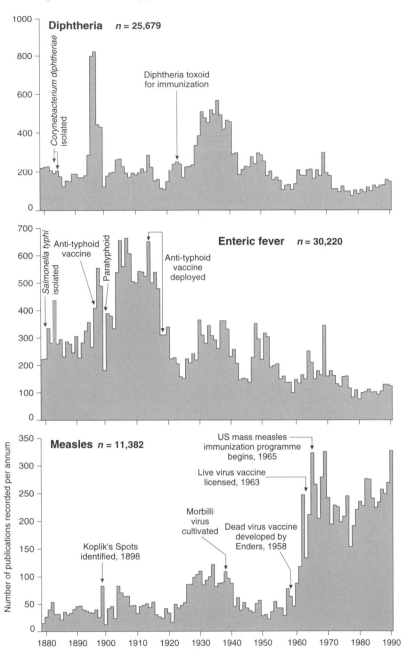

Figure 7.14. Intensity of medical writing on the six marker diseases. Number of publications annually, 1879–1990, for each of the six diseases as recorded in *Index Medicus*. Significant advances in prevention or treatment are marked.

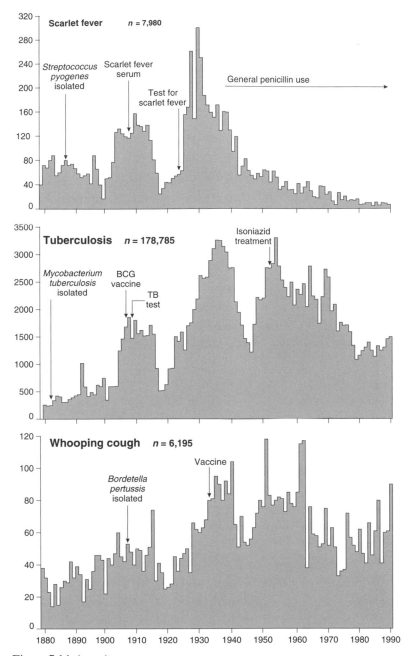

Figure 7.14. (*cont.*)

(ii) The *prevention hypothesis* states that mortality decline arises from those conditions which prevent cases of the disease arising in the first place; *ceteris paribus*, a decline in mortality follows. The preventive conditions may include both medical factors (for example, vaccination) and non-medical (for example, reduced virulence, improved social conditions, diet, knowledge). Successful prevention of cases of a disease should be reflected in a decline in the number of reported cases per unit of population. We capture this here by studying the number of reported cases per 100,000 population.

We now consider how the importance of these two classes of factors – treatment and prevention – in accounting for mortality decline may be assessed. We take the indices defined above and apply them to two case studies: (i) changes in measles mortality in a single country (the United States, 1960–88) and (ii) changes in mortality from four diseases (diphtheria, measles, scarlet fever, and whooping cough) in four developed countries (Australia, Ireland, Japan, and the United States) between 1930 and 1990.

Case study I: measles in the United States, 1960–88: To provide a benchmark for testing the two hypotheses, we have graphed in figure 7.15 the annual crude mortality rate for measles alongside the case–fatality ratio (a measure of the treatment hypothesis) and incidence (a measure of the prevention hypothesis). The basic data have already been given in table 7.2. Because the three time series are in radically different units, they have been converted to index numbers (1960=100), and a log scale has been used for the vertical axis. The implication of the log scale is that deaths from measles per unit of population (bar graph) fell exponentially over the period, and this trend is followed faithfully by the line trace for cases per 100,000 population (prevention hypothesis). In contrast, the time series for deaths per 1,000 cases (treatment hypothesis) oscillates about a constant mean over the period.

We conclude that there is *prima facie* evidence to suggest that the prevention of cases of measles in the population achieved more than treatment of actual cases in contributing to the decline of measles mortality in the United States over this period.

Case study II: diphtheria, measles, scarlet fever in four developed countries, 1930–90: To extend our evaluation of the treatment and prevention hypotheses as possible explanations of twentieth-century trends in mortality, we took yearly data from WHO's *World Health Statistics Annual* (and its precursors) for the period 1930–90 on reported deaths, cases, and total populations for four countries (Australia, Ireland, Japan, and the United States) and for four of our marker diseases – diphtheria, measles, scarlet fever, and whooping cough. The choice of countries and the absence of enteric fever and tuberculosis were dictated solely by data availability. As described earlier in this

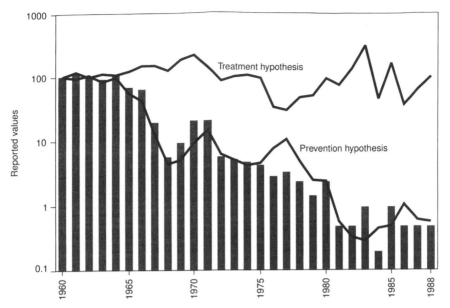

Figure 7.15. Measles mortality in the United States, 1960–1988. Time trends in indices of the treatment and prevention hypotheses (line traces) benchmarked against the crude reported death rate (histogram). For plotting purposes, the series have been expressed as index numbers (1960=100).

section, the raw data were used to construct annual time series for prevention, treatment, and crude deaths for each disease and country.

To check for possible time changes in the relative importance of treatment and prevention over the sixty-year period, each time series was divided into a series of ten-year windows (1930–9; 1940–9; 1950–9; 1960–9; 1970–9; 1980–9). For each window, disease, and country, we computed the simple Pearson correlation coefficient between (i) deaths per million population and deaths per 1,000 cases (treatment), and (ii) deaths per million population and cases per 100,000 population (prevention); this yielded potentially 144 correlation coefficients for study. We regarded ten-year windows as the absolute minimum size for which it was reasonable to calculate correlations. We would have preferred bigger windows but, even at this size, randomly occurring missing observations meant that in practice our potential 144 coefficients were reduced to only twenty-six with a full complement of data and which we used for further work.

Given the way the analysis has been structured, a positive influence of either prevention or treatment upon death rates will yield a positive correlation coefficient. Figure 7.16 plots the results obtained. The correlations defined in the previous paragraph were used as x (treatment) and y (prevention) coordinates to plot each time window/disease/country observation on graph A; the disease

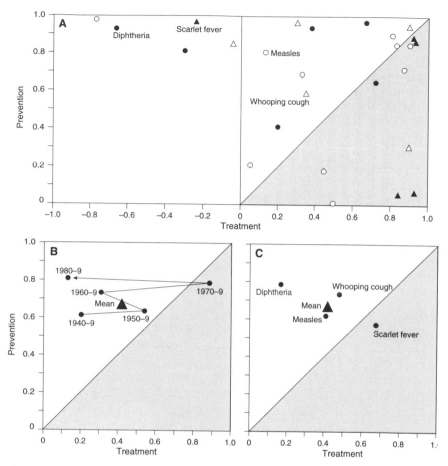

Figure 7.16. Time changes in mortality from four diseases (diphtheria, measles, scarlet fever, and whooping cough), 1930–1990, attributable to prevention and treatment. (A) Scattergram of diseases on measures of prevention and treatment irrespective of time window and geographical location. (B) Average prevention/treatment position by time periods. (C) Average prevention/treatment position by disease. Shaded regions mark chart areas in which the treatment hypothesis is more important than the prevention hypothesis.

information associated with each point has been retained. Graphs 7.16B and C have been derived from A. On 7.16B, the average coordinate position of each time window irrespective of disease and country is recorded, along with the grand mean over all twenty-six observations. On 7.16C, the average coordinate position of each disease, ignoring time window and country, is plotted, along with the grand mean. The 45° line marks equality between the treatment and prevention hypotheses. Below the line (shaded), treatment is more important than prevention and vice versa.

Graph 7.16B shows that it was only in the decade 1970–9 that treatment was more important than prevention, and then only by a small margin. The vectors linking the points show that, over this sixty-year period, the evidence in favour of the prevention rather than the treatment hypothesis systematically strengthened. Graph 7.16C indicates that this was true for three of the four diseases studied. The exception was scarlet fever and, given the period studied here, Lancaster's work (1990, pp. 114–15) suggests why (see earlier in this section):

The decline in death rates from scarlet fever has occurred in many countries; it cannot be ascribed to progress in medical science, with the possible exception of the improvement about 1940 that may have been partly due to the use of the sulphonamide drugs.

Summary: We recognise the provisional nature of our attempt to assess the relative importance of prevention as opposed to treatment (or, as Lancaster describes it, 'progress in medical science') in accounting for post-1930 trends in mortality decline from our marker diseases. In particular, our analysis suffers from sample size limitations in terms of countries and time periods. But the preliminary evidence is consistent: prevention has been better than cure in reducing mortality, a truism that has increased in force over the course of the century.

7.4 The changing disease environment

In section 1.2.3, we commented upon the growing range of infectious diseases, some capable of generating outbreaks, some epidemics, and some, such as HIV, pandemics. The diseases which we examined in chapters 2–6 have largely been the 'classic' epidemic generators: diseases which have been associated with the human population for in excess of 1,000 years and, in some cases, over 5,000 years. But these are only part of the overall epidemic disease burden and, in closing this book, it is important to look forward briefly at the factors which are shaping the geographical patterns of all diseases, both old and emerging, at the end of the twentieth century.

Diseases spread in a specific historical and geographical context. In the late twentieth century, the environmental context within which disease control is set is evolving at a faster rate than at any time in human history. Table 7.4 summarises some of the geographical changes that have disease implications. We illustrate here the impact of four of these: (1) demographic growth and migration of the host population, (2) the collapse of geographical space, (3) global land-use changes, and (4) global warming.

Table 7.4. *Geographical changes and virus emergence*

Geographical change	Disease	Probable mechanism	Location
Increased spatial interaction: migration and travel	Dengue	Disseminated by travel and migration	Worldwide
	Yellow fever	Both virus and major vector (*Aedes aegypti*)	Africa, Caribbean
	Seoul-like viruses	Infected rats carried in ships	United States
Land use change: (A) Agricultural	Influenza	Integrated pig–duck farming	China
	Hantaan	Contract with rodents during rice harvest	China
	Argentine haemorrhagic fever	Agriculture favours natural rodent host; human contact during harvest	South America
	Bolivian haemorrhagic fever	Contact with rodent host during harvest	South America
	Oropouche	Cacao hulls encouraged breeding of insect vector	South America
	Monkeypox	Subsistence agriculture and forest hunting; increased contact with rodent host	Tropical Africa
(B) Forests and woodland	Kyasanur forest	Tick vector increased as forest land replaced by sheep grazing	India
	Lyme disease	Tick vectors increased as fields replaced by woodland	Northeast United States
(C) Water	Dengue, dengue haemorrhagic fever, yellow fever	Water containers encourage breeding of mosquito vector	Asia, Africa, South America, Caribbean
	Venezuelan equine encephalitis, Rift Valley fever	Building of dams and irrigation favour increase in vector	Panama, Africa
Military operations	Leishmaniasis	Military campaigns in new environment (e.g., Operation Desert Storm)	Gulf, United Kingdom, United States
Global warming	Malaria	Extension of thermal range into middle latitudes	Worldwide

Source: Haggett (1994), tab. 2, p. 97; based partly on Morse (1994), tab. 3, p. 330.

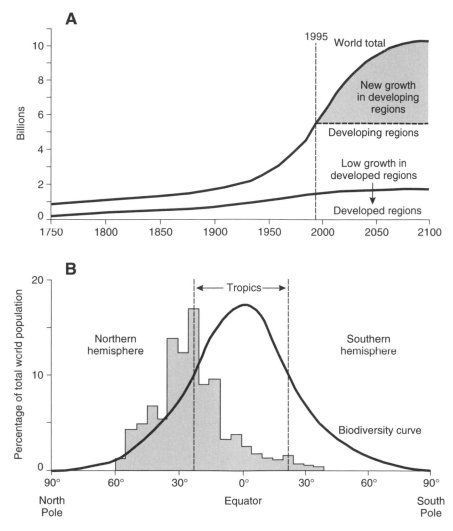

Figure 7.17. Global population growth. (A) Course of global population growth for the period from 1750 and projected forward to 2100. (B) Geographical distribution of population distribution (stippled histogram) in terms of 5° latitudinal bands north and south of the equator. The biodiversity curve is approximate and does not make allowances for the global distribution of humidity. Source: Haggett (1995).

(a) Rapid growth and relocation of the human population

Whatever the rate of past disease emergence, there are reasons to consider the late twentieth century as one of special significance for the human host population. Figure 7.17A shows the historical pattern of growth in the human population from 1750, with a forward projection to 2100. Three aspects of this change call for comment. First, the rapid acceleration in growth is very recent. In the past four decades, the world's population has more than doubled, from 2.5 billion in 1950 to 5 billion in 1988. On the United Nations' 'medium-growth' assumptions, this total is expected to reach 6.3 billion by the end of the century and 8.5 billion by the year 2025 (Sadik, 1991). Although that rate of growth is now decelerating (its peak was at 2.1 per cent per annum in the quinquennium from 1965 to 1970), the multiplier of resource use per capita continues to increase, with evident environmental implications.

Secondly, a geographical redistribution of world population is accompanying this growth. For example, it is expected that some 94 per cent of population growth over the next twenty years will occur in the developing countries. Figure 7.17B illustrates the present geographical distribution of population, with its marked concentration in northern mid-latitudes. Present and future growth will shift the balance of world population towards the tropics and low latitudes. As a result of this shift, Haggett (1991) has estimated that the average temperature experienced by the global population will rise by around +1 °C, from 17 °C to 18 °C. Figure 7.17B also shows that this latitudinal shift in the concentration of population will place more people than at any time in the world's previous history in areas of high microbiological diversity, potentially exposing a greater share of the world's population to conventional tropical diseases.

Thirdly, the world's growing population is increasingly concentrated in cities. In 1800, less than 2 per cent of the world's population lived in urban communities. By 1970, this had risen to one-third and, by 2000, the fraction will have reached one-half. Along with the increasing proportion of urban population, the number of large cities and their average density will also have increased. On United Nations' estimates, the number of cities with a million or more inhabitants is expected to rise from 200 in 1985 to 425 by the end of the century. At that date there are likely to be twenty-five cities with populations in excess of 11 million.

The disease implications of urbanisation are complex (B. Williams, 1989). Positive effects from improved sanitation or better access to health care facilities have to be set against the negative effects from increased risk of disease contacts through crowding and pollution. Crompton and Savioli (1993) have shown that where rural–urban migration in developing countries results in peri-urban shanty settlements, high rates of intestinal parasitic infections (notably amoebiasis, giardiasis, ascariasis, and trichuriasis) can result. Each is a common intestinal infection caused by protozoan parasites or helminths transferred from human to human by the faecal–oral route. They pose an increasing health burden as the share of urban population in developing countries rises towards one-half of all population. In a long-term historical context, Haggett (1992) has indicated that the aggregation of human populations into high-density urban 'islands' has had important effects in providing the host reservoirs necessary to maintain infection chains for many diseases. The implications of urbanisation for measles have been discussed by Cliff, Haggett, and Smallman-Raynor (1993, pp. 7, 47–8) and, for a wide range of other infectious diseases, by Fine (1993).

(b) The collapse of geographical space
The second main environmental change has come from the collapse (in terms of both time and cost) of geographical space, and the increased spatial mobility of the human population which has accompanied this collapse. We look first at the evidence for such change and then at its disease implications.

(i) Changes in travel patterns: The manner in which travel patterns have changed for the host population over recent generations has been illustrated in an interesting way by the distinguished epidemiologist, D. J. Bradley. Bradley (1988) has compared the travel patterns of his great-grandfather, his grandfather, his father, and himself. The lifetime travel track of his great-grandfather around a village in Northamptonshire could be contained within a square of only 40 km side. His grandfather's map was still limited to southern England, but it now ranged as far as London and could easily be contained within a square of 400 km side. If we compare these maps with those of Bradley's father (who travelled widely in Europe) and Bradley's own sphere of travel, which is worldwide, then the enclosing square has to be widened to sides of 4,000 km and 40,000 km respectively. In broad terms, the spatial range of travel has increased tenfold in each generation, so that Bradley's own range is one thousand times wider than that of his great-grandfather.

Against this individual cameo, we can set some general statistical trends from recent years. One indicator of the dramatic increase in spatial mobility is shown in figure 7.18. This plots for France over a 200-year period the average kilometres travelled daily both by transport mode and by all modes. Since the vertical scale is logarithmic the graph shows that, despite changes in the mode used, average travel has increased exponentially, a trend broken only by the two world wars. Over the whole period, mobility has increased by more than 1,000. The precise rates of flux or travel of population both within and between countries are difficult to catch in official statistics. But most available evidence suggests that the flux over the last few decades has increased at an accelerating rate. While world population growth rate since the middle of this century has been running at between 1.5 and 2.5 per cent per annum, the growth in international movements of passengers across national boundaries has been between 7.5 and 10 per cent per annum. One striking example is provided by Australia: over the last four decades its resident population has doubled, while the movement of people across its international boundaries (that is, into and out of Australia) has increased nearly a hundredfold.

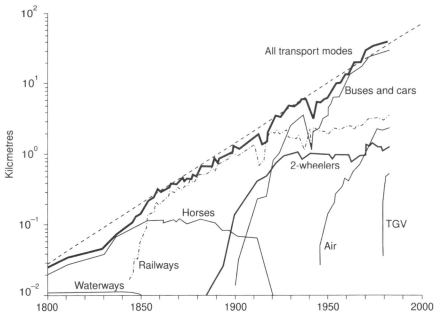

Figure 7.18. Increased spatial mobility of the population of France over a 200-year period, 1800–2000. Curves give the average kilometres travelled daily by mode. Note that the vertical scale is logarithmic so that increases in average travel distance increase exponentially over time. Source: Haggett (1994), fig. 7.4, p. 101; based on data in Grubler and Nakicenovic (1991).

(ii) Disease implications of increased travel: The implications of increased travel are twofold: short-term and long-term. First, an immediate and important effect is the exposure of the travelling public to a range of diseases not encountered in their home country. The relative risks met in tropical areas by travellers coming from Western countries (data mainly from North America and Western Europe) have been estimated by the World Health Organization (1995a, p. 56) and are illustrated in figure 7.19. These suggest a spectrum of risks from unspecified 'traveller's diarrhoea' (a high risk of 20 per cent) to paralytic poliomyelitis (a very low risk of less than 0.001 per cent). Another way in which international aircraft from the tropics can cause the spread of disease to a non-indigenous area is seen in the occasional outbreaks of tropical diseases around mid-latitude airports. Typical are the malaria cases that appeared within 2 km (1 1/4 m) of a Swiss airport, Geneva–Cointrin, in the summer of 1989 (Bouvier, Pittet, Loutan, and Starobinski, 1990). Cases occurred in late summer when high temperatures allowed the in-flight survival of infected *anopheles* mosquitoes that had been inadvertently introduced into

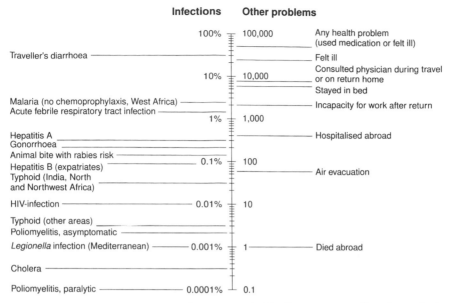

Figure 7.19. Relative threats posed by communicable diseases to travellers in tropical areas. Note that the scale is logarithmic. Source: WHO (1995a), fig. 7.1, p. 56.

the aircraft while at an airport in a malarious area. The infected mosquitoes escaped when the aircraft landed at Geneva to cause malaria cases among several local residents, none of whom had visited a malarious country.

A second short-term factor with modern aircraft is their increasing size. D. J. Bradley (1988) postulates a hypothetical situation in which a person in the travelling population is assumed to have a chance of 1 in 10,000 of being in the infectious stage of a given communicable disease. With a 200-seat aircraft, the probability of having an infected passenger on board (x) is 0.02 and the number of potential contacts (y) is 199. If we assume homogeneous mixing, this gives a combined risk factor (xy) of 3.98. If we double the aircraft size to 400 passengers, then the corresponding figures are $x=0.04$, $y=399$, and $xy=15.96$. In other words, *ceteris paribus*, doubling the aircraft size increases the risk from the flight fourfold. Thus the new generation of wide-bodied jets presents fresh possibilities for disease spread, not only through their flying range and their speed, but also from their size.

On a longer time scale, increased travel brings some possible long-term genetic effects. With more travel and longer-range migration, there is an enhanced probability of partnerships being formed and reproduction arising from unions between individuals from formerly distant populations. As Khlat and Khoury (1991) have shown, this can bring advantages from the viewpoint of some diseases. For example, the probability of occurrence of conditions such as cystic fibrosis or spinal muscular atrophy is reduced; the risk of these is somewhat higher in children of consanguineous unions. Conversely, inherited disorders such as sickle cell anaemia might become more widely dispersed.

(c) Changing global land use

The combination of population growth and technological change has given mankind the capacity to alter environments in ways which are unprecedented in human history. We illustrate the disease implications of three such changes.

(i) Agricultural colonisation   Accelerated world population growth has put pressure on food supplies in tropical areas and has led to the colonisation of new environments in the search for expanded food production. Venezuelan haemorrhagic fever is a severe and often fatal zoonotic virus disease only recently identified in the Guanarito area in central Venezuela. Cases were not found in the cities but were confined to rural inhabitants of the area who were largely engaged in farming or cattle ranching. Major outbreaks in 1989 and again in 1990–1 had fatality rates of around one-quarter. First diagnosed as due to dengue haemorrhagic fever, the disease is now known to be due to a separate virus, named the Guaranito virus, which is associated with rodent reservoirs.

Guaranito appears to be one of a family of arenaviruses known to cause haemorrhagic fevers in humans. They include the Junin and Machupo viruses, the cause of haemorrhagic fever outbreaks in Argentina and Bolivia. In each case, transfer appears to be from a wild rodent host (*Akodon azarae* and *Calomys musculinus* in Argentina and *C. callosus* in Bolivia); the main risk of transfer occurs during the corn harvesting season. Similar seasonal risks from epidemics of haemorrhagic fevers are associated with the family of Hantaan viruses in China which appear to be spread to humans during the rice harvest. Field mice, rats, and bank voles are involved in fever transmission in different parts of the world.

(ii) Deforestation and reforestation   Changes in the global forest cover also appear to be linked to disease changes. The deforestation of the tropical rain forests has been spatially complex, with a fern-like pattern of new logging roads being driven into the forests to abstract the highest-quality timber. New settlers following the logging roads into Amazonia encountered heavy malarial infections. This is partly because the land-use changes have greatly increased the forest-edge environments suitable for certain mosquito species.

Disease changes can also result from an opposite process in which abandoned farmland reverts to woodland. The classic case is the emergence of Lyme disease, caused by the spirochetal bacterium *Borrelia burgorferi* (Schmid, 1985). Lyme disease is now the most common vector-borne disease in the United States, but retrospective studies suggest it was not reported there until 1962 in the Cape Cod area of New England. The link between Lyme disease and 'Lyme arthritis' was not established until the 1970s, when an endemic focus was recognised around Old Lyme in south-central Connecticut. The critical land-use change which precipitated the emergence or re-emergence of the disease appears to have been the abandonment of farmland fields to woodland growth. The new woodland proved an ideal habitat for deer populations, the definitive host for certain Ixodes ticks which spread the bacterium through bites. The complex seasonal cycle of the vectors, which involves the ticks, the deer, the white-footed mouse (the reservoir for the pathogen), and human visitors using the forest, illustrates how sensitive is the ecological balance in which disease and environment is held. Epidemic Lyme disease is now a growing problem in Europe, fuelled by reversion of farmland to woodland (partly due to EU set-aside land policies), deer proliferation, and increased recreational use of forested areas. Lyme disease has now been reported from most temperate parts of the world in both northern and southern hemispheres.

(iii) Water control and irrigation   Until recently, Rift Valley fever was primarily a disease of sheep and cattle. It was confined to Africa south of the Sahara, with periodic outbreaks in East Africa, South Africa, and, in the mid-1970s, Sudan. The first major outbreak as a human disease occurred in Egypt in 1977 when there were 200,000 cases and 600 deaths; the deaths were usually associated with acute haemorrhagic fever and hepatitis.

The Egyptian epidemic has been provisionally linked to the construction of the Aswan Dam on the Nile. Completed in 1970, the dam created a 800,000-hectare water body and stabilised water tables so that its surface water provided breeding sites for mosquitoes. Whether the mosquito population provided a corridor that allowed the virus to enter Egypt from southern Sudan has yet to be proved. But the possibility led to concern for the epidemiological implications of other dam-building schemes in the African tropics. Completion of the Diama Dam on the Senegal River in 1987 was followed by a severe outbreak of Rift Valley fever upstream from the new dam. Over 1,200 cases and 244 deaths resulted. But, in contrast to Egypt, immunological studies demonstrated that Rift Valley fever was already endemic in people and livestock in a wide area of the Senegal River basin. Ecological changes favouring the vector and associated with dam building seem to be implicated in allowing both (i) invasion of the virus into a previously virgin population and (ii) severe flare-ups in a population with low-level endemicity.

(d) Global warming
Of the many global scenarios for disease and the environment in the early part of the next century, it is the health implications of global warming that have

caught the attention of governments and press worldwide. There have already been major studies of this issue in at least three countries: the United States (H. B. Smith and Tirpak, 1989), Australia (Ewan, Bryant, and Calvert, 1990), and the United Kingdom (Bannister, 1991). The World Health Organization also has a committee looking at the topic.

It has been postulated that a number of health effects will follow from a worldwide increase in average temperature from global warming. For infectious diseases, the main effects relate to changes in the geographical range of pathogens, vectors, and reservoirs. So far, few attempts have yet been made to compute the relative burden of morbidity and mortality that would be yielded by these effects. Any such calculation would also need to offset losses against gains that might accrue (for example, reductions in hypothermia against increases in hyperthermia).

The magnitude and spatial manifestations of global warming are still speculative. One of the main conclusions of the report of the Intergovernmental Panel on Climate Change (IPCC) in 1990 was how far research still had to go before reliable estimates of global warming could be made. But some rough orders of magnitude can be computed from the estimates of the different models that have been used. In global terms, warming appears to range from 'a predicted rise from 1990 to the year 2030 of 0.7 °C to 1.5 °C with a best estimate of 1.1 °C' (Intergovernmental Panel on Climatic Change, 1990).

We can obtain some idea of the implications of the predicted shift for local mean temperatures with reference to the United Kingdom. Current differences between the coldest (Aberdeen, latitude 57.10° N) and warmest (Portsmouth, latitude 50.48° N) of its major cities is 2.4 °C; this is well beyond the postulated IPCC warming effect by the year 2030. Climate is a much more complex matter than average temperature, but – if the global warming models carry over to the UK – then, by 2030, Edinburgh might have temperatures something like those of the English Midlands and London something like those of the Loire valley in central France. If we accept the much higher estimate of +4.8 °C warming over eighty years, this brings London into the temperature bands of southern France and northern Spain. Provided that these projections are sensible, something might be gained by comparative studies of disease incidence within the UK and adjacent EU countries, and disease incidence in warmer climates that match those predicted for the UK.

The biological diversity of viruses and bacteria is partly temperature-dependent, and it is much greater in lower than higher latitudes (see figure 7.17). Conditions of higher temperature would favour the expansion of malarious areas, not just for the more adaptable *Plasmodium vivax* but also for *P. falciparum*. Rising temperatures might also allow the expansion of the endemic areas of other diseases of human importance: these include, for example, leishmaniasis and arboviral infections such as dengue and yellow fever. Higher temperatures also favour the rapid replication of food-poisoning organisms. Warmer climates might also encourage the number of people going barefoot in poorer countries, thereby increasing exposure to hookworms, schistosomes, and Guinea worm infections. But not all effects would be negative. Warmer external air temperatures might reduce the degree of indoor crowding and lower the transmission of influenza, pneumonias, and 'winter' colds.

While modest rises in average temperatures are the central and most probable of any greenhouse effects, they are likely to be accompanied by three other main changes: (a) sea level rises of up to a metre; (b) increased seasonality in rainfall, thus reducing the level of water available for summer use; and (c) storm frequency increases (Henderson-Sellars and Blong, 1989).

7.5 Controlling epidemic spread

Efforts to prevent the spatial spread of communicable diseases lie deep in human history. While archaeological investigations from Peru to China provide evidence of disease control only by extensive civil engineering works (to supply safe water and to dispose of human and animal wastes), later historical accounts show increasing concerns about imported diseases. By the thirteenth century, most Italian cities were posting gatemen to identify potential sources of infection from visitors to the city. Venice, with its widespread trading links with the Levant and the Oriental lands beyond, pioneered the idea of quarantine. Its tiny Dalmatian colony, Ragusa (now Dubrovnik) saw the first recorded attempt, in 1377, to place a moratorium on travel and trade. Originally a thirty-day waiting period (a *trentino*), it was widely adopted by port cities as a defence against the plague and was later extended to forty days (a *quarantino*), the familiar quarantine period (Carmichael, 1993b, p. 198). As we have seen in chapter 2, it was just such an idea of protecting the United States by isolation that lay behind the generation of the foreign cities data in the *Weekly Abstract*.

The story of the steps by which the early Venetian quarantine measures were extended to become the International Quarantine Regulations of today has been told in detail elsewhere (Roemer, 1993). Highlights included the earliest sanitary conference at Venice in 1576, the first International Sanitary Conference convened in Paris in 1851, and the formation of key international control bodies: the Pan American Sanitary Bureau (1902), the International Office of Public Hygiene (1907), the Health Section of the League of Nations (1922), and the World Health Organization (1946). For the medieval world, the main threat came from imported plague but, by the nineteenth century, it was concern about cholera and yellow fever that drove the need for regulations. Smallpox, louse-born typhus, and relapsing fever were not added to the international list of regulated diseases until 1922.

In this section, we set out a schema for the different control strategies. We then examine the prime achievement of international public health this century – the global eradication of smallpox – and ask how far this provides a model for the eradication of other communicable diseases. In conclusion, we note briefly some of the problems which are likely to affect disease control in the next few decades.

7.5.1 Evolving control strategies

It is helpful to consider the problem of control strategies for communicable diseases by setting it within a modelling framework. We look here at a very simple model of disease transmission, at its implications for endemic reservoirs, and at how it may be translated into general control and forecasting frameworks.

(a) A simple transmission model

As we described in section 1.3.2, the ways in which diseases are transmitted have attracted mathematical interest from Bernoulli onwards: the classic account is given by Bailey (1975) in his *Mathematical Theory of Infectious Diseases*. To give a flavour of this approach, a very simplified diagram of the spread of measles infection through a human population is illustrated in the upper part of figure 7.20. Here, the stock of individuals at risk, S, is added to by births at some rate γ. The chains of infection necessary for an epidemic to be maintained are created by mixing between the susceptibles and those with the disease, I, at a rate β. Infectives recover (or die) from the disease at a rate μ.

As shown in the lower part of the figure, protection against the spread of infection can be taken at two points in the flow diagram. Method A, a geographical strategy, is to interrupt the mixing of infectives and susceptibles with protective spatial barriers. This may take the form of isolating an individual or community or of restricting the geographical movements of infected individuals through quarantine requirements; another approach is by locating populations in supposedly safe areas. For animal populations, there exists a third possibility: the creation of a *cordon sanitaire* by the wholesale evacuation of areas or by the destruction of those infected. The second approach (B) is to short-circuit the route from susceptibles to recovereds by the establishment of immunity through some variant of immunisation; see the reviews by Hinman (1966) and Spink (1978).

(b) Disease reservoirs and population thresholds

To be maintained endemically, each of the infectious diseases studied in chapters 4–6 must exceed what is known as the *critical community size* for that disease. We have explored the relationship between city size, levels of mortality, and epidemic frequency for our six marker diseases at several points in those chapters.

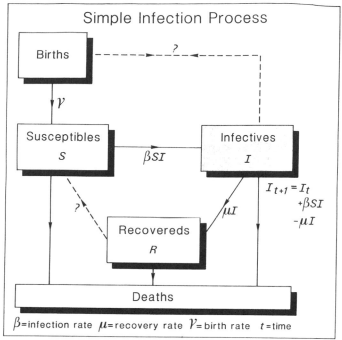

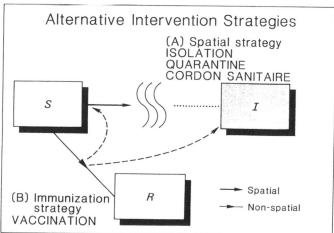

Figure 7.20. Simplified model of control strategies for an infection process. (Top) Main components of an *SIR* (*Susceptible–Infective–Recovered*) model for the spread of a human transmissible disease such as measles. (Bottom) Alternative intervention strategies: spatial intervention based on (A) blocking links between infectives and susceptibles and (B) opening of new pathways through immunisation which outflanks the infectives (*I*) box. Source: Cliff, Haggett, and Smallman-Raynor (1993), fig. 16.1, p. 414.

For the infectious disease most commonly used in modelling studies (measles), the critical community size required to sustain endemicity has been studied in detail in two classic papers by Bartlett (1957) and Black (1966). Bartlett plotted the mean period (time interval) between epidemics (in weeks) for a sample of nineteen English towns. The time interval was found to be inversely related to the population size of the community. Given the reporting rates for measles at the time, the work implied that a population of around 250,000 to 300,000 is required to ensure continuous transmission chains of infection.

Black extended Bartlett's work by examining the relationship between measles endemicity and population size in eighteen island communities. Black plotted, on logarithmic scales, the percentage of months with notified cases against population size; the population size with 100 per cent reporting denotes the endemicity threshold. Of the islands studied by Black, only Hawaii with a total population (then) of 550,000 displayed clear endemicity. Other islands close to Bartlett's 250,000 value just failed to display endemicity. This may, of course, reflect the difference between the isolation of islands as opposed to the mainland location of Bartlett's cities.

The basic notion of a threshold population, below which an infectious disease becomes naturally self-extinguishing, is paramount in articulating control strategies (Greenhalgh, 1986). It suggests that vaccination may be employed to reduce the susceptible population below some critical mass so that biological processes may achieve the rest. As a result, attempts have been made to establish the endemicity thresholds for a variety of transmissible diseases (see below). Once the population size of an area falls below the threshold then, when the disease concerned is eventually extinguished, it can only recur by reintroduction from other reservoir areas.

Thus the generalised persistence of disease implies geographical transmission between regions as shown in figure 7.21.

Taking measles for illustrative purposes, in large cities above the size threshold, like community **A**, a continuous trickle of cases is reported. These provide the reservoir of infection which sparks a major epidemic when the susceptible population, S, builds up to a critical level. Since clinical measles confers subsequent lifelong immunity to the disease, this build-up occurs only as children are born, lose their mother-conferred immunity, and escape vaccination or the disease. Eventually the S population will increase sufficiently for an epidemic to occur. When this happens, the S population is diminished and the stock of infectives, I, increases as individuals are transferred by infection from the S to the I population. This generates the D-shaped relationship over time between sizes of the S and I populations shown on the end plane of the block diagram.

If the total population of a community falls below the 250,000 size threshold, as in settlements **B** and **C** of figure 7.21, measles epidemics can, as noted above, arise only when the virus is reintroduced by the influx of infected

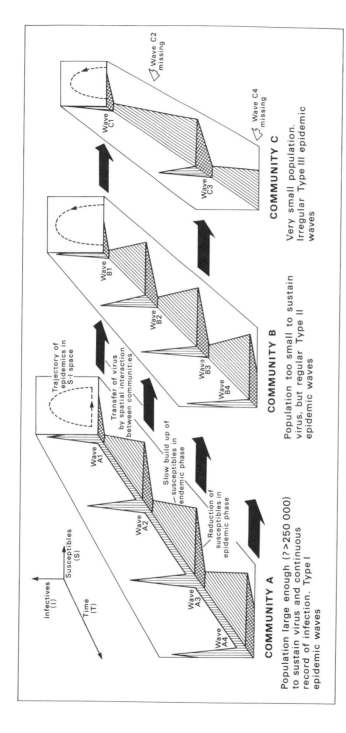

Figure 7.21. Conceptual view of spread of a communicable disease (measles) in communities of different population sizes. Stages in spread according to the Bartlett model. Source: Cliff and Haggett (1988), fig. 6.5A, p. 246.

Table 7.5. *Critical population sizes for endemicity of selected infectious diseases*

Disease	Infectious period (days)	Theshold population for endemicity (thousands)	
		Theoretical	From Icelandic data
Measles	4–9	300–500	290
Enteric fever	7–14	?	?
Scarlet fever	10–21	?	64
Whooping cough	14–21	?	186
Diphtheria	14–28	?	54
Tuberculosis	Very long	?	?

Source: Partly from Cliff and Haggett (1990), tab. 1, p. 98.

individuals from reservoir areas. These movements are shown by the broad arrows in figure 7.21. In such smaller communities, the S population is insufficient to maintain a continuous record of infection. The disease dies out and the S population grows in the absence of infection. Eventually the S population will become big enough to sustain an epidemic when infection arrives. Given that the total population of the community is insufficient to renew by births the S population as rapidly as it is diminished by infection, the epidemic will eventually die out.

It is the repetition of this basic process which generates the successive epidemic waves witnessed in most communities. Of particular significance is the way in which the continuous infection and regular Type I epidemic waves of endemic communities break down, as population size diminishes, into first, discrete but regular Type II waves in community **B** and then, secondly, into discrete and irregularly spaced Type III waves in community **C**. Thus disease-free windows will automatically appear in both time and space whenever population totals are small and densities are low.

This model enhances our understanding of the relative importance of population size and distance effects in accounting for the propagation of the six marker diseases in the cities of the North American and British Isles regions (sections 6.3 and 6.4). Spatial interaction effects only become significant in maintaining the chains of infection for cities below the population size required to sustain endemic disease. Table 7.5 lists the endemicity thresholds for some of our markers, estimated by the authors from Icelandic data in the manner described in Cliff and Haggett (1990). Given the infectious periods of the marker diseases whose thresholds were not calculated, as compared with the remainder, the population thresholds for all six are likely to be in the range

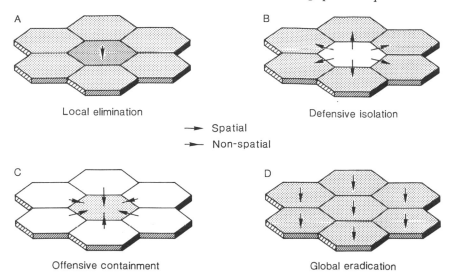

Figure 7.22. Schematic diagram of four spatial and aspatial control strategies to prevent epidemic spread. Infected areas are stippled; disease-free areas left white. Geographical areas shown arbitrarily as hexagons. Source: Cliff, Haggett, and Smallman-Raynor (1993), fig. 16.9, p. 423.

c. 50,000–300,000. As shown in figures 6.12 and 6.22, most of the North American and British cities are above these figures, and this accounts for the dominance of size effects detected in the analyses of sections 6.3 and 6.4.

(c) Spatial strategies for disease control
If we look at the strategy by which smallpox was finally eradicated (see later in this chapter), we can see the control process as one of progressive spatial reduction in the areas of the world in which the disease was endemic. Cliff and Haggett (1989) discuss a stage-by-stage schema of possible reduction strategies, stressing the ways in which geographical considerations impinge upon control by vaccination. These different spatial control strategies are illustrated in figure 7.22; in each of the four maps, infected areas have been stippled, while disease-free areas have been left blank.

In the first stage, *local elimination*, the emphasis is on breaking, in some particular location, the disease chain by vaccination. The programmes aimed at eliminating indigenous measles in countries such as the United States, Czechoslovakia, and Australia illustrate this phase. Such vaccination programmes may themselves be variable within a country and have a geographical component.

Once an area is cleared of the disease in question, then there is a need for a second stage, *defensive isolation*, which entails the building of a spatial barrier around a disease-free area. Attempts to erect such barriers were made in the nineteenth century but may be impractical today. We have already noted the difficulties that mass air travel causes for the use of quarantine to prevent infectious cases from gaining access to susceptible populations; the United States's experience with its measles elimination programme, discussed in section 7.2.3, illustrates the point.

A third stage, *offensive containment*, is a more appropriate approach in these circumstances. This is the reverse of the second case in that the spread of a local outbreak within a larger disease-free area is halted and progressively eliminated by a combination of vaccination and isolation. Tinline (1972) has explored the use of such ring-control strategies for foot-and-mouth disease, a contagious virus disease of livestock.

The fourth and final stage of *global eradication* would arise in principle from the combination of the previous three methods: infected areas would be progressively reduced in size, and the coalescence of such disease-free areas would lead, eventually, to the elimination of the disease on a worldwide basis. Thus the ultimate extinction of a bacillus or virus from the planet rests on a global control programme to reduce the sizes of the geographically distributed populations that are at risk to levels at which the chains of infection cannot be maintained. In terms of the Bartlett model, this means systematically reducing the wave order of different communities from I to II, and from II to III, eventually bringing the Type III waves into phase so that the fade-out of all the remaining active areas coincides.

As we have seen in figure 7.20, for those diseases for which vaccination is a possibility, this is one of the main approaches that can be deployed to create and maintain disease-free areas. For measles, the impact of vaccination policies upon the size and spacing of recurrent epidemics has been considered in Griffiths (1973), R. M. Anderson and Grenfell (1986), and R. M. Anderson and May (1983). Figure 7.23 shows the predicted effect of partial immunisation, sustained over fifteen years, at 80 per cent of the one- to two-year-olds in a theoretical population.

The slow damping of epidemic amplitude is evident as the cumulative impact of vaccination is felt and, eventually, the endemic cycle is broken and whole epidemics are missed.

Work by Griffiths relates figure 7.23 back to our earlier discussion of measles thresholds. He examined the long-run effect upon a community of a continuing partial vaccination programme. If x denotes the proportion of children not artificially immunised by vaccination ($0 \leq x \leq 1$), Griffiths found that the critical community size for measles endemicity is multiplied by $1/x^2$. So, taking Bartlett's threshold estimate of 250,000, 50 per cent immunisation will increase the critical community size to 1 million, while 90 per cent immunisation will increase the threshold to 25 million. Thus, with vaccination, natural fade-out will become very widespread, enhancing the possibility of

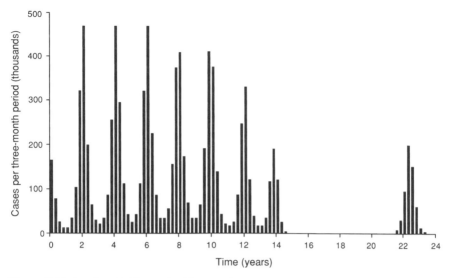

Figure 7.23. Predicted effects of widespread measles immunisation. Application of the Anderson and May model with the level of immunisation held constant for fifteen years at 80 per cent of one- to two-year-olds. Source: Cutts (1990), fig. 10, p. 23.

eradication. In principle, this might apply to any disease controllable by vaccination.

(d) Spatial forecasts of spread
Spatial forecasting models using mathematical formulations to estimate the likely spread of an infectious disease are increasingly being used in epidemiological studies. One case study which illustrates the potential for modelling global disease transmission is provided by the work of Gould (1995). He took the largest 102 urban centres in the conterminous United States and used air passenger origin–destination data to compute a weighted 102×102 transition (contact) probability matrix. Contact probabilities were particularly high amongst the five largest cities which in 1992 'exchanged' by air travel some 13 million people every year; likewise, probabilities were low amongst smaller and distant centres with small volumes of population exchange. In mathematical terms, the matrix forms an operator capable of multiplying a state vector. The state vector in Gould's case was the distribution of AIDS cases on a city-by-city basis at a particular year (1986). After a series of probabilistic multiplications the 'projected' AIDS distribution for 1990 was calculated.

The results of the projections are shown in figure 7.24A. The projected values from the Gould model (horizontal axis) show a close approximation to the observed AIDS rates (vertical axis), with a correlation of about 80 per

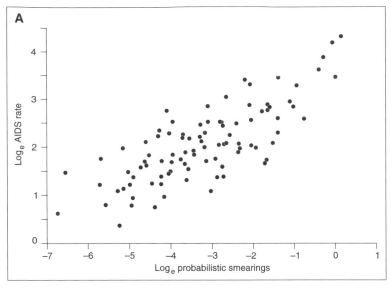

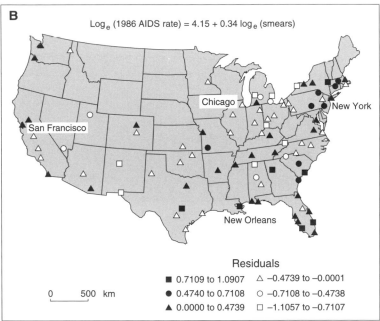

Figure 7.24. Projective modelling of AIDS epidemic in the United States. (A) Actual AIDS rates for 102 United States cities on the vertical axis plotted against the probabilistic estimates on the horizontal axis. (B) Maps of residuals to show which cities were overpredicted (white symbols) and which were underpredicted (black symbols) by the model. Source: Gould (1995), p. 27.

cent. Figure 7.24B maps the residuals from the projection; that is, those cities under- and overpredicted by the model. Many of the negative residuals (towns with AIDS rates overpredicted) lie in the older 'rustbelt' towns of the northeast United States with many blue-collar workers of Catholic and recent immigrant backgrounds. Many southern cities which are tourist destinations come out as positive residuals: they have AIDS rates higher than the model would predict.

Models of this kind, where they can be calibrated on historical data from recent epidemic events, can be used to predict the spread of communicable diseases in the future. Russian workers have used such models on a world network of cities to project the spread of a new strain of influenza (Rvachev and Longini, 1985). Cliff and Haggett (1988, pp. 102–7) have used similar models to predict the likelihood of measles imports into the several regions of the United States. The construction of global early warning systems for the transmission of communicable diseases is in prospect.

7.5.2 Global control programmes

When the epidemiological history of the twentieth century comes to be written, the outstanding success that historians will be able to record is the global eradication of smallpox. The complex story which culminated in the last recorded natural case in October 1977 (there were to be two subsequent laboratory deaths) has been superbly told and in massive detail by Fenner, Henderson, Arita, Jesek, and Ladnyi (1988). The success has inevitably raised questions as to whether other infectious diseases, measles among them, can also be eradicated. We look briefly at the smallpox eradication programme and compare its success with the prospects for poliomyelitis.

(a) The global eradication of smallpox

Although WHO has from time to time conducted major campaigns against infectious disease (notably malaria and yaws), only one disease – smallpox – has so far been globally eradicated. The practical reality of devising, coordinating, and financing a field programme involving more than thirty national governments, as well as some of the world's most complex cultures and demanding environments, proved to be of heroic proportions. Until the mid-1960s, control of smallpox was based primarily upon mass vaccination to break the chain of transmission between infected and susceptible individuals by eliminating susceptible hosts. Although this approach had driven the disease from the developed world, the developing world remained a reservoir area. Thus between 1962 and 1966, some 500 million people in India were vaccinated, but the disease continued to spread. Between 5 and 10 per cent of the population always escaped the vaccination drives, concentrated especially in the vulnerable under-fifteen age group. Nevertheless, the susceptibility of the

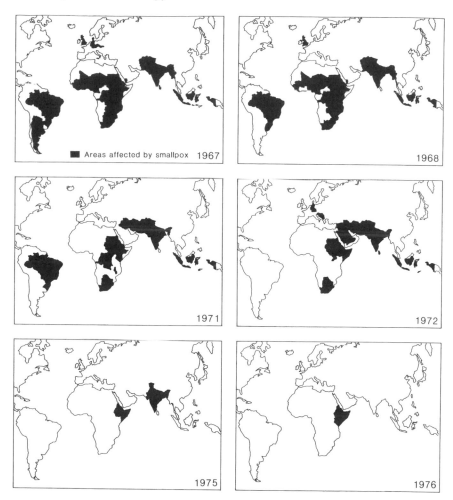

Figure 7.25. Global eradication of smallpox under the WHO Intensified Programme, 1967–1977. Countries with smallpox cases for the year in question marked in black. Source: redrawn from maps and graphs in Fenner, Henderson, Arita, Jesek, and Ladnyi (1988), fig. 10.4, plates 10.42–10.51, pp. 516–37.

virus to concerted action had been demonstrated and led to critical decisions at the Nineteenth World Health Assembly in 1966.

This Assembly embarked upon a ten-year global smallpox eradication programme, which was launched in 1967. It started with mass vaccination, but rapidly recognised the importance of selective control. Contacts of smallpox cases were traced and vaccinated, as well as the other individuals in those locations where the cases occurred. The success of the four-phase programme

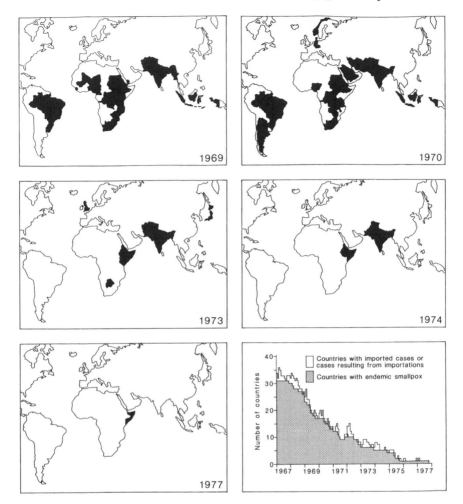

Figure 7.25. (*cont.*)

(*preparatory, attack, consolidation*, and *maintenance*) may be judged from the maps and graphs in figure 7.25. By 1970, retreat was in progress in Africa. By 1973, the disease had been eliminated in Latin America and the Philippines; a few strongholds remained in Africa, but most of the Indian subcontinent remained infected. Despite a major flare-up of the disease in 1973 and 1974, the hunt by WHO for cases and case contacts continued. By 1976 the disease had been eradicated in South and East Asia and only a part of East Africa remained to be cleared. The world's last recorded smallpox case was a 23-year-old man of Merka town, Somalia, on 26 October 1977. After a two-year period during which no other cases (other than laboratory accidents) were

recorded, WHO formally announced at the end of 1979 that the global eradication of smallpox was complete.

(b) The poliomyelitis elimination campaign

The dramatic success of the WHO smallpox programme has inevitably raised
the prospect and hope that other virus-borne diseases can be eradicated. In
1974, WHO established its Expanded Programme on Immunization (EPI)
with the objective of greatly reducing the incidence of six other crippling diseases: diphtheria, measles, neonatal tetanus, pertussis, poliomyelitis, and
tuberculosis (plate 7.1). Two further diseases (hepatitis B and yellow fever)
were later added. Historical mortality trends for four of these diseases (diphtheria, measles, pertussis, and tuberculosis) have, of course, been examined in
previous chapters of this book. With the exception of yellow fever, table 7.6
summarises some of the characteristics of the diseases and indicates in the
final two columns the continental variation in vaccination levels achieved to
date for two areas of the world, Africa and Europe. Very high levels are being
reached in Europe holding out the prospect of elimination of some of our
marker diseases from these regions. Indeed, some countries, like Finland, are
already free of measles.

Comprehensive reviews of the impact of such vaccination programmes
upon world health appear in Cutts and Smith (1994) and in WHO's
Immunization Policy (WHO, Global Programme for Vaccines and
Immunization, 1995). An important consideration is how far smallpox is a
useful control model for other communicable diseases. For, whatever the huge
difficulties in practice, in principle smallpox was well suited (perhaps uniquely
well suited) to global eradication: Fenner (1986) has summarised the special
characteristics of smallpox which allowed global eradication. Fenner also
recognised that the biological features of smallpox, while a necessary pre-con-
dition for global eradication, were not in themselves sufficient to ensure
success. For example, Fenner has demonstrated that the disease was economically significant in the West. Quite apart from the disease and death from
smallpox itself, the cost of vaccination, plus that of maintaining quarantine
barriers, is calculated to have been about US$ 1,000 million per annum in the
last years of the virus's existence in the wild. These costs disappear completely
if, and only if, *global* eradication is achieved.

Eleven years after the close of its successful smallpox campaign, the 41st
World Health Assembly, meeting in Geneva in 1988, committed WHO to the
global eradication of a second disease, poliomyelitis. Like smallpox, this
target involves not only eliminating the disease, but totally eradicating the
causative virus. The goal was made possible by forty years of research and
vaccine development since Enders, Weller, and Robbins succeeded in growing
poliovirus in cell culture. The licensing of the Salk inactivated (1955) and
Sabin attenuated live vaccine (1961) was reinforced by the early success of the

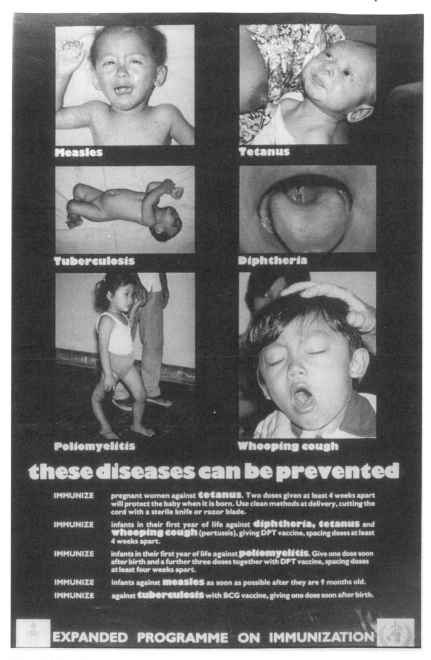

Plate 7.1. The Expanded Programme on Immunization. One of several posters produced by WHO to publicise its immunisation campaign. Source: Dr John Clements, Expanded Programme on Immunization, World Health Organization, Geneva.

Table 7.6. *Target diseases in the WHO Expanded Programme on Immunization*

Disease	Infectious agent	Reservoir	Spread	Nature of vaccine	Form of vaccine (doses)	Immunisation coverage (%), Africa	Immunisation coverage (%), Europe
Diphtheria	Toxin-producing bacterium (*C. diphtheriae*)	Humans	Close contact respiratory or cutaneous	Toxoid	Fluid (1)	50.0	86.0
Hepatitis B	Virus	Humans	Perinatal; child–child; blood; sexual spread	HBsAg	Fluid (3)	0.15	12.0
Measles	Virus	Humans	Close respiratory contact and aerosolised droplets	Attenuated live virus	Freeze-dried (1)	49.0	78.0
Pertussis	Bacterium (*B. pertussis*)	Humans	Close respiratory contact	Killed whole cell pertussis bacterium	Fluid (3)	50.0	86.0
Poliomyelitis	Virus (serotypes 1, 2, and 3)	Humans	Faecal–oral; close respiratory contact	Attenuated live viruses of three types	Fluid (4)	50.0	92.0
Tetanus (neonatal)	Toxin-producing bacterium (*Cl. tetani*)	Animal intestines; soil	Spores enter body through wounds, umbilical cord	Toxoid	Fluid (3)	35.0	N/A
Tuberculosis	*Mycobacterium tuberculosis*	Humans	Airborne droplet nuclei from sputum-positive person	Attenuated *M. bovis*	Freeze-dried (1)	68.0	81.0
Yellow fever	Virus	Humans; monkeys	Mosquito-borne	Attenuated live virus	Freeze-dried (1)	6.0	N/A

Note:
Immunisation coverage at March 1994. Africa excludes South Africa.
Source: WHO, Global Programme for Vaccines and Immunization (1995); based on data in tabs. 1–3, pp. 2–5.

countries of the Pan American Health Organization which had agreed in 1985 to eradicate the wild poliovirus from the Americas.

The level of global success achieved by 1993 is mapped in figure 7.26. The map indicates that no country in the Americas reported cases and that Europe, Japan, Australia, and New Zealand were free of cases. Tropical Africa and South and East Asia remained major zones where disease incidence remained high. Overall, the level of vaccination worldwide has risen from less than 5 per cent of children in 1974 to over 80 per cent in 1994. Over the same period the number of reported cases worldwide has fallen from a peak of over 70 million to fewer than 7 million.

WHO has warned against complacency. Declining polio incidence mostly reflects individual protection from immunisation, and not wild virus eradication. For although surveillance is improving, less than 15 per cent of cases are being officially reported. The global strategy has five components: (a) high immunisation coverage with oral polio vaccine, (b) sensitive disease surveillance detecting all suspected cases of poliomyelitis, (c) national or subnational immunisation days, (d) rapid, expertly managed outbreak response when suspected cases are detected, and (e) 'mopping-up' immunisation in selected high-risk areas where wild virus transmission may persist.

The major cost of eradicating poliomyelitis will be borne by the endemic countries themselves but donor country support will be required for vaccine, laboratories, personnel, and research. Of these, the most urgent need is for vaccine: although each dose of oral vaccine currently costs only 7¢, over two billion doses will be required per year for routine and mass immunisation. In the longer run, the economic benefits of disease eradication far exceed the cost. Since its own last case in 1977, the USA has saved its total contribution once every twenty-six days. If present progress is maintained, the global initiative will start to pay for itself by the year 1998, produce savings of half a billion dollars by the year 2000. These savings will increase to US$3 billion annually by the year 2015.

7.6 Controlling future epidemics

At the close of a book which has largely been concerned with establishing global baselines for epidemic diseases in the past, it is important to look to the future. Here we see a series of trends which will influence control measures for infectious diseases in the coming decades. On the credit side, we expect to see positive improvements in vaccine power and efficiency, but on the debit side, we expect these to be balanced in some instances by increased microbiological resistance – disease-causing organisms are also in the survival business. We see five contextual trends which will affect our ability to exert global control.

(1) Disease control is likely to rely and less and less on spatial barriers. The
   speed of modern air transport (most of the world's cities are now within

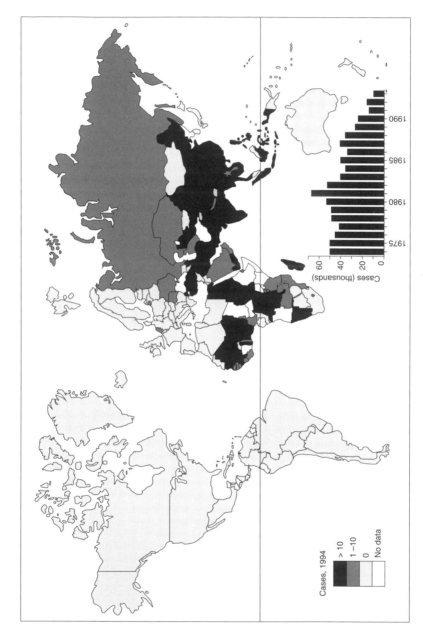

Figure 7.26. World incidence of indigenous poliomyelitis in 1993. (Inset) Annual number of cases of poliomyelitis notified in the world, 1974–93. Source: map included in pamphlet, WHO (1995b).

thirty-six hours of each other) and the complexity of air connections (there are now 4,028 airports in the world with regular scheduled services) make the traditional 'drawbridge' strategy increasingly irrelevant. The quarantine barriers first set up by the earliest international sanitary conferences were modelled to fit a slower mode of travel, notably ships, and fewer connection points.

(2) Rapid reporting and surveillance are likely to be increasingly critical in control. The use of electronic reporting (such as the United States's NETSS (National Electronic Telecommunications Surveillance System)) is likely to be extended worldwide through the Internet. Weekly bulletins such as WHO's *Weekly Epidemiological Record* or CDC's *Morbidity and Mortality Weekly Report* will be regularly updated on an on-line basis.

(3) Ever-widening lists of communicable diseases and the high cost of surveillance will make sampling essential. The legal requirement to notify certain infectious diseases is tending to be replaced by sampling systems in which sentinel practices are used to pick up trends in disease prevalence. This will intensify the legal problems associated with vaccination, identification, and constraints on freedom of movement (Matthews and Churchill, 1994).

(4) Mathematical methods will increasingly supplement other epidemiological tools in global control. As well as the increased use of spatial models like those discussed earlier in this chapter in forecasting, there will be the need to scan regularly the torrent of international and local data for 'aberrant' behaviour. Traditional CPE (current/previous experience) graphs will be replaced by automatic monitoring in which anomalous events will be highlighted for the epidemiologist to consider (Stroup, Wharton, Kafadar, and Dean, 1993). Such anomalies may well range, for example, from clinical reports of resistant malaria strains, to unusual clusters of meningitis cases, to higher-than-average influenza reports.

(5) Disease control and socio-economic development are likely to be ever more closely tied together. In his *World Health Report* for 1995, the director-general of WHO stated that: 'The world's most ruthless killer and the greatest cause of suffering on earth is listed in the latest edition of WHO's International Classification of Diseases under the code Z59.5. It stands for extreme poverty' (1995c, p. 1). The number of extreme poor has been rising over the last decade at a rate above gross population growth and, in 1990, was estimated at over 1.1 billion, or over one-fifth of humanity. For communicable diseases, the links between poverty and disease come through many channels: absence of knowledge of protective measures, poor diet, and lack of vaccination, clean water, and sanitation. The correlation runs the gamut of geographical scales, from the global North–South contrast between the developed and developing worlds, to

the local contrast between the affluent suburbs and deprived inner-city ghettos of a Western city.

We may argue that little changes. We have seen how the same factors – absence of knowledge of protective measures, poor diet, and lack of vaccination, clean water, and sanitation – affected mortality rates from our six marker diseases a century ago. Many of the causes have been substantially reduced or eliminated in certain regions, and globally there has been the century-long decline in mortality from the six diseases which we have illustrated in this book. But, especially in the developing world and among the urban poor, our marker diseases remain major killers, a fact to which the WHO Expanded Programme bears witness. The five trends we have described highlight some of the more important contexts of change against which disease control is likely to be set. Each century, public health has had to fight disease with the tools available and the constraints imposed at the time. The twenty-first century will be no exception as it prepares to fight old diseases causing old problems and old diseases causing new problems (for example, drug resistance), as well as wholly new diseases.

Postscript

We opened the preface to this book by referring to the most familiar journal in the epidemiological world, the *Morbidity and Mortality Weekly Report*, and linked this back to the *Weekly Abstract* which preceded it more than a century before. Surveying and monitoring the ever-changing disease world has been a constant concern which spans from medieval Japanese monks, through Lutheran parish priests in Iceland, to eighteenth-century Massachusetts tavern keepers. We like to think that in this volume we have kept faith with at least one generation of such observers. We hope that John Maynard Woodworth (see plate 2.1), his small staff in the Marine Hospital Service, and the hundreds of US consuls in large and small outposts across the world would be pleased that the figures they so patiently collected then could play some small part in assembling the complex jigsaw that will need to be in place if we are ever going to be able to decipher world epidemics. Their generation forms part of a chain which stretches through the *MMWR* and its modern equivalents around the world to the sophisticated electronic networks that are now replacing them. For the past observers, as for the present, continual vigilance is the first barrier against the disease-bearing microbes and plagues that seem likely to threaten humanity for the foreseeable future.

Appendices

These appendices are intended as a guide to the main sources of commentary and of epidemiological and demographic data for the countries whose cities have been analysed in this book. The work described in chapters 2–6 has been based upon data published in the United States's *Weekly Abstract*, 1888–1912, cross-checked against selected records of the United Kingdom's registrar general. Accordingly, appendix A lists in detail these primary sources of information. For completeness, the relevant sources are outlined for the entire life of the foreign city tables, 1878–1912.

But we have examined material in detail for only a relatively brief window of time from 1888 to 1912. Accordingly, the sources listed in appendices B–D cover both earlier source material and run through to the present day. Appendix B deals with international sources and appendix C with national sources. Names and addresses of international and national epidemiological agencies responsible for collecting and publishing disease data at these levels appear in appendix D. We do not claim to have been exhaustive in our coverage. Whilst we hope we have captured the most important sources, readers will be able to complement our lists from their own knowledge, and we would be pleased to receive details of such additions.

Appendix A

Primary data sources

1. United States marine hospital service / public health service

Weekly Abstract

The National Quarantine Act of 1878 granted the US Marine Hospital Service, fore-runner of the US Public Health Service, powers of quarantine against vessels from infected ports overseas. As described in chapter 2, the Service prepared weekly abstracts of sanitary reports received from foreign locations to assist in the exercise of the quarantine powers, and these were begun as *Bulletins of the Public Health* in 1878. The publication was subsequently renamed twice, first in 1887 (*Weekly Abstract of Sanitary Reports*) and then in 1896 (*Public Health Reports*), and it was to remain a prin-cipal weekly source of international (and domestic) morbidity and mortality statistics until 1912. Thereafter, international statistics continued in reduced form until 1951. In these appendices, all general references to the publication under its various aliases are as the *Weekly Abstract*.

The structure and content of the *Weekly Abstract* is outlined in chapter 2. In brief, a typical edition from the turn of the century was divided into two parts along geo-graphical lines: United States; and Foreign and Insular. Each section was further divided into tabular and written reports. *United States section*: This consisted of tabu-lated statistics of: immigration at major ports during the week; the transactions of national, state, and municipal quarantine and inspection stations; reports of cases and deaths from quarantine diseases by state and county; estimated population and deaths from all causes, and selected infectious diseases (cholera, diphtheria, enteric fever, measles, scarlet fever, smallpox, tuberculosis, typhus fever, variola, yellow fever, and whooping cough) by city; and meteorological conditions for major cities. These tabular statistics were supplemented by state-by-state sanitary reports of Service personnel and miscellaneous reprints of items pertaining to the public health under the jurisdic-tion of the Service. *Foreign and Insular section*: This consisted of tabulated statistics of morbidity and mortality overseas as reported by various officials (consuls, diplomats, chargés d'affaires, and officers of the Service). Two tables were published on a regular weekly basis: cases and deaths from quarantine diseases (cholera, plague, smallpox, and yellow fever) by country and subdivision; estimated population and deaths from all causes, and selected infectious diseases (cholera, diphtheria, enteric fever, measles,

384

plague, scarlet fever, smallpox, tuberculosis, typhus fever, yellow fever, and whooping cough) by foreign city. In addition to the tabulated statistics were written reports from those locations where information was either not available on a weekly basis, or where extra information was available. Supplementary information was provided in the form of occasional statistical tables, especially during the course of major health events. Reprints of topical articles from European medical journals were occasionally included.

Details of bound editions of the *Weekly Abstract* in which mortality statistics in overseas cities appeared, 1878–1912, are as follows: **Bulletins of the Public Health** (Washington, DC: Government Printing Office), 1878–9 (vol. I, nos. 1–46, 13 July 1878 to 24 May 1879);[1] **Weekly Abstract of Sanitary Reports** (Washington, DC: Government Printing Office), 1887 (vol. II, nos. 47–96, 20 January–30 December), 1888 (1889, vol. III, nos. 1–52), 1889 (1890, vol. IV, nos. 1–52), 1890 (1890, vol. V, nos. 1–52), 1891 (1892, vol. VI, nos. 1–52), 1892 (1893, vol. VII, nos. 1–53), 1893 (1894, vol. VIII, nos. 1–52), 1894 (1895, vol. IX, nos. 1–52), 1895 (1896, vol. X, nos. 1–52); **Public Health Reports** (Washington, DC: Government Printing Office), 1896 (1897, vol. XI, nos. 1–52), 1897 (1898, vol. XII, nos. 1–53), 1898 (1899, vol. XIII, nos. 1–52), 1899 (1900, vol. XIV, nos. 1–52), 1900 (1901, vol. XV, part I, nos. 1–26, and 1901, vol. XV, part II, nos. 27–52), 1901 (1902, vol. XVI, part I, nos. 1–26, and 1902, vol. XVI, part II, nos. 27–52), 1902 (1902, vol. XVII, part I, nos. 1–26, and 1903, vol. XVII, part II, nos. 27–52), 1903 (1903, vol. XVIII, part I, nos. 1–26, and 1904, vol. XVIII, part II, nos. 27–52), 1904 (1904, vol. XIX, part I, nos. 1–26, and 1905, vol. XIX, part II, nos. 27–53), 1905 (1905, vol. XX, part I, nos. 1–26, and 1906, vol. XX, part II, nos. 27–52), 1906 (1906, vol. XXI, part I, nos. 1–26, and 1907, vol. XXI, part II, nos. 27–52), 1907 (1907, vol. XXII, part I, nos. 1–26, and 1908, vol. XXII, part II, nos. 27–52), 1908 (1908, vol. XXIII, parts I and II), 1909 (1909, vol. XXIV), 1910 (1910, vol. XXV), 1911 (1911, vol. XXVI, part I, nos. 1–26, and 1912, vol. XXVI, part II, nos. 27–52), 1912 (1912, vol. XXVII, part I, nos. 1–26, and 1913, vol. XXVII, part II, nos. 27–52).

The weekly tables of mortality from major infectious diseases in foreign cities were discontinued in issue no. 51 of 1912 (*Public Health Reports*, 1913, vol. XXVII, part II, pp. 2179–80). But the weekly tables of morbidity and mortality from quarantine diseases in foreign locations continued in the *Public Health Reports* until the 1950s. These tables were begun in the *Weekly Abstract of Sanitary Reports* in 1894 (1895, vol. IX) and included running totals of cases and deaths from cholera and yellow fever. Smallpox and human plague were added to the tables in the late 1890s, with the further addition of typhus fever in 1916. The tables were later expanded to include other major infectious diseases on a country-by-country basis before they were finally discontinued in the last issue of 1951 (*Public Health Reports*, vol. 66, no. 52) when the aims of the journal were redefined.[2]

To supplement the foreign disease data in the *Weekly Abstract* between 1878 and 1912, a number of other publications of the Marine Hospital Service (renamed the Public Health and Marine Hospital Service from 1902, and the Public Health Service from 1912) ran parallel. The primary focus of these publications was domestic, but they occasionally contained information of international interest.

(1) **(Annual)** *Annual Report of the Supervising Surgeon General of the Marine Hospital Service* (and similar titles) (Washington, DC: Government Printing Office): annual volumes, 1878–1912. This was begun in 1872 as *Annual Report of the Supervising*

Surgeon of the Marine Hospital Service of the United States for the Year 1872 (US Department of the Treasury, US Marine Hospital Service, 1872. Washington, DC: Government Printing Office) to provide a complete report of the transactions, including receipts and disbursements, of the Marine Hospital Service. Included among the forty-one issues of the *Annual Report* to 1912 were annual summaries of the sanitary conditions of foreign ports and the international activity of quarantinable diseases as reported in the *Weekly Abstract*. These were supplemented by detailed reports of international disease activity commissioned by the Service, one of the most notable being: *Report of the Commission Appointed to Investigate the Cholera Epidemic and the Danger of Transmission of Contagious Diseases from Foreign Countries 1893* (US Department of the Treasury, US Marine Hospital Service, 1895. *Annual Report of the Supervising Surgeon General of the Marine Hospital Service of the United States for the Fiscal Year 1893, Volume II* (Washington, DC: Government Printing Office), pp. 175–381).

(2) **(Occasional)** *Bulletin of the Hygienic Laboratory* (Washington, DC: Government Printing Office). The Hygienic Laboratory, forerunner of the National Institutes of Health, was established by Act of Congress on 3 March 1901 to conduct investigations of infectious and contagious diseases and other matters pertaining to public health. Results of the investigations, which were largely restricted to domestic health events, were published as occasional bulletins and were restricted by law to ten editions each year.

(3) **(Occasional)** *Bulletin of the Yellow Fever Institute* (Washington, DC: Government Printing Office). The Yellow Fever Institute was established within the Public Health and Marine Hospital Service in 1901 to 'collect all facts concerning yellow fever; to designate the specific lines of investigation to be made, and to make them'.[3] The results were to be published in a maximum of five bulletins per year, with each bulletin not to exceed 5,000 copies. The publications were concerned with all aspects of yellow fever, including: transmission; aetiology; diagnosis; symptoms; domestic and overseas history and geography; and quarantine.

(4) **(Occasional)** *Public Health Bulletin* (Washington, DC: Government Printing Office). A series of publications concerned with miscellaneous subjects, from descriptions of the geographical foci of leprosy to regulations of maritime quarantine.

In addition to the above, the Service also circulated numerous other publications, including: complete copies of the quarantine laws; histories of the Service; lists of Service regulations; and medical handbooks. Finally, beginning in 1903, the Service published the annual series *Transactions of the Annual Conference of State and Territorial Health Officers*. This publication was largely concerned with discussion of domestic health events.

Readers wishing to study United States's public health data through to the present day may consult the following:

American Statistics Index: A Comprehensive Guide and Index to the Statistical Publications of the United States Government (Washington, DC: Congressional Information Service, 1974–, monthly). The 1974 edition contains retrospective information. The publication identifies statistical data published by the federal government and includes index and abstract sections.

Federal Statistical Directory (22nd edn), Executive Office of the President, Office of

Management and Budget (Washington, DC: US Government Printing Office, 1970).

Guide to US Government Statistics (4th edn), John Andriot (McLean, VA: Documents Index, 1973). This is an annotated guide to recurring statistical publications of US agencies. It is arranged by Sudocs classification scheme. While many publications of interest to scientists are included, primary emphasis is on economic and social statistics.

Statistics Sources (5th edn), Paul Wasserman and Jacqueline Bernero (Detroit, MI: Gale Research, 1977). This publication identifies primary sources of statistical data, especially in US publications, of national rather than regional scope. It includes over 20,000 citations to sources of statistical data on nearly 12,000 subjects.

Health. United States 1978, DHEW Pub. no. (HRA) 76–1232 (Rockville, MD: US Department of Health, Education, and Welfare, US Public Health Service, US Health Resources Administration, US National Center for Health Statistics, 1978). This publication consists of reports to Congress required by the Public Health Service Act. The publications consist of four parts: Part A: *Financial Aspects of the Nation's Health Care*; Part B: *Health Resources*; and Parts C and D: *Health Status and Use of Health Services*.

In the United States, the Office of Management and Budget's Statistical Policy Division exists solely for the purpose of coordinating the statistical collection and dissemination functions of the federal government. Other government agencies involved primarily in statistical activities for health and demography include the Department of Health, Education, and Welfare's (DHEW) National Center for Health Statistics and National Center for Educational Statistics, and the Department of Commerce's Bureau of the Census.

2. United Kingdom Registrar General

The registration of births and deaths in England and Wales can be traced back to the Tudor period when the reign of Henry VIII (1509–47) saw the start of parish registers in 1538. Except for a brief period in the middle of the seventeenth century, however, registration did not become statutory until the 1830s. The Births and Deaths Registration Act of 1836 provided for vital registration in England and Wales by the establishment of the General Register Office. The Act became effective in July 1837 and, from that year, tabular statistics on births, deaths, and marriages have been published regularly by the registrar general of England and Wales. The recording of births and deaths was consolidated in 1874 when the Births and Deaths Registration Act introduced death certificates and a penalty for failure to register.[4]

The publications of the registrar general, which are detailed below, are best known for their statistical summaries of births, deaths, and marriages in London and other large cities of England and Wales. Among the pages of the reports, however, are regular tables listing the population, births, deaths from all causes, and deaths from major epidemic diseases (including diphtheria, enteric fever, measles, scarlet fever, smallpox, and whooping cough) in approximately thirty overseas cities. The colonial influence in the choice of cities is readily apparent. At the turn of the century, statistics from the Indian cities of Bombay, Calcutta, and Madras and the Egyptian cities of Alexandria and

Cairo featured in the tables. But to these can be added cities of Northern and Central Europe, Scandinavia, and North America. These overseas statistics appear in three publications of the registrar general during the period 1878–1912:

1. **(Weekly)** *Weekly Return of Births and Deaths in London and in . . . Other Large Towns . . .* (and similar titles) (London: HMSO): 1878 (vol. XXXIX, no. 1)–1912 (vol. LXXIII, no. 52).

2. **(Quarterly)** *Quarterly Return of Marriages, Births, and Deaths Registered in the Divisions, Counties, and Districts of England and Wales . . .* (and similar titles) (London: HMSO): 1878 (no. 157)–1912 (no. 256).

3. **(Annual)** *Annual Summary of Births, Deaths, and Causes of Death in London and Other Large Cities* (and similar titles) (London: HMSO): 1878 (*Forty-first Report*)–1912 (*Seventy-fifth Report*).

Appendix B

International epidemiological sources

The systematic international recording of information about mortality and morbidity from disease begins with the Health Section of the League of Nations established in the aftermath of the Great War. To promote comparability of recording between nations, the *International Classification of Diseases* (ICD) has been developed. The origins of this classification system are discussed in Benjamin (1968, pp. 8–86). The first edition of the ICD list was prepared by the International Statistical Institute, and it appeared in 1911 under the title *International List of Causes of Death*. Revisions have appeared roughly decennially to keep abreast of advances in medical science. The tenth edition (1992) is currently used. Initially, the list formed a basis for the recording of mortality data alone, but it was extended to cover morbidity from 1948 when responsibility for revision of the list was passed from the International Statistical Institute to the World Health Organization. From that date, the ICD list has been entitled *International Statistical Classification of Disease, Injuries, and Causes of Death*.

The following list gives the major sources of international epidemiological data and associated information. It is arranged historically.

1. League of Nations

The first meeting of the Health Committee of the Health Section of the League of Nations took place in August 1921 to consider 'the question of organising means of more rapid interchange of epidemiological information'. To meet this need, a series of publications were instituted and are described below.

Epidemiological Intelligence

Series E.I., *Epidemiological Intelligence*, is the key epidemiological surveillance publication and contains both data and articles. It and its successors are the main source of published international data on mortality in the period between the world wars. The first issue (E.I.1), focusing upon the spread of epidemics and the epidemiological situation in Eastern Europe generally in 1921, and in Russia, Romania, the Serb–Croat–Slovene state, and Greece in particular, appeared in 1922. Five subsequent issues also centred upon this region. The titles of E.I.1–E.I.6 are: *Epidemiological*

Situation in Eastern and Central Europe in 1921 (E.I.1); *Epidemics in Russia Since 1914*: Report to the Health Committee of the League of Nations by Professor L. Tarassevitch (Moscow), Part I (E.I.2); *Epidemiological Situation in Eastern and Central Europe*, January–April 1922 (E.I.3); *Epidemiological Situation in Eastern and Central Europe*, January–June 1922 (E.I.4); *Epidemics in Russia Since 1914*: Report to the Health Committee of the League of Nations by Professor L. Tarassevitch (Moscow), Part II (E.I.5.); *Epidemiological Situation in Eastern and Central Europe*, May–December 1922 (E.I.6). In addition to reports, these publications contained limited mortality data.

The E.I. Series was retitled in 1923 as *Annual Epidemiological Report and Corrected Statistics of Notifiable Diseases*, and this appeared as an annual until the issue for the year 1938 (published in 1941). The title indicates the emphasis on notifiable diseases: data are included on causes of death from thirty-one infectious diseases, vital statistics by country, and a table showing the mortality from certain causes for individual countries. This table was updated each year and showed trends. Soon after, however, the series had evolved into a fixed format of tables of data on communicable diseases and vital statistics (monthly to 1932, bimonthly between 1932 and 1937, and monthly again from 1937–38). The *Epidemiological Report* (published monthly to the end of 1931, bimonthly between 1932 and 1936, and monthly again from January 1937) contains official statistics of cases and deaths attributed to the following diseases: (a) *plague, cholera, yellow fever, smallpox*, and *typhus*; and (b) *enteric fever, influenza, acute poliomyelitis, diphtheria, scarlet fever*, and *epidemic cerebro-spinal meningitis*. The tables for diseases of the first group are included in all issues of the *Epidemiological Report*. Tables referring to the diseases of the second group appear regularly during the season of special prevalence of the diseases in question; at other times of the year they are published at longer intervals. Statistics of certain other diseases (*relapsing fever, encephalitis lethargica, miliary fever, malaria, undulant fever, dysentery, measles, whooping cough, chickenpox, venereal diseases, anthrax, trachoma*, and *puerperal fever*) are given with a few months' interval. Monthly or four-weekly *birth, death*, and *infant mortality* rates for numerous large cities throughout the world are also published in these reports. In addition, statistics of deaths attributed to principal epidemic diseases (*tuberculosis, pneumonia, diarrhoea*, and *enteritis*) in these cities, and records of mean temperature and rainfall, are given with some months' interval. All statistics are arranged by disease. Each number of the *Epidemiological Report* contains a general review, in which either the trend of one or more of the chief epidemic diseases is described, or a study of vital statistics is provided. Population figures are given in a special table. Morbidity rates are not generally given on the grounds that they would not be comparable owing to varying degrees of accuracy in notification in different countries.

Titles of the E.I. Series, published between 1923 and 1936, are: *(Corrected) Statistics of Notifiable Diseases in European Countries, 1922* (E.I.7); *for 22 European Countries, 15 African Countries, 14 American Countries, 12 Asiatic Countries, and for Australasia for the Year 1923* (E.I.8); *for 29 European Countries, 17 African Countries, 20 American Countries, 16 Asiatic Countries, and for Australasia for the Year 1924* (E.I.9); *for 33 European Countries, 34 African Countries, 24 American Countries, 23 Asiatic Countries, and for Australasia for the Year 1925* (E.I.10); *for the Year 1926* (E.I.11); *for the Year 1927* (E.I.12); *for the Year 1928* (E.I.13); *for the Year 1929* (E.I.14);

for the Year 1930 (E.I.15); *for the Year 1931* (E.I.16); *for the Year 1932* (E.I.17); *for the Year 1933* (E.I.18); *for the Year 1934* (E.I.19). E.I.1–E.I.18 were also published as *Epidemiological Intelligence.*

A reorganisation of material involving this series and two others (*Weekly Epidemiological Record* and *Bulletin of the Health Organisation*, described below) was undertaken in 1937. From this date, the E.I. Series focused on statistical material alone, and articles and commentary were handled solely through the two other outlets. The *Annual Epidemiological Report* (the E.I. Series) continued containing: monthly tables of communicable diseases and vital statistics; data grouped by periods of four weeks, by months, or by quarters; medians for the corresponding periods of the thirteen preceding years given as bases for comparison; and epidemiological indices. The last major publication in this series (E.I.23) included crude mortality rates for the period 1911–35 for fifty-one countries for all causes, infant mortality, ten infectious diseases, puerperal sepsis, and ill-defined diseases. In addition, some material was published on deaths for fourteen causes for large cities in certain countries. Titles of E.I.20–E.I.23 are: *Corrected Statistics of Notifiable Diseases for the Year 1935* (E.I.20); *for the Year 1936* (E.I.21); *for the Year 1937* (E.I.22); *for the Year 1938* (E.I.23).

Because of the approximate two-year lag between date of data gathering and date of publication, production of the series was abandoned during the Second World War (1939–45). As described under World Health Organization below, two fill-in publications were produced by the new World Health Organization to cover the years 1939–46 and 1947–48, before the annual cycle of publication of statistical information was resumed through WHO in 1950.

To supplement the definitive data in the E.I. Series, other series ran in parallel:

(1) **Monthly Epidemiological Report** (R.E.1–R.E.225). This ran for nineteen years from 1922 to 1940 and was a statistical supplement to the *Weekly Epidemiological Record* (see below). It contains in monthly and bimonthly form, and without publication lags of two to three years, many of the uncorrected data subsequently published in final corrected form in the *Annual Epidemiological Report* (E.I. Series).

(2) **Weekly Epidemiological Record** (R.H. Series) The *Weekly Epidemiological Record*, consisting of epidemiological notes and data relating to topics of contemporary interest, was commenced in 1926. Its particular aim was to publicise current official reports on the prevalence of notifiable communicable diseases from practically all countries where such information was available, and to provide intelligence from all parts of the world on the prevalence of plague, cholera, yellow fever, smallpox, and typhus, as well as any other disease judged to constitute an international menace. Demographic data, for example birth rates for selected world cities, were also included. The series was produced continuously by the Health Section of the League as the serial R.H.1–R.H.1087 until the end of 1946, when it was continued under the auspices of the World Health Organization (see below). It is of value for epidemiological analysis for ancillary information but, as might be expected, does not provide the systematic coverage of the E.I. Series.

(3) **Bulletin of the Health Organisation**: A third series, the *(Quarterly) Bulletin of the Health Organisation of the League of Nations*, was commenced in 1932 to make available scattered documentation relating to the general work and technical committees of the Health Organisation of the League. Texts of epidemiological articles

and monographs appeared here. The publication is only of limited use as background material for the types of analyses described in this book.

Judicious use of the E.I. Series (*Epidemiological Intelligence/Epidemiological Report*) permits the construction of reasonably continuous time series of mortality for many of the world's countries and selected cities on a monthly basis for a wide range of diseases from 1922 to 1938. Supporting contextual information and commentary is available in the *Weekly Epidemiological Record* and, less frequently, the *Bulletin*.

Other relevant series of the League of Nations are the following:

(1) A critical set of *Statistical Handbooks* covering most of the countries of Europe and the Baltic republics, as well as Canada, appeared between 1924 and 1930. These handbooks detail each country's data collection procedures and sources for births, marriages, deaths, and disease from historical times into the early years of the twentieth century. Titles are: No. 1, *The Official Vital Statistics of the Kingdom of the Netherlands* (C.H. 159); No. 2, *The Official Vital Statistics of the Kingdom of Belgium* (C.H. 162); No. 3, *The Official Vital Statistics of the Kingdom of England and Wales* (C.H. 270); No. 4, *The Official Vital Statistics of the Kingdom of Spain* (C.H. 271); No. 5, *The Official Vital Statistics of the Republic of Austria* (C.H. 272); No. 6, *The Official Vital Statistics of the Scandinavian Countries and the Baltic Republics* (C.H. 428) (Ser. L.o.N.P. 1926 III.8); No. 7, *The Official Vital Statistics of the Republic of Portugal* (C.H.445) (Ser. L.o.N.P. 1926 III.8); No. 8, *The Official Vital Statistics of the Republic of Czechoslovakia* (C.H.524) (Ser. L.o.N.P. 1926 III.27); No. 9, *The Official Vital Statistics of the French Republic* (C.H.530) (Ser. L.o.N.P. 1927 III.2); No. 10, *The Official Vital Statistics of the Kingdom of Hungary* (C.H.565) (Ser. L.o.N.P. 1927 III.3); No. 11, *The Official Vital Statistics of Ireland: The Irish Free State and Northern Ireland* (C.H.741) (Ser. L.o.N.P. 1928 III.14); No. 12, *The Official Vital Statistics of Switzerland* (C.H.669) (Ser. L.o.N.P. 1927 III.16); No. 13, *The Official Vital Statistics of the Kingdom of Scotland* (C.H.771) (Ser. L.o.N.P. 1929 III.2); No. 14, *The Official Vital Statistics of the Dominion of Canada* (C.H.834) (Ser. L.o.N.P. 1930 III.1).

(2) *International Health Year-Book*: This series consists of complete monographs on the public health organisation of various countries, and it also gives details of the International Health Year-Books of the following geographical areas: Africa; Africa, French Possessions; America; Argentine Republic; Australia; Austria; Belgian Congo; Belgium; British India; British Somaliland; Bulgaria; Canada; Ceylon; China; Czechoslovakia; Denmark; Egypt; Eire; Estonia; Far East; Federated Malay States; Finland; France; French Colonies; French Indo-China; Germany; Greece; Hungary; Iran; Italian Colonies; Italy; Japan; Kenya (Colony and Protectorate); Latvia; Lithuania; Luxemburg; Mexico; Netherlands; New Zealand; Norway; Panama; Persia (see Iran); Philippines; Poland; Portuguese India; Romania; Salvador; Spain; Straits Settlements; Sweden; Switzerland; Tanganyika (British Mandate); Turkey; United Kingdom: England and Wales, Scotland, Northern Ireland; United States; Uruguay; USSR; Yugoslavia. Titles of the series are: 1924 *Reports on the Public Health Progress of Twenty-two Countries* (C.H. 349); 1925 (C.H.477); 1927 *Reports on the Public Health Progress of Twenty-seven Countries in 1926* (C.H.599); 1928 *Reports on the Public Health Progress of Twenty-nine Countries (Thirty-five Public Health Administrations) in 1927* (C.H.733); 1929 *Reports (with Vital and Public Health Statistics) on the Public*

Health Progress of Forty Countries and Colonies in 1928 (C.H.838); 1930 *Reports (with Vital and Public Health Statistics) on the Public Health Progress of Thirty-four Countries and Colonies in 1929* (C.H.951).

Full particulars of all League of Nations publications are given in: *General Catalogue*, 1935 (1920–May 1935); *First Supplement to General Catalogue* (June 1935–December 1936); *Second Supplement to General Catalogue* (January–December 1937); *Third Supplement to General Catalogue* (January–December 1938); *Fourth Supplement to General Catalogue* (January–December 1939); *Publications of the League of Nations, January 1st 1940–December 31st 1945*; *Publications of the League of Nations, January–December 1946*. All the publications listed above are available in the libraries of (a) United Nations, Palais des Nations, 1211 Geneva 10, Switzerland, and the World Health Organization, 1211 Geneva 27, Switzerland. A further important bibliographic source is *A Repertoire of League of Nations Serial Documents, 1919–1947, Volume II* (Victor Yves and Catherine Ghebali. The Carnegie Endowment for International Peace/Oceana Publications, Inc., Dobbs Ferry, New York, 1973).

2. World Health Organization

As described above, the *Annual Epidemiological Report* (E.I. Series), issued by the Health Organisation of the League of Nations since 1922, is the main source of epidemiological data at an international level for the period between the two world wars. The last volume in this series (E.I.23) contained statistics for the year 1938 and appeared in 1941. The publication of the World Health Organization (WHO) that links to the E.I. Series is *Annual Epidemiological and Vital Statistics*, first published by WHO in 1951 for the years 1939–46. The second volume covers the years 1947–49. It continued annually from 1950 under the same title until 1962 when it was renamed *World Health Statistics Annual*, a title which has carried through to the present day. This yearbook, which was published in three parts until the 1980s, summarises vital statistics and causes of death in both English and French, and contains statistical data on morbidity and mortality from infectious diseases as well as the number of immunisations performed. It also reports on the number of persons working in various health occupations as well as the ratio of medical personnel to the population of various countries. Titles are as follows: *Part I: Vital Statistics and Causes of Death*; *Part II: Infectious Diseases: Cases, Deaths and Vaccinations*; *Part III: Health Personnel and Hospital Establishments* (from 1954). The collection of information on morbidity from communicable diseases, health manpower, and health establishments (information which comprises Parts II and III of the yearbook) was discontinued in 1982, and subsequent editions appeared as a single volume.

While this serial is the main international *printed* source of epidemiological data, computer-based records of mortality and morbidity became available after 1977. Driven by developments in computing, an outline of an Information Service on World Health Statistics was published in 1974, positing the electronic storage and publishing of mortality and morbidity data by countries. The data bank went on-line in 1977 (*World Health Statistics Annual, 1973–1976*, WHO (1976; Geneva), vol. I, pp. v–vi, 784–8). The data bank provides, upon request, relevant health statistical information in a standardised content-fixed and form-fixed record layout. Requests should be addressed to: Global Epidemiological Surveillance and Health Situation Assessment, World Health Organization, 1211 Geneva 27, Switzerland.

Mortality data bank file

(a) Sources of data: Mortality data are drawn exclusively from civil registration systems in each country. While data quality varies from nation to nation, WHO relies on the existence of a universal vital registration system with reasonably complete certification of death according to the ICD list.

(b) Content: Country name, revision of ICD list used to classify deaths, year of death, amount of detail in cause of death data, age distribution of death details, age, sex, and cause of death. Special files, for example relating to cancer mortality, are also held.

Past records have been added to the file, the earliest being for the year 1950. Inevitably, the data matrix is incomplete, but time series of over forty years' duration are increasingly available for mortality for many of the world's countries. Appendix B gives the country-by-country details of mortality data held in the bank.

Morbidity data bank file

In parallel with the mortality data bank, a morbidity data bank was also established. This was a much more ambitious project than the mortality data bank. First, data had to be gathered from a variety of sources, such as: annual WHO questionnaires sent to member states; annual reports and other publications of national health administrations; and periodic reports (weekly, monthly, and quarterly) sent to WHO by national public health services. Secondly, whereas the mortality data are annual, the morbidity data give the seasonal breakdown of reported cases by months, four-week, or quarterly periods wherever possible, as well as year of report. Content otherwise parallels that of the mortality database and is retrospective. Regretfully, the logistic difficulties of acquiring the necessary data and changes of policy at WHO (associated with the needs of its Health for All by the Year 2000 Global Strategy) led to freezing of the data base in 1982 (*World Health Statistics Annual*, 1993 (Geneva: World Health Organization), p. xviii). But a unique window of morbidity data at a global scale covering the period c. 1950–1980 is available therein. Country-by-country details are given in this book in appendix C.

The changes introduced simultaneously enabled the focus of *World Health Statistics Report* to be shifted from data presentation to the interpretation of data as a means of improving the utilisation of quantitative information for administrative and research purposes.

Other relevant WHO series are the following:

(1) *Epidemiological and Vital Statistics Report* (1947–66); renamed as *World Health Statistics Report* (1967–77); renamed again as *World Health Statistics Quarterly* (1978 to present). This publication appeared first in 1947 to fulfil a function inherited from the League of Nations and covered by the League's *Monthly Epidemiological Report*. It provides current health guidance based on analysis of statistical data, rather than raw data themselves.

(2) *Weekly Epidemiological Record* (1947 to present). This is a continuation of the same-named League of Nations publication (see above) and is concerned with epidemiological data used in disease surveillance at an international level. Priority is

given to diseases and risk factors known to threaten international health. These range from diseases requiring official notification under International Health Regulations (plague, cholera, and yellow fever, 1994) through to major communicable diseases.

(3) *Bulletin of the World Health Organization* (1947–present) This represents a continuation in style and content of the *Bulletin* of the League of Nations described above. It includes review articles and original papers on scientific research in the laboratory and field.

(4) *Epidemiological Information Bulletin* (1945–) A semi-monthly publication providing summaries and analyses of official notifications received of certain dangerous diseases (quarantine diseases) as agreed by the International Sanitary Conventions of 1944.

3. Other international sources

1. United Nations

To complement WHO epidemiological data, a basic source of demographic data is the United Nations' *Demographic Yearbook* (New York: Statistical Office of the United Nations). This publication has appeared annually since 1948 and provides, in addition to basic vital statistics on a country-by-country basis, an in-depth treatment of a different aspect of demographic statistics each year. Topics are covered on a cyclical rotation pattern and include, for example, historical trends of population size and characteristics, population censuses, natality statistics, and mortality statistics.

2. General

Bunle (1954) has reviewed the 'movement of population' in the world from 1906 to 1936, using a short-list of thirty causes of death for thirty-one countries; the number of deaths by cause and country were presented for persons of all ages combined.

A major series of articles examining the mortality for European countries was published in the first few years after the formation of WHO (Pascua 1949, 1950, 1951). Subsequently, a number of other WHO reports have presented data on specific causes of death, providing trends over various time periods.

Appendix C

National epidemiological sources

The following alphabetical list details the major epidemiological sources for the countries of the world in which our 100 cities are located (see tables 3.3 and 3.4). Within each country, the material is arranged under three headings: (a) sources of morbidity data, (b) sources of mortality data, and (c) sources of population data. Information is listed under the current (1995) names and jurisdictions of the respective countries. Where necessary, these are cross-referenced with the 1888–1912 names and jurisdictions indicated in tables 3.3 and 3.4.

The countries listed fall in one of six World Health Organization regions, viz. (a) European Region, (b) Eastern Mediterranean Region, (c) South East Asian Region, (d) Western Pacific Region, (e) African Region, and (f) American Region. Readers should refer to the WHO Regional Offices or to the national epidemiological agencies whose addresses are given in appendix D for recent changes.

AUSTRALIA. Commonwealth of Australia. WHO Western Pacific Region (WPR). Area: 2,974,581 miles^2. Population: 18.3 million (1995). European colonisation from late eighteenth century with the six colonies federated into the Commonwealth of Australia from 1901. **(a) Sources of morbidity data:** Reported cases of notifiable infectious diseases are regularly reported in: *Notification Diseases Report* (weekly); *Communicable Diseases Intelligence* (fortnightly). Annual information on the incidence and immunisation coverage of eight vaccine-preventable diseases (diphtheria, measles, pertussis, poliomyelitis, tetanus, neonatal tetanus, tuberculosis, and yellow fever) from 1974 is given in the *Information System Summary Volume, WHO Western Pacific Region* (WHO, Expanded Programme on Immunization (EPI), Geneva, annual). **(b) Sources of mortality data:** Standardised mortality tables giving 178 causes of death for males and females are given for Australia by quinquennial periods for the period 1906 to 1975 in *International Mortality Statistics* (Alderson, 1981, tabs. 1–178, pp. 113–477). Mortality data for Australia with causes of deaths classified by age, sex, and ICD code are available on computer tape from WHO for the forty-three years between 1950 and 1992 (WHO (1994), Annex I). Annual totals and crude mortality rates of deaths from infectious diseases for Australia for the years 1939 through 1946 are reported in *Annual Epidemiological and Vital Statistics*

1939–1946 (WHO (1952), part II, tab. 40, p. 70) and for the two cities of Melbourne and Sydney for ten infectious diseases (tabs. 48–57, pp. 88–108). Trends in mortality in Australia are discussed in *Expectations of Life* (Lancaster, 1990, pp. 414–22). **(c) Sources of population data:** The first census taken in Australia was held in 1828 in New South Wales. There were further censuses for *New South Wales* in 1933, 1841, 1846(5)1861, 1871(10)1901. Other provincial censuses include: *Queensland* (included in New South Wales censuses 1828–56), 1861, 1864, 1868, 1871(5)1886, 1897, 1901; *South Australia*, 1844, 1846, 1851, 1855, 1860, 1861(5)1881, 1891, 1901; *Tasmania* (included in New South Wales censuses 1833–6), 1841(1)1843, 1848, 1851, 1857, 1861, 1870, 1881(10)1901; *Victoria*, (included in New South Wales censuses 1841–51), 1854, 1857, 1859, 1870, 1881(10)1901; *Western Australia*, 1848, 1854, 1859, 1870, 1881(10)1901. *National* censuses were undertaken in 1911, 1927, 1933, 1947, 1954, 1961, 1966. Full details are given *International Population Census Bibliography, No. 3, Oceania* (University of Texas, 1966, pp. 2.1–2.34). Population estimates for Australia by age (five-year groups up to age eighty), sex, and quinquennia for the period 1906 to 1975 are given in *International Mortality Statistics* (Alderson, 1981, tab. 180, p. 484).

AUSTRIA-HUNGARY. *See* Austria, Czechoslovakia, Hungary, Yugoslavia.

AUSTRIA. *Republik Österreich.* WHO European Region (EUR). Area: 32,370 miles². Population: 7.9 million (1995). Central European country formed out of the Austro-Hungarian Empire in 1918; part of Germany for the period 1938–45. **(a) Sources of morbidity data:** Reported cases of notifiable infectious diseases are regularly reported in *Monatsausweis über angezeighte falle . . .* (monthly). Annual information on the incidence and immunisation coverage of eight vaccine-preventable diseases (diphtheria, measles, pertussis, poliomyelitis, tetanus, neonatal tetanus, tuberculosis, and yellow fever) from 1974 is given in the *Information System Summary Volume, WHO European Region* (WHO, Expanded Programme on Immunization (EPI), Geneva, annual). **(b) Sources of mortality data:** Standardised mortality tables giving 178 causes of death for males and females are given for Austria by quinquennial periods for the period 1901 to 1975 in *International Mortality Statistics* (Alderson, 1981, tabs. 1–178, pp. 113–477). Annual totals and crude mortality rates of deaths from infectious diseases for Austria for the years 1939 through 1946 are reported in *Annual Epidemiological and Vital Statistics 1939–1946* (WHO (1952), part II, tab. 20, p. 49) and for the city of Vienna for ten infectious diseases (tabs. 48–57, pp. 88–108).[1] Mortality data for Austria with causes of deaths classified by age, sex, and ICD code are available on computer tape from WHO for the thirty-eight years between 1955 and 1992 (WHO (1994), Annex I). **(c) Sources of population data:** Annotated estimates for decennial death rates for Austria by cause of death for the period 1821 to 1901 are published in *Statistique générale de la France* (France, Bureau de la Statistique Générale; appendix, pp. 83–594). The first census for Austria was held in 1857 with subsequent censuses conducted in 1869, 1880(10)1920, 1923, 1934, 1951, 1961. A full listing appears in the *International Population Census Bibliography, No. 6, Europe* (University of Texas, 1967c, pp. 3.1–3.15). Population estimates for Austria by age (five-year groups up to age eighty), sex, and quinquennia for the period 1901 to 1975 are given in *International Mortality Statistics* (Alderson, 1981, tab. 180, p. 485).

BELGIUM. *Royaume de Belgique*. WHO European Region (EUR). Area: 11,780 miles². Population: 10.0 million (1995). Independent nation since 1831. **(a) Sources of morbidity data:** Reported cases of notifiable infectious diseases are regularly reported in *Epidemiologische Opgave* (monthly). Annual information on the incidence and immunisation coverage of eight vaccine-preventable diseases (diphtheria, measles, pertussis, poliomyelitis, tetanus, neonatal tetanus, tuberculosis, and yellow fever) from 1974 is given in the *Information System Summary Volume, WHO European Region* (WHO, Expanded Programme on Immunization (EPI), Geneva, annual). **(b) Sources of mortality data:** Standardised mortality tables giving 178 causes of death for males and females are given for Belgium by quinquennial periods for the period 1901 to 1975 in *International Mortality Statistics* (Alderson, 1981, tabs. 1–178, pp. 113–477).² Annotated estimates for decennial death rates for Belgium by cause of death for the period 1841 to 1901 are published in *Statistique générale de la France* (France, Bureau de la Statistique Générale; appendix, pp. 83–594). Annual totals and crude mortality rates of deaths from infectious diseases for Belgium for the years 1939 through 1946 are reported in *Annual Epidemiological and Vital Statistics 1939–1946* (WHO (1952), part II, tab. 21, p. 50) and for the two cities of Antwerp and Brussels for ten infectious diseases (tabs. 48–57, pp. 88–108). Trends in mortality in Belgium are discussed in *Expectations of Life* (Lancaster, 1990, p. 393). **(c) Sources of population data:** The first census for Belgium was held in 1831–40 (*Population. Relevé décennal–1831 à 1840. Mouvement de l'état civil de 1840*). Subsequent censuses were conducted in 1846(10)1876, 1880, 1890(10)1920, 1926, 1934, 1946, 1944–7, 1961. A full listing appears in the *International Population Census Bibliography, No. 6, Europe* (University of Texas, 1967c, pp. 4.1–4.16). Population estimates for Belgium by age (five-year groups up to age eighty), sex, and quinquennia for the period 1926 to 1975 are given in *International Mortality Statistics* (Alderson, 1981, tab. 180, p. 487).

BRAZIL. WHO American Region (AMR). Area: 3,286,169 miles². Population: 161.4 million (1995). **(a) Sources of morbidity data:** Reported cases of notifiable infectious diseases are regularly reported in *Boletim epidemiologico semanal* (weekly). Annual information on the incidence and immunisation coverage of eight vaccine-preventable diseases (diphtheria, measles, pertussis, poliomyelitis, tetanus, neonatal tetanus, tuberculosis, and yellow fever) from 1974 is given in the *Information System Summary Volume, WHO American Region* (WHO, Expanded Programme on Immunization (EPI), Geneva, annual). **(b) Sources of mortality data:** Mortality data for Brazil with causes of deaths classified by age, sex, and ICD code are available on computer tape from WHO for the eleven years between 1979 and 1989 (WHO (1994), Annex I). **(c) Sources of population data:** The first census was held in 1872 (*Recenseamento de população do imperio de Brazil a que se Procedeu no dia 1° de agosto de 1872*). Subsequent censuses were conducted in 1890(10)1960. There were also state and city censuses. Full details are given in *International Population Census Bibliography, No. 1, Latin America and the Caribbean* (University of Texas, 1965a, pp. 6.1–6.26).

BURMA. *See* Myanmar.

CEYLON. *See* Sri Lanka.

COLOMBIA. WHO American Region (AMR). Area: 439,825 miles². Population:

35.1 million (1995). **(a) Sources of morbidity data:** Reported cases of notifiable infectious diseases are regularly reported in *Informe semanal de enfermedades* (weekly); *Boletin epid. de antioquia* (quarterly). Annual information on the incidence and immunisation coverage of eight vaccine-preventable diseases (diphtheria, measles, pertussis, poliomyelitis, tetanus, neonatal tetanus, tuberculosis, and yellow fever) from 1974 is given in the *Information System Summary Volume, WHO American Region* (WHO, Expanded Programme on Immunization (EPI), Geneva, annual). **(b) Sources of mortality data:** Mortality data for Colombia with causes of deaths classified by age, sex, and ICD code are available on computer tape from WHO for the thirty-two years between 1953 and 1990 (WHO (1994), Annex I). **(c) Sources of population data:** The first (colonial) census for Colombia was held in 1770. Subsequent censuses were conducted in 1778, 1782, 1803, 1810, 1825, 1835 (the first national census, *Censo de población de la República de la Nueva Grenada, levantado con arreglo a las disposiciones de la lei de 2 de junio de 1834 en los meses de enero, febrero, i marzo del año de 1835 en las diferentes provincias que comprende su territorio*), 1843, 1851, 1864, 1870, 1905, 1912, 1918(10)1938, 1951. Full details are given in *International Population Census Bibliography, No. 1, Latin America and the Caribbean* (University of Texas, 1965a, pp. 11.1–11.7).

CUBA. WHO American Region (AMR). Area: 44,164 miles^2. Population: 11.1 million (1995). **(a) Sources of morbidity data:** Reported cases of notifiable infectious diseases are regularly reported in *Informe semanal de enfermedades transm.* (weekly). Annual information on the incidence and immunisation coverage of eight vaccine-preventable diseases (diphtheria, measles, pertussis, poliomyelitis, tetanus, neonatal tetanus, tuberculosis, and yellow fever) from 1974 is given in the *Information System Summary Volume, WHO American Region* (WHO, Expanded Programme on Immunization (EPI), Geneva, annual). **(b) Sources of mortality data:** Mortality data for Cuba with causes of deaths classified by age, sex, and ICD code are available on computer tape from WHO for the twenty-six years between 1959 and 1990 (WHO (1994), Annex I). **(c) Sources of population data:** The first census for Cuba was held in 1768. Subsequent censuses were conducted in 1774, 1792, 1817, 1841, 1846, 1861, 1877, 1887, 1899, 1907, 1919, 1931, 1943, 1953. Full details are given in *International Population Census Bibliography, No. 1, Latin America and the Caribbean* (University of Texas, 1965a, pp. 13.1–13.7).

CZECHOSLOVAKIA (Czech Republic & Slovak Republic). *Ceska a Slovenska Federativni Republika.* WHO European Region (EUR). Area: 49,373 miles^2. Population: 15.6 million (1995). Central European country formed in 1918 from Austro-Hungarian Empire. Parts ceded to Germany and Hungary in late 1930s. **(a) Sources of morbidity data:** Reported cases of notifiable infectious diseases are regularly reported in *Monthly Epidemiological Report* (monthly). Annual information on the incidence and immunisation coverage of eight vaccine-preventable diseases (diphtheria, measles, pertussis, poliomyelitis, tetanus, neonatal tetanus, tuberculosis, and yellow fever) from 1974 is given in the *Information System Summary Volume, WHO European Region* (WHO, Expanded Programme on Immunization (EPI), Geneva, annual). **(b) Sources of mortality data:** Standardised mortality tables giving 178 causes of death for males and females are given for Czechoslovakia by quinquennial periods for the period 1916 to 1975 in

International Mortality Statistics (Alderson, 1981, tabs. 1–178, pp. 113–477). Annual totals and crude mortality rates of deaths from infectious diseases for Bohemia–Moravia–Silesia and Slovakia for the years 1939 through 1946 are separately reported in *Annual Epidemiological and Vital Statistics 1939–1946* (WHO (1952), part II, tabs. 39A and 39B, pp. 68–9). Trends in mortality in Czechoslovakia are discussed in *Expectations of Life* (Lancaster, 1990, p. 393). Mortality data for Czechoslovakia with causes of deaths classified by age, sex, and ICD code are available on computer tape from WHO for the thirty-nine years between 1953 and 1991 (WHO (1994), Annex I). Mortality data for the Czech Republic with causes of deaths classified by age, sex, and ICD code are available on computer tape from WHO for the year 1992 (WHO (1994), Annex I). **(c) Sources of population data:** The first census for Czechoslovakia was held in 1850. Subsequent censuses were conducted in 1880(10)1920, 1921, 1930, 1939, 1947, 1950, 1960. A full listing appears in the *International Population Census Bibliography, No. 6, Europe* (University of Texas, 1967c, pp. 6.1–6.19). Population estimates for Czechoslovakia by age (five-year groups up to age eighty), sex, and quinquennia for the period 1916 to 1975 are given in *International Mortality Statistics* (Alderson, 1981, tab. 180, p. 490).

DENMARK. *Kongeriget Danmark*. WHO European Region (EUR). Area: 16,629 miles². Population: 5.2 million (1995). Independent country from 1815; also historically the southern provinces of Schleswig and Holstein, now part of Germany. **(a) Sources of morbidity data:** Reported cases of notifiable infectious diseases are regularly reported in *Epi-nyt Weekly* (weekly). Annual information on the incidence and immunisation coverage of eight vaccine-preventable diseases (diphtheria, measles, pertussis, poliomyelitis, tetanus, neonatal tetanus, tuberculosis, and yellow fever) from 1974 is given in the *Information System Summary Volume, WHO European Region* (WHO, Expanded Programme on Immunization (EPI), Geneva, annual). **(b) Sources of mortality data:** Standardised mortality tables giving 178 causes of death for males and females are given for Denmark by quinquennial periods for the period 1901 to 1975 in *International Mortality Statistics* (Alderson, 1981, tabs. 1–178, pp. 113–477).[3] Annotated estimates for decennial death rates for Denmark by cause of death for the period 1801 to 1901 are published in *Statistique générale de la France* (France, Bureau de la Statistique Générale; appendix, pp. 83–594). Annual totals and crude mortality rates of deaths from infectious diseases for Denmark for the years 1939 through 1946 are reported in *Annual Epidemiological and Vital Statistics 1939–1946* (WHO (1952), part II, tab. 23, p. 52) and for the capital city of Copenhagen for ten infectious diseases (tabs. 48–57, pp. 88–108). Trends in mortality in Denmark are discussed in *Expectations of Life* (Lancaster, 1990, p. 402). Mortality data for Denmark with causes of deaths classified by age, sex, and ICD code are available on computer tape from WHO for the forty-two years between 1951 and 1992 (WHO (1994), Annex I). **(c) Sources of population data:** The first census for Denmark was held in 1769 (*Folketaellingen 15. August 1769*). Subsequent censuses were conducted in 1787, 1801–34, 1837, 1840(5)1860, 1870(10)1890, 1901(5)1921, 1925(5)1960. A full listing appears in the *International Population Census Bibliography, No. 6, Europe* (University of Texas, 1967c, pp. 7.1–7.11). Population estimates for Denmark by age (five-year groups up to age eighty), sex, and quinquennia for the period 1901 to 1975 are given in *International Mortality Statistics* (Alderson, 1981, tab. 180, p. 491).

ECUADOR. WHO American Region (AMR). Area: 104,510 miles². Population: 11.8 million (1995). **(a) Sources of morbidity data:** Reported cases of notifiable infectious diseases are regularly reported in *Boletim epidemiologico semanal* (weekly). Annual information on the incidence and immunisation coverage of eight vaccine-preventable diseases (diphtheria, measles, pertussis, poliomyelitis, tetanus, neonatal tetanus, tuberculosis, and yellow fever) from 1974 is given in the *Information System Summary Volume, WHO American Region* (WHO, Expanded Programme on Immunization (EPI), Geneva, annual). **(b) Sources of mortality data:** Mortality data for Ecuador with causes of deaths classified by age, sex, and ICD code are available on computer tape from WHO for the twenty-eight years between 1961 and 1990 (WHO (1994), Annex I). **(c) Sources of population data:** The first census for Ecuador was held in 1825. The data were included in a report to the Colombian Congress of 1827 (Ecuador was not separated from Colombia until 1832), entitled *Memoria, esposición que el secretario de estado del despacho ... al Congreso de 1827*. Subsequent censuses were conducted in 1861, 1906, 1950, 1962. Full details are given in *International Population Census Bibliography, No. 1, Latin America and the Caribbean* (University of Texas, 1965a, pp. 15.1–15.4).

EGYPT. WHO Eastern Mediterranean Region (EMR). Area: 386,198 miles². Population: 58.5 million (1995). **(a) Sources of morbidity data:** Reported cases of notifiable infectious diseases are regularly reported in *Newsletter* (monthly). Annual information on the incidence and immunisation coverage of eight vaccine-preventable diseases (diphtheria, measles, pertussis, poliomyelitis, tetanus, neonatal tetanus, tuberculosis, and yellow fever) from 1974 is given in the *Information System Summary Volume, WHO Eastern Mediterranean Region* (WHO, Expanded Programme on Immunization (EPI), Geneva, annual). **(b) Sources of mortality data:** Annual totals and crude mortality rates of deaths from infectious diseases for Egypt for the years 1939 through 1946 are reported in *Annual Epidemiological and Vital Statistics 1939–1946* (WHO (1952), part II, tab. 9, p. 38) and for the cities of Alexandria and Cairo for ten infectious diseases (tabs. 48–57, pp. 88–108). Mortality data for Egypt with causes of deaths classified by age, sex, and ICD code are available on computer tape from WHO for the twenty-six years between 1954 and 1987 (WHO (1994), Annex I). **(c) Sources of population data:** The first census was taken in 1882. Subsequent censuses were taken in 1897(10)1957, 1960. Full details are given in *International Population Census Bibliography, No. 2, Africa* (University of Texas, 1965b, pp. 56.1–56.4).

EIRE. *See* Ireland.

ENGLAND AND WALES. WHO European Region (EUR). Constituent part of the United Kingdom of Great Britain and Northern Ireland. Area: 58,825 miles². Population: 51.6 million (1995). **(a) Sources of morbidity data:** Reported cases of notifiable infectious diseases are regularly reported in *CDR, Communicable Diseases Report* (weekly); *OPCS Monitor* (quarterly). Annual information on the incidence and immunisation coverage of eight vaccine-preventable diseases (diphtheria, measles, pertussis, poliomyelitis, tetanus, neonatal tetanus, tuberculosis, and yellow fever) from 1974 is given in the *Information System Summary Volume, WHO European Region* (WHO, Expanded Programme on Immunization (EPI),

Geneva, annual). **(b) Sources of mortality data:** Standardised mortality tables giving 178 causes of death for males and females are given for England and Wales by quinquennial periods for the period 1901 to 1975 in *International Mortality Statistics* (Alderson, 1981, tabs. 1–178, pp. 113–477). Mortality data for the United Kingdom with causes of deaths classified by age, sex, and ICD code are available on computer tape from WHO for the forty-three years between 1950 and 1992 (WHO (1994), Annex I).[4] Annotated estimates of decennial death rates for England and Wales by cause of death for the period 1841 to 1901 are published in *Statistique générale de la France* (France, Bureau de la Statistique Générale; appendix, pp. 83–594). Annual totals and crude mortality rates of deaths from infectious diseases for England and Wales for the years 1939 through 1946 are reported in *Annual Epidemiological and Vital Statistics 1939–1946* (WHO (1952), part II, tab. 34, p. 63) and for the four cities of Birmingham, Cardiff, Liverpool, and London for ten infectious diseases (tabs. 48–57, pp. 88–108). Trends in mortality in England and Wales are discussed in *Expectations of Life* (Lancaster, 1990, pp. 373–81). Mortality data for England and Wales with causes of deaths classified by age, sex, and ICD code are available on computer tape from WHO for the forty-three years between 1950 and 1992 (WHO (1994), Annex I). **(c) Sources of population data:** The first census for England and Wales was held in 1801 (*Abstract of Answers and Returns Made Pursuant to an Act, Passed in the Forty-first Year of His Majesty King George III Entitled 'An Act for Taking an Account of the Population of Great Britain, and the Increase or Diminution Thereof'. Enumeration, Part I, England*). Subsequent censuses were conducted in 1811(10)1931, 1951, 1961. A full listing appears in the *International Population Census Bibliography, No. 6, Europe* (University of Texas, 1967c, pp. 8.1–8.20). Population estimates for England and Wales by age (five-year groups up to age eighty), sex, and quinquennia for the period 1901 to 1975 are given in *International Mortality Statistics* (Alderson, 1981, tab. 180, p. 510).

FRANCE. *La Republique Française.* WHO European Region (EUR). Area: 211,208 miles[2]. Population: 57.8 million (1995). **(a) Sources of morbidity data:** Reported cases of notifiable infectious diseases are regularly reported in *BEH, Bulletin épidémiologique hebdomadaire* (weekly). Annual information on the incidence and immunisation coverage of eight vaccine-preventable diseases (diphtheria, measles, pertussis, poliomyelitis, tetanus, neonatal tetanus, tuberculosis, and yellow fever) from 1974 is given in the *Information System Summary Volume, WHO European Region* (WHO, Expanded Programme on Immunization (EPI), Geneva, annual). **(b) Sources of mortality data:** Standardised mortality tables giving 178 causes of death for males and females are given for France by quinquennial periods for the period 1901 to 1975 in *International Mortality Statistics* (Alderson, 1981, tabs. 1–178, pp. 113–477).[5] Annotated estimates for decennial death rates for France by cause of death for the period 1811 to 1901 are published in *Statistique générale de la France* (France, Bureau de la Statistique Générale; appendix, pp. 83–594). Annual totals and crude mortality rates of deaths from infectious diseases for France for the years 1939 through 1946 are reported in *Annual Epidemiological and Vital Statistics 1939–1946* (WHO (1952), part II, tab. 26, p. 55) and for the cities of Lyon and Paris for ten infectious diseases (tabs. 48–57, pp. 88–108). Trends in mortality in France are discussed in *Expectations of Life* (Lancaster,

1990, pp. 388–93). Mortality data for France with causes of deaths classified by age, sex, and ICD code are available on computer tape from WHO for the forty-two years between 1950 and 1991 (WHO (1994), Annex I). **(c) Sources of population data:** The first census for France was held in 1831. Subsequent censuses were conducted in 1846(5)1866 (*Dénombrements des années 1841, 1846, et 1851*, etc.), 1872, 1876(5)1911, 1921(5)1936, 1946, 1950, 1951, 1954, 1962. A full listing appears in the *International Population Census Bibliography, No. 6, Europe* (University of Texas, 1967c, pp. 11.1–11.28). Population estimates for France by age (five-year groups up to age eighty), sex, and quinquennia for the period 1901 to 1975 are given in *International Mortality Statistics* (Alderson, 1981, tab. 180, p. 494).

GERMANY. *Bundesrepublik Deutschland*. WHO European Region (EUR). Area: 138,000 miles^2. Population: 81.3 million (1995). From 1990 unified from the German Democratic Republic (East Germany) and the German Federal Republic (West Germany). **(a) Sources of morbidity data:** Reported cases of notifiable infectious diseases in the German Democratic Republic were regularly reported in *Übersicht Ausgewahller Meldep . . .* (weekly) and in the German Federal Republic in *Bundesgesundheitsblatt* (monthly). Annual information on the incidence and immunisation coverage of eight vaccine-preventable diseases (diphtheria, measles, pertussis, poliomyelitis, tetanus, neonatal tetanus, tuberculosis, and yellow fever) from 1974 is given in the *Information System Summary Volume, WHO European Region* (WHO, Expanded Programme on Immunization (EPI), Geneva, annual). **(b) Sources of mortality data:** Mortality data for the German Democratic Republic with causes of deaths classified by age, sex, and ICD code are available on computer tape from WHO for the twenty-one years between 1969 and 1990 and for the German Federal Republic for the thirty-nine years between 1952 and 1990 (WHO (1994), Annex I). Annotated estimates for decennial death rates for Germany by cause of death for the period 1841 to 1901 (and for the states of Bavaria 1831–1901, Prussia 1821–1901, and Saxony 1831–1901) are published in *Statistique générale de la France* (France, Bureau de la Statistique Générale; appendix, pp. 83–594). Trends in mortality in Germany are discussed in *Expectations of Life* (Lancaster, 1990, p. 393). Mortality data for Germany with causes of deaths classified by age, sex, and ICD code are available on computer tape from WHO for the two years between 1990 and 1991 (WHO (1994), Annex I). **(c) Sources of population data:** The first census for Germany was held in 1821. Subsequent censuses were conducted in 1831, 1832, 1834, 1837, 1840, 1843, 1846, 1849, 1852, 1858, 1861, 1864, 1867, 1871, 1875, 1880(5)1910, 1919, 1925, 1933, 1935, 1939, 1945, 1946, 1950, 1951, 1961, 1964. A full listing appears in the *International Population Census Bibliography, No. 6, Europe* (University of Texas, 1967c, pp. 12.1–12.78).

GREAT BRITAIN. *See* England and Wales, Northern Ireland, and Scotland.

GREECE. *Elliniki Dimokratia*. WHO European Region (EUR). Area: 50,994 miles^2. Population: 10.3 million (1995). **(a) Sources of morbidity data:** Reported cases of notifiable infectious diseases are regularly reported in *Bulletin of Repo. Cases of Infectious Diseases* (monthly). Annual information on the incidence and immunisation coverage of eight vaccine-preventable diseases (diphtheria, measles, pertussis, poliomyelitis, tetanus, neonatal tetanus, tuberculosis, and yellow fever) from 1974 is given in the *Information System Summary Volume, WHO European Region* (WHO, Expanded Programme on Immunization (EPI), Geneva, annual). **(b) Sources of mortality data:** Standardised mortality tables giving 178 causes of death for males and females are given for Greece by quinquennial periods for the period 1921 to 1975 in *International Mortality Statistics* (Alderson, 1981, tabs. 1–178, pp. 113–477). Mortality data for Greece with causes of deaths classified by age, sex, and ICD code are available on computer tape from WHO for the thirty-six years between 1956 and 1991 (WHO (1994), Annex I). **(c) Sources of population data:** The first census for Greece was held in 1828. The results were published on p. 211 of Mansolas (1867), *Renseignements statistiques sur l'Etat de la Grèce.* Subsequent censuses were conducted in 1838–45, 1853, 1856, 1861, 1870, 1879, 1889, 1896, 1907, 1913, 1920, 1923, 1928, 1936, 1940, 1947, 1951, 1961. A full listing appears in the *International Population Census Bibliography, No. 6, Europe* (University of Texas, 1967c, pp. 14.1–14.12). Population estimates for Greece by age (five-year groups up to age eighty), sex, and quinquennia for the period 1921 to 1975 are given in *International Mortality Statistics* (Alderson, 1981, tab. 180, p. 495).

HAITI. WHO American Region (AMR). Area: 10,850 miles^2. Population: 7.2 million (1995). **(a) Sources of morbidity data:** Reported cases of notifiable infectious diseases are regularly reported in *Rapport heb. des maladies transm.* (weekly). Annual information on the incidence and immunisation coverage of eight vaccine-preventable diseases (diphtheria, measles, pertussis, poliomyelitis, tetanus, neonatal tctanus, tuberculosis, and yellow fever) from 1974 is given in the *Information System Summary Volume, WHO American Region* (WHO, Expanded Programme on Immunization (EPI), Geneva, annual). **(b) Sources of mortality data:** Mortality data for Haiti with causes of deaths classified by age, sex, and ICD code are available on computer tape from WHO for the three years between 1980 and 1983 (WHO (1994), Annex I). **(c) Sources of population data:** The first census for Haiti was held in 1950 (*Recensement général de la Republique d'Haiti: août 1950*). Full details are given in *International Population Census Bibliography, No. 1, Latin America and the Caribbean* (University of Texas, 1965a, p. 21.1).

HOLLAND. *See* Netherlands.

HUNGARY. *Magyar Koztarsasag.* WHO European Region (EUR). Area: 35,920 miles^2. Population: 10.5 million (1995). **(a) Sources of morbidity data:** Reported cases of notifiable infectious diseases are regularly reported in *Notified Diseases – Half Yearly* (half yearly). Annual information on the incidence and immunisation coverage of eight vaccine-preventable diseases (diphtheria, measles, pertussis, poliomyelitis, tetanus, neonatal tetanus, tuberculosis, and yellow fever) from 1974 is given in the *Information System Summary Volume, WHO European Region* (WHO, Expanded Programme on Immunization (EPI), Geneva, annual). **(b) Sources of mortality data:** Standardised mortality tables giving 178 causes of death for males and females are given for Hungary by quinquennial periods for the period 1916 to 1975 in *International Mortality Statistics* (Alderson, 1981, tabs. 1–178, pp. 113–477).[6] Annotated estimates for decennial death rates for Hungary by cause of death for the period 1871 to 1901 are published in *Statistique générale de la France* (France, Bureau de la Statistique Générale; appendix, pp. 83–594). Trends in mortality in Hungary are discussed in *Expectations of Life* (Lancaster,

1990, p. 393). Mortality data for Hungary with causes of deaths classified by age, sex, and ICD code are available on computer tape from WHO for the forty-eight years between 1955 and 1992 (WHO (1994), Annex I). **(c) Sources of population data:** The first census for Hungary was held in 1784–7 (*Az elsõ Magyarországi Népszámlálás, 1784–1787*). Subsequent censuses were conducted in 1851–5, 1857, 1870, 1881, 1891, 1893, 1900, 1910, 1917, 1920, 1930, 1938, 1941, 1949, 1960. City censuses for Budapest are available from 1857 and regional censuses from 1880. A full listing appears in the *International Population Census Bibliography, No. 6, Europe* (University of Texas, 1967c, pp. 15.1–15.20). Population estimates for Hungary by age (five-year groups up to age eighty), sex, and quinquennia for the period 1916 to 1975 are given in *International Mortality Statistics* (Alderson, 1981, tab. 180, p. 496).

INDIA. WHO South East Asia Region (SEAR). Area: 1,581,410 miles². Population 931.0 million (1995). **(a) Sources of morbidity data:** Reported cases of notifiable infectious diseases are regularly reported in *Epidemiological Bulletin Quarterly* (quarterly); *Weekly Epidemiological Report (Cholera Only)* (weekly). Annual information on the incidence and immunisation coverage of eight vaccine-preventable diseases (diphtheria, measles, pertussis, poliomyelitis, tetanus, neonatal tetanus, tuberculosis, and yellow fever) from 1974 is given in the *Information System Summary Volume, WHO South East Asian Region* (WHO, Expanded Programme on Immunization (EPI), Geneva, annual). **(b) Sources of mortality data:** Trends in mortality in India are discussed in *Expectations of Life* (Lancaster, 1990, pp. 412–13). **(c) Sources of population data:** The first census for India was held in 1872 (*Census of India 1872*). Subsequent censuses were conducted in 1881(10)1961. A full listing appears in the *International Population Census Bibliography, No. 5, Asia* (University of Texas, 1967b, pp. 14.1–14.108).

IRELAND (for the period after partition in 1922, see also Northern Ireland). *Republic of Ireland (Poblacht Na hEireann)*. WHO European Region (EUR). Area: 27,136 miles². Population: 3.5 million (1995). **(a) Sources of morbidity data:** Reported cases of notifiable infectious diseases are regularly reported in *Infectious Disease Monitoring* (weekly and quarterly). Annual information on the incidence and immunisation coverage of eight vaccine-preventable diseases (diphtheria, measles, pertussis, poliomyelitis, tetanus, neonatal tetanus, tuberculosis, and yellow fever) from 1974 is given in the *Information System Summary Volume, WHO European Region* (WHO, Expanded Programme on Immunization (EPI), Geneva, annual). **(b) Sources of mortality data:** Standardised mortality tables giving 178 causes of death for males and females are given for Ireland by quinquennial periods for the period 1921 to 1975 in *International Mortality Statistics* (Alderson, 1981, tabs. 1–178, pp. 113–477).[7] Annotated estimates for decennial death rates for Ireland by cause of death for the period 1861 to 1901 are published in *Statistique générale de la France* (France, Bureau de la Statistique Générale; appendix, pp. 83–594). Annual totals and crude mortality rates of deaths from infectious diseases for Ireland for the years 1939 through 1946 are reported in *Annual Epidemiological and Vital Statistics 1939–1946* (WHO (1952), part II, tab. 27, p. 56) and for the capital city of Dublin for ten infectious diseases (tabs. 48–57, pp. 88–108). Trends in mortality in Ireland are discussed in *Expectations of Life* (Lancaster, 1990, pp. 385–7). Mortality data for Ireland with causes of deaths classified by age, sex, and ICD code are available on computer tape from WHO for the forty-two years between 1950 and 1991 (WHO (1994), Annex I). **(c) Sources of population data:** The first census for Ireland was held in 1659 (*A Census of Ireland, Circa 1659 with Supplementary Material from the Poll Money Ordinances (1660–1661)*). Subsequent censuses were conducted in 1821(10)1911, 1926, 1936(5)1961. A full listing appears in the *International Population Census Bibliography, No. 6, Europe* (University of Texas, 1967c, pp. 17.1–17.14). Population estimates for Ireland by age (five-year groups up to age eighty), sex, and quinquennia for the period 1921 to 1975 are given in *International Mortality Statistics* (Alderson, 1981, tab. 180, p. 492).

ITALY. *Repubblica Italiana*. WHO European Region (EUR). Area: 116,304 miles². Population: 57.9 million (1995). Separate states until unification in 1870; small territorial adjustments in northern Italy in present century. **(a) Sources of morbidity data:** Reported cases of notifiable infectious diseases are regularly reported in *BEN, Bolletino epidemiologico nazionale* (monthly). Annual information on the incidence and immunisation coverage of eight vaccine-preventable diseases (diphtheria, measles, pertussis, poliomyelitis, tetanus, neonatal tetanus, tuberculosis, and yellow fever) from 1974 is given in the *Information System Summary Volume, WHO European Region* (WHO, Expanded Programme on Immunization (EPI), Geneva, annual). **(b) Sources of mortality data:** Standardised mortality tables giving 178 causes of death for males and females are given for Italy by quinquennial periods for the period 1901 to 1975 in *International Mortality Statistics* (Alderson, 1981, tabs. 1–178, pp. 113–477). Annotated estimates for decennial death rates for Italy by cause of death for the period 1871 to 1901 are published in *Statistique générale de la France* (France, Bureau de la Statistique Générale; appendix, pp. 83–594). Annual totals and crude mortality rates of deaths from infectious diseases for Italy for the years 1939 through 1946 are reported in *Annual Epidemiological and Vital Statistics 1939–1946* (WHO (1952), part II, tab. 29, p. 58) and for the four cities of Milan, Naples, Palermo, and Rome for ten infectious diseases (tabs. 48–57, pp. 88–108). Trends in mortality in Italy are discussed in *Expectations of Life* (Lancaster, 1990, p. 393). Mortality data for Italy with causes of deaths classified by age, sex, and ICD code are available on computer tape from WHO for the forty years between 1951 and 1990 (WHO (1994), Annex I). **(c) Sources of population data:** The first full population census for Italy was held in 1838. Subsequent censuses were conducted in 1846, 1857–8, 1861, 1871, 1881, 1901, 1911, 1921, 1930, 1931, 1936, 1944, 1951, 1961. Early state censuses, for example for Milano (1774), Mantova, Parma, Stati Estensi, Stati Pontifico e Roma, Ducato di Toscana and Trieste, are also available. A full listing appears in the *International Population Census Bibliography, No. 6, Europe* (University of Texas, 1967c, pp. 18.1–18.33). Population estimates for Italy by age (five-year groups up to age eighty), sex, and quinquennia for the period 1901 to 1975 are given in *International Mortality Statistics* (Alderson, 1981, tab. 180, p. 488).

JAPAN. WHO Western Pacific Region (WPR). Area: 142,007 miles². Population: 125.9 million (1995). **(a) Sources of morbidity data:** Reported cases of notifiable infectious diseases are regularly reported in *Monthly Report of Communicable Diseases* (monthly). Annual information on the incidence and immunisation coverage of eight vaccine-preventable diseases (diphtheria, measles, pertussis, poliomyelitis, tetanus, neonatal tetanus, tuberculosis, and yellow fever) from 1974 is given in the *Information System Summary Volume, WHO Western Pacific Region* (WHO, Expanded Programme on Immunization (EPI), Geneva, annual). **(b) Sources of mortality data:** Standardised mortality tables giving 178 causes of death for males and females are given for Japan by quinquennial periods for the period 1901 to 1975 in *International Mortality Statistics* (Alderson, 1981, tabs. 1–178, pp. 113–477). Annual totals and crude mortality rates of deaths from infectious diseases for Japan for the years 1939 through 1946 are reported in *Annual Epidemiological and Vital Statistics 1939–1946* (WHO (1952), part II, tab. 19, p. 48). Trends in mortality in Japan are discussed in *Expectations of Life* (Lancaster, 1990, pp. 410–12). Mortality data for Japan with causes of deaths classified by age, sex, and ICD code are available on computer tape from WHO for the forty-three years between 1950 and 1992 (WHO (1994), Annex I). **(c) Sources of population data:** Although rough counts of families were taken between 1721 and 1850, the first full census occurred in 1872 (*Meiji 5 nen (1872) Nihon Zenkoku Koseki-hyô – Table of Household Registration for All Japan*). Subsequent censuses were conducted in 1873(1)1898, 1903(5)1918, 1920, 1930, 1935, 1940, 1944(1)1948, 1950, 1954, 1955, 1960, 1965. A full listing appears in the *International Population Census Bibliography, No. 5, Asia* (University of Texas, 1967b, pp. 19.1–19.42). Population estimates for Japan by age (five-year groups up to age eighty), sex, and quinquennia for the period 1901 to 1975 are given in *International Mortality Statistics* (Alderson, 1981, tab. 180, p. 499).

MALAYA. *See* Malaysia

MALAYSIA. WHO Western Pacific Region (WPR). Area: 50,841 miles². Population: 20.1 million (1995). **(a) Sources of morbidity data:** Reported cases of notifiable infectious diseases are regularly reported in *Weekly Epidemiological Record* (weekly). Annual information on the incidence and immunisation coverage of eight vaccine-preventable diseases (diphtheria, measles, pertussis, poliomyelitis, tetanus, neonatal tetanus, tuberculosis, and yellow fever) from 1974 is given in the *Information System Summary Volume, WHO Western Pacific Region* (WHO, Expanded Programme on Immunization (EPI), Geneva, annual). **(b) Sources of mortality data:** Mortality data for Malaysia with causes of deaths classified by age, sex, and ICD code are available on computer tape from WHO for the three years between 1977 and 1979 (WHO (1994), Annex I). **(c) Sources of population data:** The first census, for Sarawak, was held in 1871 (*Sarawak Gazette*). Subsequent censuses were conducted in 1891 (British North Borneo and Labnan), 1901 (the first full census of the Federated Malay States, published as *Census of the Population, 1901*), 1909, 1911(10)1931, 1947, 1957, 1960. A full listing appears in the *International Population Census Bibliography, No. 5, Asia* (University of Texas, 1967b, pp. 27.1–27.6).

MEXICO. WHO American Region (AMR). Area: 763,944 miles². Population: 93.7 million (1995). **(a) Sources of morbidity data:** Reported cases of notifiable infectious diseases are regularly reported in *Epidemiologia bol. mensual* (monthly). Annual information on the incidence and immunisation coverage of eight vaccine-preventable diseases (diphtheria, measles, pertussis, poliomyelitis, tetanus, neonatal tetanus, tuberculosis, and yellow fever) from 1974 is given in the *Information System Summary Volume, WHO American Region* (WHO, Expanded

Programme on Immunization (EPI), Geneva, annual). **(b) Sources of mortality data:** Annual totals and crude mortality rates of deaths from infectious diseases for Mexico for the years 1939 through 1946 are reported in *Annual Epidemiological and Vital Statistics 1939–1946* (WHO (1952), part II, tab. 15, p. 44) and for the two cities of Guadalajara and Mexico City for ten infectious diseases (tabs. 48–57, pp. 88–108). Mortality data for Mexico with causes of deaths classified by age, sex, and ICD code are available on computer tape from WHO for the thirty-seven years between 1955 and 1991 (WHO (1994), Annex I). **(c) Sources of population data:** The first national census for Mexico was held in 1895 (*Censo general de la República Mexicana verificado el 20 de octubre de 1895*). Subsequent censuses were conducted in 1900, 1910, 1921, 1930(10)1960. Full details are given in *International Population Census Bibliography, No. 1, Latin America and the Caribbean* (University of Texas, 1965a, pp. 26.1–26.21).

MYANMAR. WHO South East Asia Region (SEAR). Area: 261,610 miles^2. Population: 46.6 million (1995). **(a) Sources of morbidity data:** Annual information on the incidence and immunisation coverage of eight vaccine-preventable diseases (diphtheria, measles, pertussis, poliomyelitis, tetanus, neonatal tetanus, tuberculosis, and yellow fever) from 1974 is given in the *Information System Summary Volume, WHO South East Asian Region* (WHO, Expanded Programme on Immunization (EPI), Geneva, annual). **(b) Sources of mortality data:** Mortality data for Myanmar with causes of deaths classified by age, sex, and ICD code are available on computer tape from WHO for the two years between 1977 and 1978 (WHO (1994), Annex I). **(c) Sources of population data:** The first census of Burma was held in 1872 (*Report on the Census of British Burma Taken in August 1872*). Subsequent censuses were conducted in 1881(10)1941, 1953, 1954. The censuses between 1872 and 1931 were combined with those of India. A full listing appears in the *International Population Census Bibliography, No. 5, Asia* (University of Texas, 1967b, pp. 7.1–7.4).

NETHERLANDS. *Koninkrijk der Nederlanden.* WHO European Region (EUR). Area: 13,433 miles^2. Population: 15.5 million (1995). **(a) Sources of morbidity data:** Cases of notifiable infectious diseases are regularly reported in *Maambericht Gezondheisstatstiek* (monthly); *Staatstoezicht op Fe volgesondheid* (monthly). Annual information on the incidence and immunisation coverage of eight vaccine-preventable diseases (diphtheria, measles, pertussis, poliomyelitis, tetanus, neonatal tetanus, tuberculosis, and yellow fever) from 1974 is given in the *Information System Summary Volume, WHO European Region* (WHO, Expanded Programme on Immunization (EPI), Geneva, annual). **(b) Sources of mortality data:** Standardised mortality tables showing 178 causes of death for males and females are given for the Netherlands by quinquennial periods for the period 1901 to 1975 in *International Mortality Statistics* (Alderson, 1981, tabs. 1–178, pp. 113–477).[8] Annotated estimates for decennial death rates for the Netherlands by cause of death for the period 1841 to 1901 are published in *Statistique générale de la France* (France, Bureau de la Statistique Générale; appendix, pp. 83–594). Annual totals and crude mortality rates of deaths from infectious diseases for the Netherlands for the years 1939 through 1946 are reported in *Annual Epidemiological and Vital Statistics 1939–1946* (WHO (1952), part II, tab. 32, p. 61). Trends in mortality in the Netherlands are discussed in *Expectations of Life*

(Lancaster, 1990, p. 395). Mortality data for the Netherlands with causes of deaths classified by age, sex, and ICD code are available on computer tape from WHO for the forty-two years between 1950 and 1991 (WHO (1994), Annex I). **(c) Sources of population data:** The first census for the Netherlands was held in 1795. Subsequent censuses were conducted in 1830, 1840, 1849(10)1909, 1920, 1930, 1947, 1960. A full listing appears in the *International Population Census Bibliography, No. 6, Europe* (University of Texas, 1967c, pp. 23.1–23.15). Population estimates for the Netherlands by age (five-year groups up to age eighty), sex, and quinquennia for the period 1901 to 1975 are given in *International Mortality Statistics* (Alderson, 1981, tab. 180, p. 500).

NORTHERN IRELAND (for the period prior to partition in 1922, see Ireland). Constituent part of the United Kingdom of Great Britain and Northern Ireland. WHO European Region (EUR). Area: 5,238 miles². Population: 1.6 million (1995). Separate identity within the United Kingdom since 1921. **(a) Sources of morbidity data:** Reported cases of notifiable infectious diseases are regularly reported in *Communicable Diseases N. Ireland* (monthly); *Return of Infectious Diseases Notified* (quarterly). Annual information on the incidence and immunisation coverage of eight vaccine-preventable diseases (diphtheria, measles, pertussis, poliomyelitis, tetanus, neonatal tetanus, tuberculosis, and yellow fever) from 1974 is given in the *Information System Summary Volume, WHO European Region* (WHO, Expanded Programme on Immunization (EPI), Geneva, annual). **(b) Sources of mortality data:** Standardised mortality tables giving 178 causes of death for males and females are given for Northern Ireland by quinquennial periods for the period 1921 to 1975 in *International Mortality Statistics* (Alderson, 1981, tabs. 1–178, pp. 113–477).[9] Annual totals and crude mortality rates of deaths from infectious diseases for Northern Ireland for the years 1939 through 1946 are reported in *Annual Epidemiological and Vital Statistics 1939–1946* (WHO (1952), part II, tab. 36, p. 65) and for the city of Belfast for ten infectious diseases (tabs. 48–57, pp. 88–108). Trends in mortality in Northern Ireland are discussed in *Expectations of Life* (Lancaster, 1990, p. 385). Mortality data for Northern Ireland with causes of deaths classified by age, sex, and ICD code are available on computer tape from WHO for the forty-three years between 1950 and 1992 (WHO (1994), Annex I). **(c) Sources of population data:** The first census in Northern Ireland was held in 1659 (*A Census of Ireland, Circa 1659 with Supplementary Material from the Poll Money Ordinances, 1660–1661*). Subsequent censuses were conducted in 1821(10)1911, 1926, 1937, 1939, 1951, 1960. A full listing appears in the *International Population Census Bibliography, No. 6, Europe* (University of Texas, 1967c, pp. 24.1–24.12). Population estimates for Northern Ireland by age (five-year groups up to age eighty), sex, and quinquennia for the period 1921 to 1975 are given in *International Mortality Statistics* (Alderson, 1981, tab. 180, p. 511).

NORWAY. *Kongeriket Norge*. WHO European Region (EUR). Area: 149,300 miles². Population: 4.4 million (1995). Sweden and Norway united from 1815 until 1905. **(a) Sources of morbidity data:** Reported cases of notifiable infectious diseases are regularly reported in *SIFF–MSIS* (weekly); *Notified Cases of Communicable Diseases* (monthly). Annual information on the incidence and immunisation coverage of eight vaccine-preventable diseases (diphtheria, measles, pertussis, poliomyelitis, tetanus, neonatal tetanus, tuberculosis, and yellow fever) from 1974 is given in the *Information System Summary Volume, WHO European Region* (WHO, Expanded Programme on Immunization (EPI), Geneva, annual). **(b) Sources of mortality data:** Standardised mortality tables giving 178 causes of death for males and females are given for Norway by quinquennial periods for the period 1901 to 1975 in *International Mortality Statistics* (Alderson, 1981, tabs. 1–178, pp. 113–477). Annotated estimates for decennial death rates for Norway by cause of death for the period 1801 to 1901 are published in *Statistique générale de la France* (France, Bureau de la Statistique Générale; appendix, pp. 83–594). Annual totals and crude mortality rates of deaths from infectious diseases for Norway for the years 1939 through 1946 are reported in *Annual Epidemiological and Vital Statistics 1939–1946* (WHO (1952), part II, tab. 31, p. 60) and for the capital city of Oslo for ten infectious diseases (tabs. 48–57, pp. 88–108). Trends in mortality in Norway are discussed in *Expectations of Life* (Lancaster, 1990, pp. 400–2). Mortality data for Norway with causes of deaths classified by age, sex, and ICD code are available on computer tape from WHO for the forty-one years between 1951 and 1991 (WHO (1994), Annex I). **(c) Sources of population data:** The first census for Norway was held in 1769 (*The Census of Population in Norway, August 15th, 1769*). Subsequent censuses were conducted in 1801, 1815(10)1835, 1855, 1866, 1876, 1885, 1891, 1900(10)1930, 1946, 1950, 1960. A full listing appears in the *International Population Census Bibliography, No. 6, Europe* (University of Texas, 1967c, pp. 25.1–25.12). Population estimates for Norway by age (five-year groups up to age eighty), sex, and quinquennia for the period 1901 to 1975 are given in *International Mortality Statistics* (Alderson, 1981, tab. 180, p. 502).

POLAND (see also Russia). *Rzeczpospolita Polska.* WHO European Region (EUR). Area: 120,700 miles². Population: 38.7 million (1995). Poland emerged as an independent country (from Russia) in 1919 but boundaries were redrawn in 1920–1 and shifted again in 1945. **(a) Sources of morbidity data:** Reported cases of notifiable infectious diseases are regularly reported in *Informations épidemiologiques* (half-yearly). Annual information on the incidence and immunisation coverage of eight vaccine-preventable diseases (diphtheria, measles, pertussis, poliomyelitis, tetanus, neonatal tetanus, tuberculosis, and yellow fever) from 1974 is given in the *Information System Summary Volume, WHO European Region* (WHO, Expanded Programme on Immunization (EPI), Geneva, annual). **(b) Sources of mortality data:** Standardised mortality tables giving 178 causes of death for males and females are given for Poland by quinquennial periods for the period 1951 to 1975 in *International Mortality Statistics* (Alderson, 1981, tabs. 1–178, pp. 113–477). Mortality data for Poland with causes of deaths classified by age, sex, and ICD code are available on computer tape from WHO for the thirty-four years between 1959 and 1992 (WHO (1994), Annex I). **(c) Sources of population data:** The first census for Poland was held in 1897 as part of *The First General Census of the Russian Empire, 1897.* Subsequent censuses were conducted in 1921 (the first general census of Poland), 1931, 1946, 1950, 1960. City censuses for Danzig (Gdansk) were held from 1923, and for Gdynia in 1936. A full listing appears in the *International Population Census Bibliography, No. 6, Europe* (University of Texas, 1967c, pp. 26.1–26.18). Population estimates for Poland by age (five-year groups up to age eighty), sex, and quinquennia for the period 1951 to 1975 are given in *International Mortality Statistics* (Alderson, 1981, tab. 180, p. 503).

RUSSIA (see also Poland). *Rossiiskaya Federatsiya, Russian Federation.* WHO European Region (EUR). Area: 6,593,000 miles². Population: 149.7 million (1995). Former Russian Soviet Federal Socialist Republic within the Soviet Union; since 1991 the major member of the Commonwealth of Independent States (CIS). **(a) Sources of morbidity data:** Annual information on the incidence and immunisation coverage of eight vaccine-preventable diseases (diphtheria, measles, pertussis, poliomyelitis, tetanus, neonatal tetanus, tuberculosis, and yellow fever) from 1974 is given in the *Information System Summary Volume, WHO European Region* (WHO, Expanded Programme on Immunization (EPI), Geneva, annual). **(b) Sources of mortality data:** Trends in mortality in the Soviet Union are discussed in *Expectations of Life* (Lancaster, 1990, p. 395). Mortality data for parts of the former Soviet Union with causes of deaths classified by age, sex, and ICD code are available on computer tape from WHO for Armenia (1988–90), Belorus (1985–90), Kyrgyzstan (1981–90), Russian Federation (1988–91), and Ukraine (1985–90) (WHO (1994), Annex I). **(c) Sources of population data:** The first census for Russia was held in 1678–1721 (*The Population of Russia Under Peter the Great According to Censuses of That Time, 1678–1721*). Subsequent censuses were conducted in 1851, 1897, 1920, 1922, 1923, 1925, 1926, 1930, 1934, 1935, 1937, 1939, 1959. A full listing appears in the *International Population Census Bibliography, No. 6, Europe* (University of Texas, 1967c, pp. 34.1–34.8).

SCOTLAND. Constituent part of the United Kingdom of Great Britain and Northern Ireland. WHO European Region (EUR). Area: 29,794 miles². Population: 5.1 million (1995). **(a) Sources of morbidity data:** Reported cases of notifiable infectious diseases are regularly reported in *Vital Statistics Return* (every three weeks); *Communicable Diseases Scotland* (weekly). Annual information on the incidence and immunisation coverage of eight vaccine-preventable diseases (diphtheria, measles, pertussis, poliomyelitis, tetanus, neonatal tetanus, tuberculosis, and yellow fever) from 1974 is given in the *Information System Summary Volume, WHO European Region* (WHO, Expanded Programme on Immunization (EPI), Geneva, annual). **(b) Sources of mortality data:** Standardised mortality tables giving 178 causes of death for males and females are given for Scotland by quinquennial periods for the period 1901 to 1975 in *International Mortality Statistics* (Alderson, 1981, tabs. 1–178, pp. 113–477).[10] Annotated estimates for decennial death rates for Scotland by cause of death for the period 1851 to 1901 are published in *Statistique générale de la France* (France, Bureau de la Statistique Générale; appendix, pp. 83–594). Annual totals and crude mortality rates of deaths from infectious diseases for Scotland for the years 1939 through 1946 are reported in *Annual Epidemiological and Vital Statistics 1939–1946* (WHO (1952), part II, tab. 35, p. 64) and for the two cities of Edinburgh and Glasgow for ten infectious diseases (tabs. 48–57, pp. 88–108). Trends in mortality in Scotland are discussed in *Expectations of Life* (Lancaster, 1990, pp. 380–5). Mortality data for Scotland with causes of deaths classified by age, sex, and ICD code are available on computer tape from WHO for the forty-three years between 1950 and 1992 (WHO (1994), Annex I). **(c) Sources of population data:** The first census for

Scotland was held in 1801 (*Abstract of Answers and Returns Made Pursuant to an Act, Passed in the Forty-first year of His Majesty King George III Entitled 'An Act for Taking an Account of the Population of Great Britain, and the Increase or Diminution Thereof'. Enumeration, Part II, Scotland*). Subsequent censuses were conducted in 1811(10)1931, 1939, 1951, 1961. A full listing appears in the *International Population Census Bibliography, No. 6, Europe* (University of Texas, 1967c, pp. 30.1–30.14). Population estimates for Scotland by age (five-year groups up to age eighty), sex, and quinquennia for the period 1901 to 1975 are given in *International Mortality Statistics* (Alderson, 1981, tab. 180, p. 512).

SOUTH AFRICA. WHO African Region (AFR). Area: 472,550 miles^2. Population: 42.7 million (1995). **(a) Sources of morbidity data:** Reported cases of notifiable infectious diseases are regularly reported in *Health Statistics Monthly Bulletin* (monthly). Annual information on the incidence and immunisation coverage of eight vaccine-preventable diseases (diphtheria, measles, pertussis, poliomyelitis, tetanus, neonatal tetanus, tuberculosis, and yellow fever) from 1974 is given in the *Information System Summary Volume, WHO African Region* (WHO, Expanded Programme on Immunization (EPI), Geneva, annual). **(b) Sources of mortality data:** Annual totals and crude mortality rates of deaths from infectious diseases for South Africa for the years 1939 through 1946 are reported in *Annual Epidemiological and Vital Statistics 1939–1946* (WHO (1952), part II, tab. 11, p. 40) and for the cities of Cape Town, Johannesburg, and Pretoria for ten infectious diseases (tabs. 48–57, pp. 88–108). **(c) Sources of population data:** The first *Colonial censuses*, 'Cape of Good Hope' 1687–1785, 1823–56, 1865, 1875, 1891, 1904, *Natal*, 1891–, *Orange River Colony*, 1880, *Transvaal*, 1890, *Union census*, 1911 (*Census of the Union of South Africa, 1911: Annexures to General Report, Union of South Africa, 1911*), 1918, 1921(5)1951, 1960. Full details are given in *International Population Census Bibliography, No. 2, Africa* (University of Texas, 1965b, pp. 46.1–46.8).

SPAIN. *España*. WHO European Region (EUR). Area: 194,900 miles^2. Population: 39.3 million (1995). **(a) Sources of morbidity data:** Reported cases of notifiable infectious diseases are regularly reported in *Boletin microbiologico semanal* (weekly). Annual information on the incidence and immunisation coverage of eight vaccine-preventable diseases (diphtheria, measles, pertussis, poliomyelitis, tetanus, neonatal tetanus, tuberculosis, and yellow fever) from 1974 is given in the *Information System Summary Volume, WHO European Region* (WHO, Expanded Programme on Immunization (EPI), Geneva, annual). **(b) Sources of mortality data:** Standardised mortality tables giving 178 causes of death for males and females are given for Spain by quinquennial periods for the period 1901 to 1975 (incomplete series) in *International Mortality Statistics* (Alderson, 1981, tabs. 1–178, pp. 113–477).[11] Annotated estimates for decennial death rates for Spain by cause of death for the period 1861 to 1901 are published in *Statistique générale de la France* (France, Bureau de la Statistique Générale; appendix, pp. 83–594). Annual totals and crude mortality rates of deaths from infectious diseases for Spain for the years 1939 through 1946 are reported in *Annual Epidemiological and Vital Statistics 1939–1946* (WHO (1952), part II, tab. 24, p. 53) and for the three cities of Barcelona, Madrid, and Seville for ten infectious diseases (tabs. 48–57, pp. 88–108). Trends in mortality in Spain are discussed in *Expectations of Life*

(Lancaster, 1990, p. 395). Mortality data for Spain with causes of deaths classified by age, sex, and ICD code are available on computer tape from WHO for the forty years between 1951 and 1990 (WHO (1994), Annex I). **(c) Sources of population data:** The first census for Spain was held in 1787 (*Censo español ejecutado de orden del Rey, comunicada por el excmo. Sr. Conde de —, primer secretario de estado y del despacho, en el año 1787*). Subsequent censuses were conducted in 1797, 1857, 1860, 1877(10)1897, 1900(10)60. A full listing appears in the *International Population Census Bibliography, No. 6, Europe* (University of Texas, 1967c, pp. 31.1–31.12). Population estimates for Spain by age (five-year groups up to age eighty), sex, and quinquennia for the period 1901 to 1975 are given in *International Mortality Statistics* (Alderson, 1981, tab. 180, p. 506).

SRI LANKA. *Sri Lanka Prajatantrika Samajawadi*. WHO South East Asia Region (SEAR). Area: 25,330 miles². Population: 18.4 million (1995). **(a) Sources of morbidity data:** Reported cases of notifiable infectious diseases are regularly reported in *Weekly Epidemiological Report* (weekly). Annual information on the incidence and immunisation coverage of eight vaccine-preventable diseases (diphtheria, measles, pertussis, poliomyelitis, tetanus, neonatal tetanus, tuberculosis, and yellow fever) from 1974 is given in the *Information System Summary Volume, WHO South East Asian Region* (WHO, Expanded Programme on Immunization (EPI), Geneva, annual). **(b) Sources of mortality data:** Mortality data for Sri Lanka with causes of deaths classified by age, sex, and ICD code are available on computer tape from WHO for the twenty-seven years between 1950 and 1986 (WHO (1994), Annex I). Annual totals and crude mortality rates of deaths from infectious diseases for Ceylon for the years 1939 through 1946 are reported in *Annual Epidemiological and Vital Statistics 1939–1946* (WHO (1952), part II, tab. 18, p. 47) and for the city of Colombo for ten infectious diseases (tabs. 48–57, pp. 88–108). **(c) Sources of population data:** An early Dutch census was taken in 1789, while British censuses were conducted in 1814, 1821, 1824, 1827, 1871 (the first decennial census, published as *General Report 1871*), then every ten years until 1937, 1946, 1953. A full listing appears in the *International Population Census Bibliography, No. 5, Asia* (University of Texas, 1967b, pp. 9.1–9.5).

SWEDEN. *Konungariket Sverige*. WHO European Region (EUR). Area: 173,700 miles². Population: 8.8 million (1995). **(a) Sources of morbidity data:** Reported cases of notifiable infectious diseases are regularly reported in *Epid. Aktuellt* (weekly). Annual information on the incidence and immunisation coverage of eight vaccine-preventable diseases (diphtheria, measles, pertussis, poliomyelitis, tetanus, neonatal tetanus, tuberculosis, and yellow fever) from 1974 is given in the *Information System Summary Volume, WHO European Region* (WHO, Expanded Programme on Immunization (EPI), Geneva, annual). **(b) Sources of mortality data:** Standardised mortality tables giving 178 causes of death for males and females are given for Sweden by quinquennial periods for the period 1901 to 1975 in *International Mortality Statistics* (Alderson, 1981, tabs. 1–178, pp. 113–477). Annotated estimates for decennial death rates for Sweden by cause of death for the period 1801 to 1901 are published in *Statistique générale de la France* (France, Bureau de la Statistique Générale; appendix, pp. 83–594). Annual totals and crude mortality rates of deaths from infectious diseases for Sweden for the years 1939 through 1946 are reported in *Annual Epidemiological and Vital Statistics*

1939–1946 (WHO (1952), part II, tab. 37, p. 66) and for the two cities of Gothenburg and Stockholm for ten infectious diseases (tabs. 48–57, pp. 88–108). Trends in mortality in Sweden are discussed in *Expectations of Life* (Lancaster, 1990, pp. 402–7). Mortality data for Sweden with causes of deaths classified by age, sex, and ICD code are available on computer tape from WHO for the forty years between 1951 and 1990 (WHO (1994), Annex I). **(c) Sources of population data:** The first census for Sweden was held in 1749. Subsequent censuses were conducted in 1750, 1751(3)1775(5)1860(10)1930, 1935–6, 1940(5)1950, 1960, 1965. A full listing appears in the *International Population Census Bibliography, No. 6, Europe* (University of Texas, 1967c, pp. 32.1–32.18). Population estimates for Sweden by age (five-year groups up to age eighty), sex, and quinquennia for the period 1911 to 1975 are given in *International Mortality Statistics* (Alderson, 1981, tab. 180, p. 507).

SWITZERLAND. *Swiss Confederation, Schweizerische Eidgenossenschaft.* WHO European Region (EUR). Area: 15,940 miles^2. Population: 7.0 million (1995). Long-standing confederation of cantons from fourteenth century; no major boundary changes since Helvetian Confederation formed in 1815. **(a) Sources of morbidity data:** Cases of notifiable infectious diseases are regularly reported in *Bulletin de l'Off. Fed. de Santé Publiq* (weekly). Annual information on the incidence and immunisation coverage of eight vaccine-preventable diseases (diphtheria, measles, pertussis, poliomyelitis, tetanus, neonatal tetanus, tuberculosis, and yellow fever) from 1974 is given in the *Information System Summary Volume, WHO European Region* (WHO, Expanded Programme on Immunization (EPI), Geneva, annual). **(b) Sources of mortality data:** Standardised mortality tables giving 178 causes of death for males and females are given for Switzerland by quinquennial periods for the period 1901 to 1975 in *International Mortality Statistics* (Alderson, 1981, tabs. 1–178, pp. 113–477).[12] Annotated estimates of decennial death rates for Switzerland by cause of death for the period 1881 to 1901 are published in *Statistique générale de la France* (France, Bureau de la Statistique Générale; appendix, pp. 83–594). Annual totals and crude mortality rates of deaths from infectious diseases for Switzerland for the years 1939 through 1946 are reported in *Annual Epidemiological and Vital Statistics 1939–1946* (WHO (1952), part II, tab. 38, p. 67) and for the two cities of Berne and Zurich for ten infectious diseases (tabs. 48–57, pp. 88–108). Trends in mortality in Switzerland are discussed in *Expectations of Life* (Lancaster, 1990, p. 395). Mortality data for Switzerland with causes of deaths classified by age, sex, and ICD code are available on computer tape from WHO for the forty-two years between 1951 and 1992 (WHO (1994), Annex I). **(c) Sources of population data:** The first census for Switzerland was held in 1860 (*Bevölkerung. Eidgenössische volkszählung vom 10. Dezember 1860*). Subsequent censuses were conducted in 1870, 1880, 1888, 1900(10)1930, 1941, 1950, 1960. A full listing appears in the *International Population Census Bibliography, No. 6, Europe* (University of Texas, 1967c, pp. 33.1–33.11). Population estimates for Switzerland by age (five-year groups up to age eighty), sex, and quinquennia for the period 1901 to 1975 are given in *International Mortality Statistics* (Alderson, 1981, tab. 180, p. 508).

TURKEY. *Turkiye Cumhuriyeti.* WHO European Region (EUR). Area: 294,416 miles^2. Population: 62.0 million (1995). Turkey has been a republic since 1923.

Before the First World War, it was part of the Ottoman Empire. **(a) Sources of morbidity data:** Reported cases of notifiable infectious diseases are regularly reported in *Monthly Bulletin of Infectious Diseases* (monthly). Annual information on the incidence and immunisation coverage of eight vaccine-preventable diseases (diphtheria, measles, pertussis, poliomyelitis, tetanus, neonatal tetanus, tuberculosis, and yellow fever) from 1974 is given in the *Information System Summary Volume, WHO European Region* (WHO, Expanded Programme on Immunization (EPI), Geneva, annual). **(b) Sources of mortality data:** Standardised mortality tables giving 178 causes of death for males and females are given by quinquennial periods for the period 1901 to 1975 in *International Mortality Statistics* (Alderson, 1981, tabs. 1–178, pp. 113–477). Mortality data for Turkey with causes of deaths classified by age, sex, and ICD code are available on computer tape from WHO for seven years between 1978 and 1987 (WHO (1994), Annex I). **(c) Sources of population data:** The first census for Turkey was held in 1927 (*28 Tesrinievel 1927 Umumî Nüfus Tahriri. Recensement Général de la population au octobre 1927*). Subsequent censuses were conducted in 1935(5)1965. A full listing appears in the *International Population Census Bibliography, No. 5, Asia* (University of Texas, 1967b, pp. 43.1–43.14). Population estimates for Turkey by age (five-year groups up to age eighty), sex, and quinquennia for the period 1931 to 1975 are given in *International Mortality Statistics* (Alderson, 1981, tab. 180, p. 509).

UNITED KINGDOM. *See* England and Wales, Northern Ireland and Scotland.

UNITED STATES OF AMERICA. WHO American Region (AMR). Area: 3,615,211 miles². Population: 263.1 million (1995). **(a) Sources of morbidity data:** Reported cases of notifiable infectious diseases are regularly reported in *Morbidity and Mortality Weekly Report* (weekly). Annual information on the incidence and immunisation coverage of eight vaccine-preventable diseases (diphtheria, measles, pertussis, poliomyelitis, tetanus, neonatal tetanus, tuberculosis, and yellow fever) from 1974 is given in the *Information System Summary Volume, WHO American Region* (WHO, Expanded Programme on Immunization (EPI), Geneva, annual). **(b) Sources of mortality data:** Standardised mortality tables showing 178 causes of death for males and females are given for the United States by quinquennial periods for the period 1901 to 1975 in *International Mortality Statistics* (Alderson, 1981, tabs. 1–178, pp. 113–477).[13] Annual totals and crude mortality rates of deaths from infectious diseases for the United States for the years 1939 through 1946 are reported in *Annual Epidemiological and Vital Statistics 1939–1946* (WHO (1952), part II, tab. 14, p. 43) and for the ten cities of Boston, Chicago, Detroit, Los Angeles, New York City, New Orleans, Philadelphia, St Louis, Seattle, and Washington, DC, for ten infectious diseases (tabs. 48–57, pp. 88–108). Trends in mortality in the United States are discussed in *Expectations of Life* (Lancaster, 1990, pp. 426–35). Mortality data for the United States of America with causes of deaths classified by age, sex, and ICD code are available on computer tape from WHO for the forty-one years between 1950 and 1990 (WHO (1994), Annex I). **(c) Sources of population data:** The first census for the United States was taken in 1790 (*Return of the Whole Number of Persons Within the Several Districts of the United States, According to 'An Act Providing For The Enumeration of the Inhabitants of the United States', Passed*

March the First, Seventeen Hundred and Ninety-one). Subsequent censuses were conducted decennially thereafter. A full listing appears in the *International Population Census Bibliography, No. 4, North America* (University of Texas, 1967a, pp. 4.1–4.56). A second critical guide to US census material is the Department of Commerce, Bureau of the Census, and the United States Library of Congress, Reference Department, *Catalog of United States Census Publications, 1790–1945* (Washington, DC: Government Printing Office, 1950). Other catalogues cover the period since 1945. Population estimates for the United States by age (five-year groups up to age eighty), sex, and quinquennia for the period 1901 to 1975 are given in *International Mortality Statistics* (Alderson, 1981, tab. 180, p. 513).

URUGUAY. WHO American Region (AMR). Area: 72,172 miles^2. Population: 3.2 million (1995). **(a) Sources of morbidity data:** Reported cases of notifiable infectious diseases are regularly reported in *Informe semanal de enfermedades trans.* (weekly). Annual information on the incidence and immunisation coverage of eight vaccine-preventable diseases (diphtheria, measles, pertussis, poliomyelitis, tetanus, neonatal tetanus, tuberculosis, and yellow fever) from 1974 is given in the *Information System Summary Volume, WHO American Region* (WHO, Expanded Programme on Immunization (EPI), Geneva, annual). **(b) Sources of mortality data:** Annual totals and crude mortality rates of deaths from infectious diseases for Uruguay for the years 1939 through 1946 are reported in *Annual Epidemiological and Vital Statistics 1939–1946* (WHO (1952), part II, tab. 17, p. 46) and for the city of Montevideo for ten infectious diseases (tabs. 48–57, pp. 88–108). Mortality data for Uruguay with causes of deaths classified by age, sex, and ICD code are available on computer tape from WHO for thirty-three years between 1955 and 1990 (WHO (1994), Annex I). **(c) Sources of population data:** The first census for Uruguay was held in 1852. Subsequent censuses were conducted in 1860, 1895–6, 1900, 1908, 1963. Full details are given in *International Population Census Bibliography, No. 3, Oceania* (University of Texas, 1966, pp. 37.1–37.2).

VENEZUELA. WHO American Region (AMR). Area: 352,141 miles^2. Population: 21.5 million (1995). **(a) Sources of morbidity data:** Reported cases of notifiable infectious diseases are regularly reported in *Boletin epidemiologico semanal* (weekly); *Informe semanal de enfermedades trans.* (weekly). Annual information on the incidence and immunisation coverage of eight vaccine-preventable diseases (diphtheria, measles, pertussis, poliomyelitis, tetanus, neonatal tetanus, tuberculosis, and yellow fever) from 1974 is given in the *Information System Summary Volume, WHO American Region* (WHO, Expanded Programme on Immunization (EPI), Geneva, annual). **(b) Sources of mortality data:** Mortality data for Venezuela with causes of deaths classified by age, sex, and ICD code are available on computer tape from WHO for thirty-four years between 1955 and 1989 (WHO (1994), Annex I). **(c) Sources of population data:** While pre-census surveys had been carried out in 1825, 1838, 1844, 1846, 1847, 1854 and 1857, the first census for Venezuela was held in 1873 (*Memoria de la dirección general de estadística al presidente de los Estados Unidos de Venezuela en 1873*). Subsequent censuses were conducted in 1891, 1920, 1936, 1941, 1950, 1961. Full details are given in *International Population Census Bibliography, No. 3, Oceania* (University of Texas, 1966, pp. 38.1–38.9).

WALES. *See* England and Wales.

YUGOSLAVIA. WHO European Region (EUR). Area: 98,770 miles². Population: 24.1 million (1995). **(a) Sources of morbidity data:** Reported cases of notifiable infectious diseases are regularly reported in *Rapport sur l'incidence des maladies inf.* (weekly and monthly). Annual information on the incidence and immunisation coverage of eight vaccine-preventable diseases (diphtheria, measles, pertussis, poliomyelitis, tetanus, neonatal tetanus, tuberculosis, and yellow fever) from 1974 is given in the *Information System Summary Volume, WHO European Region* (WHO, Expanded Programme on Immunization (EPI), Geneva, annual). **(b) Sources of mortality data:** Standardised mortality tables giving 178 causes of death for males and females are given for Yugoslavia by quinquennial periods for the period 1921 to 1975 in *International Mortality Statistics* (Alderson, 1981, tabs. 1–178, pp. 113–477). Annotated estimates for decennial death rates for Serbia by cause of death for the period 1861 to 1901 are published in *Statistique générale de la France* (France, Bureau de la Statistique Générale; appendix, pp. 83–594). Mortality data for the former Yugoslavia with causes of deaths classified by age, sex, and ICD code are available on computer tape from WHO for the thirty-one years between 1960 and 1990 (WHO (1994), Annex I). **(c) Sources of population data:** The first census for Yugoslavia was held in 1875 (*La popolazione di Trieste nel 1875. Resoconto ufficiale del censimento generale della popolazione effettuato secondo lo stato del 31/12/1875*). Subsequent censuses were conducted in 1895, 1900, 1910, 1921, 1931, 1936, 1948, 1949, 1951, 1953, 1961. A full listing appears in the *International Population Census Bibliography, No. 6, Europe* (University of Texas, 1967c, pp. 36.1–36.8). Population estimates for Yugoslavia by age (five-year groups up to age eighty), sex, and quinquennia for the period 1921 to 1975 are given in *International Mortality Statistics* (Alderson, 1981, tab. 180, p. 514).

Appendix D

International and national epidemiological agencies

For the countries listed in appendix C, this appendix details the major agencies responsible for the collection and dissemination of epidemiological data. In many countries, there are also subnational agencies with data gathering responsibilities (for example, the state epidemiological services within the United States).

1. Regional offices of WHO

Regional offices of WHO produce their own statistical information on individual countries, viz.:

Africa	WHO Regional Office for Africa, PO Box 6, Brazzaville, Congo.
Americas	WHO Regional Office for the Americas, Pan American Sanitary Bureau, 525 23rd Street NW, Washington, DC, 20037, USA.
Eastern Mediterranean	WHO Regional Office for the Eastern Mediterranean, PO Box 1517, Alexandria – 21511, Egypt.
Europe	WHO Regional Office for Europe, 8 Scherfigsvej, DK-2100 Copenhagen Ø, Denmark.
South and East Asia	WHO Regional Office for South and East Asia, World Health House, Indraprastha Estate, Mahatma Gandhi Road, New Delhi – 110002, India.
Western Pacific	WHO Regional Office for the Western Pacific, PO Box 2932, Manila 2801, Philippines.

2. National agencies

Australia	Information Services, Australian Bureau of Statistics, PO Box 10, Belconnen, ACT 2616, Australia.
Austria	Head: Division of Population Statistics, Central Statistical Office, Neue Hofburg, Vienna 1014, Austria.
Belgium	Chief of Section Demographic Statistics, National Institute of Statistics, Leuvenseweg 44, 1000 Brussels, Belgium.
Czechoslovakia	Chief of International Statistics Division, Federal Statistics Bureau, Sokolovská 142, Karlin, Prague 8, Czechoslovakia.

Denmark	Chief Statistician, Board of Health, Sotre Kongensgade 1, 1264 Copenhagen K, Denmark.
Eire	*See* Ireland.
England and Wales	Chief Medical Statistician, Office of Population Censuses and Surveys, St Catherines House, 10 Kingsway, London WC2B 6JP, England.
France	Head, Section for Statistical Information on Morbidity and Mortality, National Institute for Health and Medical Research, 44 Chemin de Ronde, La Vasinet 78-110, Paris, France.
Greece	Director of Statistical Service, Department of National Health, 17 Aristotelous St, Athens, Greece.
Hungary	Head: Population Statistics Department, Central Statistical Office, 5–7 Keleti Karoly Street, Budapest H-1525, Hungary.
Ireland	The Director, General Statistics Office, Ardee Road, Dublin 6, Eire.
Italy	Chief of Health Statistics, Central Institute of Statistics, Viale Liege 11, 00198 Rome, Italy.
Japan	Director of Health and Welfare Statistics and Information Department, Ministry of Health and Welfare, Tokyo, Japan.
Netherlands	Head of the Department of Health Statistics, Central Statistics Bureau, 428 Prinses Beatrixlaan, PO Box 959, 2270 AZ Voorburg, Netherlands.
Northern Ireland	Registrar General, General Register Office, Fermanagh House, Ormeau Avenue, Belfast, BT2 8HX, Northern Ireland.
Norway	Chief: Division 1, Central Bureau of Statistics, Dronningens Gate 16, Oslo 1, Norway.
Poland	Chief: International Statistics Division, Central Statistical Office, A1. Niepodleglosci 208, 00-925 Warsaw, Poland.
Scotland	Registrar General, Registrar General's Office, New Register House, Edinburgh 2, Scotland.
Spain	Head of Division of Health Statistics, National Institute of Statistics, Avde Del Generalisimo 91, Madrid 16, Spain.
Sweden	Head: Division of Population Statistics, National Central Bureau of Statistics, Fack, S-102 50 Stockholm, Sweden.
Switzerland	Head of Division of Population Statistics, Federal Bureau of Statistics, Hallwylstrasse 15, 3003 Berne, Switzerland.
Turkey	Head of Division, Population Statistics, State Institute of Statistics, Ankara, Turkey.
United Kingdom	*See* England and Wales, Northern Ireland, Scotland.
USA	Director of National Center for Health Statistics, Public Health Service, Health Resources Administration, Department of Health, Education, and Welfare, Hyattsville, MD 29782, USA.
Wales	*See* England and Wales.
Yugoslavia	Director of Division of Health Statistics, State Institute for Statistics, Belgrade, Yugoslavia.

Chapter notes

1 Prologue: epidemics past

1 'And there, as I looked, was another horse, sickly pale; and its rider's name was Death, and Hades came close behind. To him was given power over a quarter of the earth, with the right to kill by sword and by famine, by pestilence and wild beasts' (Revelation, 6, viii).

2 The nature of the evidence

1 In the context of yellow fever, for example, see US Marine Hospital Service (1896), pp. 428–39.
2 US Marine Hospital Service (1884–94).
3 Steamships in excess of 2,000 tons (US Department of the Treasury, Bureau of Navigation (1901), appendix O, pp. 382–3).
4 We define a generation as the maximum time in days available for a disease-causing agent to be passed from an infected to a susceptible person, so preserving the chain of infection. After this interval expires, if no new infection has occurred, the chain will be broken by recovery of the infected person. So, for example, for the viral disease of measles, a generation is c. eighteen days (see Cliff, Haggett, and Smallman-Raynor, 1993, p. 6).
5 Estimated sailing times are based on the shortest navigable route in 1901 (US Department of the Treasury, Bureau of Navigation (1901), appendix N, pp. 361–81) by ships sailing at an average speed of 3.25 knots. The estimated average speed is computed from real journey times between US and foreign ports in the 1890s (US Department of the Treasury, Bureau of Statistics (1891), tab. 63, opposite p. 1174).
6 Orientations are based on bearings taken from Bartholomew's *The Times* pseudo-conical projection (*The Times Atlas of the World* (1986)).
7 US Department of the Treasury (1875).
8 *Ibid.*, p. 12.
9 Rapid transmission of weekly consular reports depended critically on the telegraph. The first submarine cable was established in 1850 between England and France, but it was 1866 (after several abortive schemes) before the first permanently successful transatlantic cable was laid. Once complex cable-laying technology was established, new submarine links were laid apace. By 1890 (near the start of our

study period), the international cable network ran from the United States to Central and Latin America, and from Western Europe south to Africa and east to India, China, South Asia, and Australia. By the end of our period, most US consular offices could send telegrams to Washington, DC, though not without frequent delays and breaks in transmission. Telephone communication was to come later. Boston and New York were connected in 1884, but it was 1915 before the first transcontinental telephone line opened between New York and San Francisco.

10 *Ibid.*, p. 13.
11 *Ibid.*
12 Barnes and Heath Morgan (1961).
13 US Department of State (1889).
14 US House of Representatives (1856–1902).
15 US Department of State (1880–1901).
16 The teething troubles were alluded to in a State Department dispatch in 1880, where the difficulties of obtaining surveillance data were summarised as 'chiefly owing to the fact that in certain foreign ports where infectious diseases have existed, or were supposed to exist, the local authorities have shown some hesitation in co-operating with the consular and medical officers of the United States in carrying out regulations deemed essential by this [US] government as a sanitary safeguard' (Despatch from the Department of State to diplomatic officers in Argentina, dated 29 July 1880; US National Archives and Records Service (1945–51)).
17 Circular of the Department of State, 29 July 1880 (US National Archives and Records Service (1945–51)).
18 US Marine Hospital Service (1878), *Bulletins of the Public Health*, No. 1.
19 US Marine Hospital Service (1878), *Bulletins of the Public Health*, No. 21.
20 The National Board of Health had been established by Act of Congress on 3 March 1879 by 'An Act to Prevent the Introduction of Infectious and Contagious Diseases into the United States, and to Establish a National Board of Health'.
21 In addition to provisions regarding interstate quarantine, the National Quarantine Act of 1893 provided that all ships headed from foreign ports to the United States must be issued with a Bill of Health signed by the US consul prior to departure. To assist in meeting this remit, officers of the Marine Hospital Service could be detailed to foreign ports to serve in the office of the consul. In this manner, officials of the Marine Hospital Service became increasingly important contributors of epidemiological information to the *Weekly Abstract* (Furman, 1973).
22 A further 600 copies of each weekly edition were held for binding and distribution as an annual volume. See US Marine Hospital Service (1901), p. 389.
23 The rationale of the surgeon general for discontinuing the foreign tables remains unclear. His annual report for the year 1912 warmly endorsed the work of the American consuls in foreign countries: 'Too much credit can not be given to the importance of the information thus obtained nor to the excellent service being rendered in this way by the State Department through its diplomatic and consular officers' (US Marine Hospital Service (1914), p. 240).
24 US Department of State (1889).
25 US Department of State (1893).
26 W. R. Estes, consul to Kingston, Jamaica, Dispatch to the State Department, 3 June 1892 (*Weekly Abstract of Sanitary Reports*, VII (1892), p. 285).

27 In June 1880 the consul to Amoy, China, informed the State Department that 'Owing to the entire absence of registration and all the sanitary precautions of civilised countries, reliable information cannot be obtained in Amoy, because the authorities have no physicians and keep no account whatever of disease or deaths' (W. E. Goldsbrough, consul to Amoy, China, Dispatch No. 32 to the State Department, 8 July 1880 (National Archives, Washington, 1947)). Consuls to sub-Saharan Africa fared little better. Consul Hollis, stationed in Mozambique, southern Africa, explained to the State Department that 'The authorities at the various ports of this province [Mozambique] pay little attention to matters pertaining to the public health; their health reports are not only incomplete, but are published so irregularly that they are of little value. The Government is so financially embarrassed that it can devote but little money to these matters' (W. Stanley Hollis, consul to Mozambique, Dispatch to the State Department, 24 April 1893 (*Weekly Abstract of Sanitary Reports*, VIII (1893), p. 484)).

28 In 1890, Eugene Baker, then consul to Buenos Aires, Argentina, provided the State Department with a lengthy summary of his efforts: 'I have to say that . . . I have used my utmost endeavours, sometimes under very great difficulties, to execute the provisions of the [Quarantine] law. At first by paying a gratuity, I succeeded in getting a municipal official to furnish me with the information; then, this was stopped by the municipality making a contract with the "Medical Review" here for the exclusive right to the publication of such returns, and then I was able to obtain them once a month by subscribing to the magazine. Subsequently, the "Review" suspended publication; and after the lapse of some time, another paper called the "Municipal Bulletin" was started, and from this, once more, I was enabled to procure, monthly, the information required. But, within the last few months, owing to the straightened finances of the city, the publication of that paper has been suspended; and now there is no publication of the returns of mortality at all' (Eugene Baker, consul to Buenos Aires, Dispatch No. 921 to the State Department, 31 July 1890 (National Archives, Washington, 1948)).

29 See, for example: T. Harper Hall, consul to Batoum, Dispatch to the State Department, 28 June 1892 (*Weekly Abstract of Sanitary Reports*, VII (1892), p. 360).

30 US consul to Amoy, China, Dispatch No. 27 to the State Department, 18 January 1895 (National Archives, Washington, 1947).

31 The geographically and demographically restricted nature of some local surveillance systems was recognised in 1892 by T. Harper Hall, acting consul to Batoum, in a report on the incidence of cholera in his jurisdiction: 'These figures . . . constitute the cases treated solely in the Baku town hospital. Besides this hospital, there are many more so-called private ones . . . from which no reports are issued for public use; consequently, it is quite safe to say that nearly as many more cases are treated in these private hospitals as are reported 'officially' from the town hospital' (T. Harper Hall, consul to Batoum, Dispatch to the State Department, 28 June 1892 (*Weekly Abstract of Sanitary Reports*, VII (1892), p. 360)).

32 Yellow fever proved particularly problematical. In 1903, for example, the US consul to La Guaira, Venezuela, reported that: 'It would . . . be unjust for a consul to give reports of existing diseases, when the nature of the diseases is in doubt and when the great medical men disagree as to the nature of the same . . . the first case of

'undoubted' yellow fever I shall report to your [State] Department' (L. Goldschmidt, consul to La Guaira, Venezuela, Dispatch No. 257 to the State Department, June 1903 (National Archives and Records Service, Washington, 1961)).

33 See, for example, consul to Amoy, China, Dispatch No. 11 to the State Department, October 1879 (National Archives, Washington, 1947); US consul to Amoy, China, Dispatch No. 27 to the State Department, 18 January 1895 (National Archives, Washington, 1947); communication from Arthur S. Hardy, Legation of the United States, Teheran, Persia, 19 January 1899 (*Public Health Reports*, XIV (1899), p. 330).

34 G. Bie Ravndal, consul to Beirut, Dispatch to the State Department, 22 April 1899 (*Public Health Reports*, XIV (1899), p. 837).

35 W. Stanley Hollis, consul to Mozambique, Dispatch to the State Department, 24 April 1893 (*Weekly Abstract of Sanitary Reports*, VIII (1893), p. 484).

36 Thomas E. Heenan, consul to Odessa, Russia, Dispatch to the State Department, 18 June 1892 (*Weekly Abstract of Sanitary Reports*, VII (1892), p. 389).

37 For example, Victor Vifquain, consul-general to Panama, reported to the State Department in 1897 that 'The authorities are not approachable on health matters; they will give no information on the contagious diseases, and that which is found out is by accident' (Victor Vifquain, consul-general to Panama, Dispatch to the State Department, 23 April 1897 (*Public Health Reports*, XII (1897), p. 486)). See also: anonymous communication with the State Department, 27 April 1896 (*Public Health Reports*, XI (1896), p. 498).

38 Thomas E. Heenan, consul to Odessa, Russia, Dispatch to the State Department, 8 June 1892 (*Weekly Abstract of Sanitary Reports*, VII (1892), p. 326).

39 Thomas E. Heenan, consul to Odessa, Russia, Dispatch to the State Department, 14 December 1893 (*Weekly Abstract of Sanitary Reports*, IX (1894), p. 24).

40 In a report on yellow fever in San Salvador, Consul John Jenkins informed the State Department that 'Every attempt is made by the authorities to keep . . . information [regarding yellow fever] as quiet as possible, and it is only by continued vigilance that the truth in regard to such matters becomes known, as interments are made by the police at night' (John Jenkins, consul to San Salvador, San Salvador, Dispatch to the State Department, 21 June 1901 (*Public Health Reports*, XVI (1901), p. 1724)).

41 Consul-general to St Petersburg, Russia, Dispatch No. 131 to the State Department, 19 February 1901 (National Archives and Records Service, Washington, 1963).

42 See, for example, P. L. Bridgers, consul to Montevideo, Uruguay, Dispatch Nos. 52, 56, and 59 to the State Department, 10 December 1886, 7 and 19 January 1887 (National Archives, Washington, 1948).

43 See, for example, Alvey A. Adee, acting secretary of state, Communication to the Public Health and Marine Hospital Service, 18 August 1902 (*Public Health Reports*, XVII (1902), p. 2006); consul-general to St Petersburg, Russia, Dispatch No. 18 to the State Department, 12 October 1887 (National Archives and Records Service, Washington, 1963).

44 A statement by the vice-consul to Antofagasta, Chile, in June 1894, is illustrative: 'I take it for granted the main interest in the weekly consular sanitary reports is

found in those from important ports . . . Such being the case, I deem a report for the last week of each quarter . . . and a sort of resume of the whole quarter . . . will be ample from this . . . port' (C. C. Greene, vice-consul to Antofagasta, Chile, Dispatch to the State Department, 30 June 1894 (*Weekly Abstract of Sanitary Reports*, IX (1894), p. 650)).

45 W. H. Edwards, consul-general to Berlin, Dispatch to the State Department, 23 August 1892 (*Weekly Abstract of Sanitary Reports*, VII (1892), p. 521).

46 In 1897, the consular agent to Hodeida assured the State Department that 'the rumour about the prevalence of smallpox in Hodeida is all a mistake'. A communication to the State Department by a reliable independent informant in Hodeida, however, confirmed the strong suspicion that 'smallpox is raging here' (William M. Masterson, consul to Aden, Arabia, Dispatch to the State Department, 25 March 1897 (*Public Health Reports*, XII (1897), p. 481)).

47 It was with a degree of injured pride that Eugene Seeger, consul-general to Rio de Janeiro, Brazil, explained to the State Department in February 1899 that 'in the circular of the Department of State, October 31st, the Consulate at Rio de Janeiro is styled as one from where the requisite weekly sanitary reports are not received, although they would be "particularly valuable". Permit me to say that the Sanitary Inspector connected with this Consulate sends detailed reports to the Supervising Surgeon General, US Marine Hospital service, with every mail, and in nearly every number of the "Public Health Reports" you find such reports published . . . I would greatly appreciate it if you would cause to be made the necessary correction in the future rating of this Consulate General as to sanitary Reports' (Eugene Seeger, consul-general to Rio de Janeiro, Brazil, Dispatch No. 64 to the State Department, 17 February 1899 (National Archives and Records Service, Washington, 1959)).

48 S. Comfort, consul to Bombay, India, Dispatch to the State Department, 14 January 1897 (*Public Health Reports*, XII (1897), pp. 189–90).

49 *Public Health Reports*, XX (1905), p. 419.

50 In 1887, the *Registrar General's Weekly Return* included mortality data for London and twenty-seven other 'Great Towns' in England and Wales. By 1892, the number of towns (including London) had grown to thirty-three, by 1902 to seventy-six, and, by 1912, to ninety-five. The listed causes of mortality remained unchanged during this period. In addition to deaths from all causes, mortality due to four diseases coincides with the data abstracted from the *Reports*, namely: diphtheria, measles, scarlet fever, and whooping cough. The estimated population of each town was also given.

51 The *Registrar General's Weekly Return* contained no missing weekly units in the relevant quarters.

3 The global sample: an overall picture

1 The coding, ICD-10-CM A36, refers to the classification given to this disease in the Tenth Revision of the International Classification of Diseases. See sections 1.2.2 and 1.3.2 for a discussion of the historical background to the classification.

2 The popular name of 'croup' was applied to obstruction of the larynx. Unfortunately, Home, writing in 1765, thought that 'croup' was a separate disease,

and this view persisted for so long that 'diphtheria' and 'croup' still appeared as separate headings in the UK registrar general's returns as late as 1910 even though we now know that they were one and the same disease (Gale, 1959, p. 88).

3 The row count does not divide simply by 52 because some years contained 53 weeks; this arises from the practice of reporting on a Friday or Saturday (see section 2.5.1).

4 Epidemic trends: a global synthesis

1 Some of the variables described in this section have already been used for other purposes in section 3.3.3.

2 Crude mortality, death rates, and deaths as a percentage of all causes.

Appendix A Primary data sources

1 In 1879, powers under the 1878 Quarantine Law temporarily passed from the Marine Hospital to the newly created National Board of Health, and publication of sanitary reports continued in the *National Board of Health Bulletin* (vol. 1, no. 1, issued 28 July 1879). Rights under the Quarantine Law returned to the Marine Hospital Service in 1883, but the sanitary reports went unpublished until the launch of the *Weekly Abstract of Sanitary Reports* in 1887.

2 See *Public Health Reports* (1952, vol. 67, no. 1; Washington, DC: Government Printing Office, 1–7).

3 US Marine Hospital Service (1902), p. 584.

4 See: Benjamin (1968); Glass (1973); Newsholme (1923).

Appendix C National epidemiological sources

1 The compulsory certification and registration of death was introduced under the General Sanitary Law of 1870 (League of Nations, 1925b).

2 The medical certification and registration of deaths became compulsory in Belgium in 1803 (League of Nations, 1924a).

3 The registration of urban mortality began in 1876, although cause of death registration was not required on a nationwide basis until 1921 (League of Nations, 1926).

4 As described in appendix A, the Births and Deaths Registration Act of 1836 provided for vital registration in England and Wales with the establishment of the General Register Office. Death registration was consolidated in 1874 when the Births and Deaths Registration Act introduced death certificates and a penalty for failure to register.

5 The compulsory registration of deaths began in 1803 although, at this time, certification of the cause of death was not a legal requirement (League of Nations, 1927). Information regarding cause of death became available for larger cities (those with over 100,000 population) from 1885 and, by 1906, the statistics covered the whole country.

6 Death registration has been compulsory in Hungary since 1894 (Alderson, 1981, p. 37).

7 Death registration, with cause of death, has been compulsory in Ireland since 1864 (League of Nations, 1929a).
8 Compulsory registration of deaths was introduced in 1815 (League of Nations, 1924b; Alderson, 1981, pp. 37–8).
9 A system paralleling that of England and Wales had been established by 1864 (Alderson, 1981, pp. 39–40).
10 Compulsory registration of the fact of death, and certification of the cause of death, was introduced in 1864 (League of Nations, 1929b).
11 Compulsory registration of the fact of death was introduced in 1871, with the requirement of a cause of death certificate (completed by the attendant physician or authorised medical officer) introduced three years later in 1874 (League of Nations, 1925a).
12 Death registration in Switzerland was decreed in 1874 (League of Nations, 1928).
13 In addition to the system described in appendix A and chapter 2, the US Bureau of the Census began the collection of (annual) mortality statistics in 1900. Initially, the system included ten participating states, the District of Columbia, and a selection of cities in non-registration states. Coverage grew rapidly in subsequent years until, by 1933, the entire country was included (Alderson, 1981, p. 40).

References

Full details of the serial publications encompassed by the title *Weekly Abstract* (*Bulletins of the Public Health, Weekly Abstract of Sanitary Reports*, and *Public Health Reports*; see section 2.3.1) are given in appendix A. Publication details of the *Registrar General's Weekly Returns* and *Quarterly Returns* are also given in appendix A.

Aaby, P., and Clements, C. J. (1989). 'Measles immunization research: a review'. *Bulletin of the World Health Organization*, 67, pp. 443–8.

Ablin, R. J., Gonder, M. J., and Immerman, R. S. (1985). 'AIDS: a disease of ancient Egypt?' *New York State Journal of Medicine*, 85, pp. 200–1.

Alderson, M. (1981). *International Mortality Statistics*. London: Macmillan.

Alewitz, S. (1989). *'Filthy Dirty': A Social History of Unsanitary Philadelphia in the Late Nineteenth Century*. New York: Garland.

Ampel, N. N. (1991). 'Plagues – what's past is present: thoughts on the origin and history of new infectious diseases'. *Reviews of Infectious Diseases*, 13, pp. 658–65.

Anderson, I. (1904). 'Några iakttagelser från difteriepidemica i Stockholm under åren 1903 och 1904'. *Hygiea*, 4, pp. 1346–62.

Anderson, R. M., and Grenfell, B. T. (1986). 'Quantitative investigations of different vaccination policies for the control of congenital rubella syndrome (CRS) in the United Kingdom'. *Journal of Hygiene*, 96, pp. 305–33.

Anderson, R. M., and May, R. M. (1983). 'Vaccination against rubella and measles: quantitative investigations of different policies'. *Journal of Hygiene*, 90, pp. 259–325.

(1991). *Infectious Diseases of Humans: Dynamics and Control*. Oxford: Oxford University Press.

Ashcroft, M. T. (1964). 'Typhoid and paratyphoid fevers in the tropics'. *Journal of Tropical Medicine and Hygiene*, 67, pp. 185–9.

Ashraf, A., and Green, L. P. (1972). 'Calcutta'. In: Robson and Regan, *Great Cities of the World, Volume I*, pp. 295–330.

Australia, National Centre in HIV Epidemiology and Clinical Research (1996). *Australian HIV Surveillance Report, No. 12*. Darlinghurst, NSW: National Centre in HIV Epidemiology and Clinical Research.

Bailey, N. T. J. (1975). *The Mathematical Theory of Infectious Diseases and Its Applications*. London: Griffin.

Bannister, B. A. (ed.) (1991). *Report of a Think Tank on the Potential Effects of Global Warming and Population Increase on the Epidemiology of Infectious Diseases.* Colindale: Public Health Laboratory Service.

Barea, I. (1992). *Vienna: Legend and Reality.* London: Pimlico.

Barnes, W., and Heath Morgan, J. (1961). *The Foreign Service of the United States: Origins, Development, and Functions.* Department of State, Historical Office. Washington, DC: Government Printing Office.

Bartlett, M. S. (1957). 'Measles periodicity and community size'. *Journal of the Royal Statistical Society A*, 120, pp. 48–70.

(1960). 'The critical community size for measles in the United States'. *Journal of the Royal Statistical Society A*, 123, pp. 37–44.

Basile, G. (1903). 'Il movimento del tifo in Catania nel settennio 1893–1899: brevi note de epidemiologia'. *Giornale di Reale Società Italiana d'Igiene*, 25, pp. 99, 161.

Bater, J. H. (1976). *St Petersburg: Industrialization and Change.* London: Edward Arnold.

(1983). 'Modernization and the municipality: Moscow and St Petersburg on the eve of the Great War'. In: J. H. Bater and R. A. French (eds.), *Studies in Russian Historical Geography, Volume II.* London: Academic Press, pp. 305–27.

(1985). 'Modernization and public health in St Petersburg, 1890–1914'. *Forschungen zur osteuropäischen Geschichte*, 37, pp. 357–72.

(1986). 'Between old and new: St Petersburg in the late imperial era'. In: Hamm, *The City In Late Imperial Russia*, pp. 43–78.

Baxter, R. S. (1976). *Computer and Statistical Techniques for Planners.* London: Methuen.

Benenson, A. S. (ed.) (1990). *Control of Communicable Diseases in Man, 15th Edition.* Washington, DC: American Public Health Association.

Benjamin, B. (1968). *Health and Vital Statistics.* London: Allen & Unwin.

Bennett, J. V., Holmberg, S. D., Rogers, M. F., and Solomon, S. L. (1987). 'Infectious and parasitic diseases'. In: R. W. Amler and H. B. Dull (eds.), *Closing the Gap: The Burden of Unnecessary Diseases.* Oxford: Oxford University Press, pp. 102–14.

Berman, S. (1991). 'Epidemiology of acute respiratory infections in children of developing countries'. *Review of Infectious Diseases*, 13 (suppl. 6), pp. S454–62.

Bienia, R. A., Stein, E., and Bienia, B. H. (1983). 'United States Public Health Service hospitals (1798–1981) – the end of an era'. *New England Journal of Medicine*, 308, pp. 166–8.

Billings, J. S. Jr (1906a). 'The relation of milk to typhoid fever in New York City'. *American Public Health Association Report 1905*, 31, pp. 304–11.

(1906b). 'Typhoid fever in the city of New York during 1905'. *Boston Medical and Scientific Journal*, 154, pp. 569–75.

(1912). *The Registration and Sanitary Supervision of Pulmonary Tuberculosis in New York City by the Department of Health.* New York: Department of Health Monograph Series, No. 1.

Black, F. L. (1966). 'Measles endemicity in insular populations: critical community size and its implications'. *Journal of Theoretical Biology*, 11, pp. 207–11.

Bloomfield, A. L. (1958). *A Bibliography of Internal Medicine: Communicable Diseases.* Chicago: University of Chicago Press.

Bolduan, C. F. (1912). *Typhoid Fever in New York City Together with a Discussion of the Methods Found Serviceable in Studying Its Occurrence.* New York: Department of Health Monograph Series, No. 3.

Bordley, J., and Harvey, A. M. (1976). *Two Centuries of American Medicine.* Philadelphia: W. B. Saunders Co.

Bouvier, M., Pittet, D., Loutan, L., and Starobinski, M. (1990). 'Airport malarias: a mini-epidemic in Switzerland'. *Schweizerin Medizin Wochenschreiber*, 120, pp. 1217–22.

Box, G. E. P., and Jenkins, G. M. (1976). *Time Series Analysis, Forecasting, and Control* (revised edn). San Francisco: Holden Day.

Boyer, J. W. (1981). *Political Radicalism in Late Imperial Vienna: Origins of the Christian Social Movement, 1848–1897.* Chicago: University of Chicago Press.

Bradley, D. J. (1988). 'The scope of travel medicine'. In: R. Steffen, *et al.*, (eds.), *Travel Medicine: Proceedings of the First Conference on International Travel Medicine,* Zurich, Switzerland, April 1988. Berlin: Springer Verlag, pp. 1–9.

Bradley, J. (1986). 'Moscow: from big village to metropolis'. In: Hamm, *The City In Late Imperial Russia*, pp. 9–41.

Brock, T. D. (ed.) (1990). *Microorganisms: From Smallpox to Lyme Disease.* New York: Freeman.

Brouardel (n. i.) (1894). 'L'étiologie de la fièvre typhoïde au Havre'. *Bulletin Académie de médecine (Paris)*, 31, pp. 376–411.

Brough, D. D. (1904). 'Two recent outbreaks of typhoid fever in Boston'. *Journal of the Massachusetts Association of Boards of Health*, 14, pp. 248–53.

Brownlee, J. (1907). 'Statistical studies in immunity: the theory of an epidemic'. *Proceedings of the Royal Society of Edinburgh*, 26, pp. 484–521.

(1916). 'The history of birth and death rates in England and Wales, taken as a whole from 1570 to present time.' *Public Health*, 29, pp. 221–2, 228–38.

Bucquoy (n. i.) (1894a). 'Sur l'épidémie actuelle de fièvre typhoïde à Paris'. *Bulletin Académie de médecine (Paris)*, 31, pp. 231, 274.

(1894b). 'Sur l'origine de l'épidémie de fièvre typhoïde des villes de Paris et de sens en février 1894'. *Bulletin Académie de médecine (Paris)*, 31, pp. 460–74.

Bunle, H. (1954). *Le mouvement naturel de la population dans le monde de 1906 à 1936.* Paris: L'Institut national d'études démographiques.

Cairns, J. (1978). *Cancer: Science and Society.* San Francisco: W. H. Freeman.

Capps, J. A., and Miller, J. L. (1912). 'The Chicago epidemic of streptococcus sore throat and its relation to the milk-supply'. *Journal of the American Medical Association*, 58, pp. 1848–52.

Carlsen, J., and Heiberg, P. (1897). 'Om Varigheden af dødelige Difteritilfaelde i den danske Bybefolking udenfor København'. *Ugeskrift for Laeger*, 4, pp. 1259–69.

(1903). 'Uber die Dauser der tödtlichen Diphtherie fälle in der dänischen Stadtbevölkerung ausserhalb Kopenhagens während der Jahre, 1895–1901'. *Zeitschrift fur Hygiene und Infectionskrankheiten*, 42, pp. 547–51.

Carmichael, A. G. (1993a). 'Diphtheria'. In: Kiple, *Cambridge World History of Human Disease*, pp. 680–3.

(1993b). 'History of public health and sanitation in the West before 1700'. In: Kiple, *Cambridge World History of Human Disease*, pp. 192–200.

(1993c). 'Plague of Athens'. In: Kiple, *Cambridge World History of Human Disease*, pp. 934–7.

Carmichael, A. G., and Silverstein, A. M. (1987). 'Smallpox in Europe before the seventeenth century: virulent killer or benign disease?' *Journal of the History of Medicine and Allied Sciences*, 42, pp. 147–68.

Caro, O. (1898). 'La diffusione della febre tifoidea in Italia e specialmente in Napoli'. *Giornale internazionale delle scienze mediche*, 20, pp. 205–24.

Caselli, G. (1991). 'Health transition and cause specific mortality'. In: Schofield, Reher, and Bideau, *Decline of Mortality in Europe*, pp. 68–96.

Catanach, I. J. (1988). 'Plague and the tensions of empire: India, 1896–1918'. In: D. Arnold (ed.), *Imperial Medicine and Indigenous Societies*. Manchester: Manchester University Press, pp. 149–71.

Chabal, H. (1904). 'La fièvre typhoïde à Paris et l'eau de rivière filtrée'. *Revue d'hygiène*, 26, pp. 436–44.

Chalmers, A. K. (1905) (ed.). *Public Health Administration in Glasgow*. Glasgow: James Maclehose & Sons.

(1930). *The Health of Glasgow, 1818–1925: An Outline*. Glasgow: Glasgow Corporation.

Chatfield, C. (1980). *The Analysis of Time Series: An Introduction (2nd Edition)*. London: Chapman & Hall.

Checkland, O., and Lamb, M. (eds.) (1982). *Health Care as Social History: The Glasgow Case*. Aberdeen: Aberdeen University Press.

Childs, C. (1898). 'History of typhoid in Munich'. *Lancet*, 1, pp. 348–54.

Choi, K., and Thacker, S. B. (1981a). 'An evaluation of influenza mortality surveillance, 1962–1979: (I) Time series forecasts of expected pneumonia and influenza deaths'. *American Journal of Epidemiology*, 113, pp. 215–26.

(1981b). 'An evaluation of influenza mortality surveillance, 1962–1979: (II) Percentage of pneumonia and influenza deaths as an indicator of influenza activity'. *American Journal of Epidemiology*, 113, pp. 227–35.

Christie, A. B. (1974). *Infectious Diseases: Epidemiology and Clinical Practice (2nd Edition)*. Edinburgh: Churchill Livingstone.

Cipolla, C. M. (1981). *Fighting the Plague in Seventeenth-Century Italy*. Madison: University of Wisconsin Press.

(1992). *Miasmas and Disease: Public Health and the Environment in the Pre-Industrial Age*. New Haven: Yale University Press.

Clark, J. E. (1910). 'Typhoid fever in Detroit'. *Journal of the American Medical Association*, 55, p. 1488.

Clerc, M. (1910). 'La prophylaxie de la fièvre typhoïde à New York'. *Hygiène générale et appliquée*, 5, pp. 65–77.

Cliff, A. D., and Haggett, P. (1985). *The Spread of Measles in Fiji and the Pacific: Spatial Components in the Transmission of Epidemic Waves Through Island Communities*. Department of Human Geography Publication No. HG/18. Canberra: Research School of Pacific Studies, Australian National University.

(1988). *Atlas of Disease Distributions: Analytical Approaches to Epidemiological Data*. Oxford: Blackwell Reference.

(1989). 'Spatial aspects of epidemic control'. *Progress in Human Geography*, 13, pp. 313–47.

(1990). 'Epidemic control and critical community size: spatial aspects of eliminating communicable diseases in human populations'. In: R. W. Thomas (ed.), *Spatial Epidemiology*. London: Pion, pp. 93–110.

Cliff, A. D., Haggett, P., and Ord, J. K. (1986). *Spatial Aspects of Influenza Epidemics*. London: Pion.

Cliff, A. D., Haggett, P., Ord, J. K., and Versey, G. R. (1981). *Spatial Diffusion: An Historical Geography of Epidemics in an Island Community*. Cambridge: Cambridge University Press.

Cliff, A. D., Haggett, P., and Smallman-Raynor, M. (1993). *Measles: An Historical Geography of a Major Human Viral Disease from Global Expansion to Local Retreat*. Oxford: Blackwell Reference.

Cliff, A. D., Haggett, P., Smallman-Raynor, M., Stroup, D. F., and Williamson, G. D. (1995). 'The application of multidimensional scaling methods to epidemiological data'. *Statistical Methods in Medical Research*, 4, pp. 102–23.

Cliff, A. D., Haggett, P., Stroup, D. F., and Cheney, E. (1992). 'The changing geographical coherence of measles morbidity in the United States, 1962–1988'. *Statistics in Medicine*, 11, pp. 1409–24.

Cliff, A. D., and Ord, J. K. (1981). *Spatial Processes: Models and Applications*. London: Pion.

Clout, H. D. (1977). *Themes in the Historical Geography of France*. London: Academic Press.

Cnopf (n. i.) (1898). 'Über die Diphtherie im Nürnberger Kinderspitale im Jahre 1896'. *Münchener medizinische Wochenschrift*, 45, p. 646.

Condran, G., and Cheney, R. (1982). 'Mortality trends in Philadelphia: age- and cause-specific death rates, 1870–1930'. *Demography*, 19, pp. 97–123.

Condran, G., Williams, H., and Cheney, R. (1985). 'The decline of mortality in Philadelphia from 1870 to 1930: the role of municipal services'. In: J. W. Leavitt and R. L. Numbers, *Sickness and Health in America: Readings in the History of Medicine and Public Health (2nd Edition)*. Madison: University of Wisconsin Press, pp. 422–36.

Cooley, W. W., and Lohnes, P. R. (1962). *Multivariate Procedures for the Behavioral Sciences*. New York: Wiley.

Cooper, D. B., and Kiple, K. F. (1993). 'Yellow fever'. In: Kiple, *Cambridge World History of Human Disease*, pp. 1100–7.

Cormack, R. M. (1971). 'A review of classification'. *Journal of the Royal Statistical Society A*, 134, pp. 321–67.

Corrsin, S. D. (1986). 'Warsaw: Poles and Jews in a conquered city'. In: Hamm, *The City In Late Imperial Russia*, pp. 123–51.

Coxon, A. P. M. (1982). *The User's Guide to Multidimensional Scaling with Special Reference to the MDS(X) Library of Computer Programs*. London: Heinemann.

Creighton, C. (1894). *A History of Epidemics in Britain*. Cambridge: Cambridge University Press.

(1965). *A History of Epidemics in Britain, Volume II*. London: Frank Cass.

Crimmins, E. (1980). 'The completeness of 1900 mortality data collected by registration and enumeration for rural and urban parts of states: estimates using the Chandra Sekar-Deming technique'. *Historical Methods*, 13, pp. 163–9.

Crompton, D. W. T., and Savioli, L. (1993). 'Terrestrial parasitic infections and urbanization'. *Bulletin of the World Health Organization*, 71, pp. 1–7.

Cruickshank, M. (1981). *Children and Industry: Child Health and Welfare in North-*

West Textile Towns During the Nineteenth Century. Manchester: Manchester University Press.

Cumpston, J. H. L. (1927). *The History of Diphtheria, Scarlet Fever, Measles, and Whooping Cough in Australia, 1788–1925*. Melbourne: Commonwealth of Australia, Department of Health Service Publication No. 37.

— (1989). *Health and Disease in Australia: A History*. Canberra: Australian Government Publishing Service.

Cunnison, J., and Gilfillan, J. B. S. (eds.) (1958). *The Third Statistical Account of Scotland: Glasgow*. Glasgow: Collins.

Cutts, F. T. (1990). *Measles Control in the 1990s: Principles for the Next Decade*. Geneva: World Health Organization.

Cutts, F. T., and Smith, P. G. (1994). *Vaccination and World Health*. London: Wiley.

D'Andrade, R. G., Quinn, N. R., Nerlove, S. B., and Romney, A. K. (1972). 'Categories of disease in American-English and Spanish-English'. In: A. K. Romney, R. N. Shepard, and S. B. Nerlove (eds.), *Multidimensional Scaling: Theory and Applications in the Behavioral Sciences, Volume II*. New York: Seminar Press, pp. 1–54.

Daunton, M. J. (1991). 'Health and housing in Victorian London'. In: W. F. Bynum and R. Porter (eds.), *Living and Dying in London*. London: Wellcome Institute for the History of Medicine (*Medical History*, suppl. 11), pp. 126–44.

Davis, K. (1959). *The World's Metropolitan Areas*. Berkeley: University of California Press for International Urban Research, Institute for International Studies.

de Bevoise, K. (1995). *Agents of Apocalypse: Epidemic Disease in the Colonial Philippines*. Princeton: Princeton University Press.

de Meirelles, C. (1897–8). 'A tuberculose e a nephrite no alto sertão da Bahia, raridade d'esta'. *Gazeta medica da Bahia*, 1, pp. 29–32.

de Pietra Santa (n. i.) (1894). 'La fièvre typhoïde à Paris périod décennale de décroissance, 1884–1893: ses exacerbations automno hivernales'. *Journale d'hygiène*, 19, pp. 349, 362, 373, 385.

Deacon, J. P. (1911). 'A report of the tuberculosis situation in Pennsylvania in 1909'. *Journal of the American Medical Association*, 56, pp. 339–43.

Debré, R., and Joannon, P. (1926). *La rougeole: épidémiologie, immunologie, prophylaxie*. Paris: Masson et Cie.

Delouvrier, P. (1972). 'Paris'. In: Robson and Regan, *Great Cities of the World, Volume II*, pp. 731–71.

Di Mattei, E. (1894). 'L'acqua potabile dell reitana il movimento del tifo in Catania dal 1887 al 1892: studio epidemiologico'. *Giornale di Reale Società Italiana d'Igiene*, 16, pp. 81–117.

Dietz, K. (1988). 'The first epidemic model: a historical note on P. D. En'ko'. *Australian Journal of Statistics*, 30A, pp. 56–65.

Dixey, F. A. (1898). 'Diphtheria in London, 1896–1898'. *British Medical Journal*, 22, pp. 611–13.

Dixon, S. G., and Royer, B. R. (1910–11). 'Typhoid fever in Pennsylvania; past, present, and future'. *Pennsylvania Medical Journal*, 14, pp. 757–63.

Donally, H. H. (1915). 'Scarlatina: morbidity and case fatality, by locality, sex, age, and season (based on the study of over a million cases)'. *Archives of Pediatrics*, 32, pp. 767–79.

Doyle, D. H. (1985). *Nashville in the New South, 1880–1930*. Knoxville: University of Tennessee Press.

Drolet, G. J., and Lowell, A. M. (1952). *A Half Century's Progress Against Tuberculosis in New York City*. New York: New York Tuberculosis and Health Association.

Duben, A., and Behar, C. (1991). *Istanbul Households: Marriage, Family, and Fertility, 1880–1940*. Cambridge: Cambridge University Press.

Dubos, R. J., and Dubos, J. (1953). *The White Plague: Tuberculosis, Man, and Society*. London: Gollancz.

Duffy, J. (1953). *Epidemics in Colonial America*. Port Washington, NY: Kennikat Press.

——— (1974). *A History of Public Health in New York City, 1866–1966*. New York: Russell Sage Foundation.

——— (1990). *The Sanitarians: A History of American Public Health*. Urbana: University of Illinois Press.

Dwork, D. (1981). 'Health conditions of immigrant Jews in the lower east side of New York, 1880–1914'. *Medical History*, 25, pp. 1–40.

English, P. C. (1985). 'Diphtheria and theories of infectious disease: centennial appreciation of the critical role of diphtheria in the history of medicine'. *Pediatrics*, 76, pp. 1–9.

En'ko, P. D. (1989). 'On the course of epidemics of some infectious diseases'. *International Journal of Epidemiology*, 18, pp. 749–55.

Erhardt, C., and Berlin, J. (eds.) (1974). *Mortality and Morbidity in the United States*. Cambridge, MA: Harvard University Press.

Evans, A. S. (1982). *Viral Infections of Humans*. New York: Plenum.

Evans, R. J. (1987). *Death in Hamburg: Society and Politics in the Cholera Years, 1830–1910*. Oxford: Clarendon Press.

Ewan, C., Bryant, E., and Calvert, D. (1990). *Health Implications of Long-Term Climate Change*. Canberra: National Health and Medical Research Council of Australia.

Fabela, O. G. (1907). 'Diphtheria bacilli in well persons in Mexico City'. *American Public Health Association Report*, 32, p. 199.

Faries, R. (1904–5). 'Typhoid fever in Philadelphia'. *Proceedings of the Philadelphia County Medical Society*, 25, pp. 287–90.

Fenner, F. (1986). 'The eradication of infectious diseases'. *South African Medical Journal*, 66 (suppl.), pp. 35–9.

Fenner, F., Henderson, D. A., Arita, I., Jesek, Z., and Ladnyi, I. D. (1988). *Smallpox and Its Eradication*. Geneva: World Health Organization.

Fine, P. E. M. (1979). 'John Brownlee and the measurement of infectiousness: an historical study in epidemic theory'. *Journal of the Royal Statistical Society A*, 142, pp. 347–62.

——— (1993). 'Herd immunity: history, theory, practice'. *Epidemiological Reviews*, 15, pp. 265–302.

Fissell, M. E. (1992). 'Health in the city: putting together the pieces'. *Urban History*, 19, pp. 251–6.

Fitz Gerald, A. O. (1897). 'Enteric fever in Rangoon, and its rational treatment'. *Indian Medical Gazette*, 32, p. 96.

Flinn, D. E. (1909). 'Report on an outbreak of enteric fever at Clontarf (Dublin County Borough)'. *Dublin Journal of Medical Science*, 128, pp. 251–80.

Flinn, M. W. (1974). 'The stabilisation of mortality in pre-industrial Western Europe'. *Journal of European Economic History*, 3, pp. 285–318.

(1981). *The European Demographic System, 1500–1820*. Brighton: Harvester.

Forbes, J. G. (1927). *The Prevention of Diphtheria*. Medical Research Council Special Report Series, No. 115. London: HMSO.

Ford, W. W., and Watson, E. M. (1911). 'The problem of typhoid fever in Baltimore'. *Johns Hopkins Hospital Bulletin*, 22, pp. 351–7.

Fox, D. M. (1975). 'Social policy and city politics: tuberculosis reporting in New York, 1889–1900'. *Bulletin of the History of Medicine*, 49, pp. 169–95.

France, Bureau de la Statistique Générale. *Statistique générale de la France: statistique annuelle du mouvement de la population, année 1904, Volume XXXIV*. Paris: Imprimerie Impériale.

Frank, J. A., Orenstein, W. A., Bart, K. J., Bart, S. W., El-Tantawy, N., David, R. M., and Hinman, A. R. (1985). 'Major impediments to measles elimination'. *American Journal of Diseases of Children*, 139, pp. 881–8.

Fraser, D. W. (1993). 'Legionnaires' disease'. In: Kiple, *Cambridge World History of Human Disease*, pp. 827–32.

Fried, R. C. (1972). 'Mexico'. In: Robson and Regan, *Great Cities of the World, Volume II*, pp. 645–87.

Frieden, N. M. (1981). *Russian Physicians in an Era of Reform and Revolution, 1865–1905*. Princeton, NJ: Princeton University Press.

Frost, W. H. (1976). 'Some conceptions of epidemics in general'. *American Journal of Epidemiology*, 103, pp. 141–51.

Frottier (n. i.) (1903). 'La fièvre typhoïde au Havre pendant l'année 1902'. *Revue médicale de Normandie*, n. n., pp. 257 9.

Furman, B. (1973). *A Profile of the United States Public Health Service, 1798–1948*. Washington, DC: Government Printing Office.

Gabriel, K. R. (1971). 'The biplot graphical display of matrices with applications to principal component analysis'. *Biometrika*, 58, pp. 453–67.

Gabriel, K. R., and Odoroff, C. L. (1990). 'Biplots in biomedical research'. *Statistics in Medicine*, 9, pp. 469–85.

Gagnière (n. i.) (1907). 'Sur les causes de l'épidémie de la scarlatine et de rougeole à Paris et dans le département de la Seine, et l'indication de quelques moyens destinés à y remédier'. *Médecine scolaire*, 1, pp. 105–44.

Gale, A. H. (1959). *Epidemic Diseases*. Harmondsworth: Penguin.

Galishoff, S. (1975). *Safeguarding the Public Health: Newark, 1895–1918*. Westport, CT: Greenwood Press.

(1988). *Newark: The Nation's Unhealthiest City, 1832–1895*. New Brunswick, NJ: Rutgers University Press.

Galloway, P. R. (1985). 'Annual variations in deaths by age, deaths by cause, prices, and weather in London, 1670–1830'. *Population Studies*, 39, pp. 487–505.

(1986). 'Long-term fluctuations in climate and population in the preindustrial era'. *Population and Development Review*, 12, pp. 1–24.

Garrett, L. (1993). 'The next epidemic'. In: J. Mann, D. J. M. Tarantola, and T. W. Netter, *AIDS in the World: A Global Report*. Cambridge, MA: Harvard University Press, pp. 825–39.

Gay, F. P. (1918). *Typhoid Fever*. New York: Macmillan.

Geary, R. C. (1954). 'The contiguity ratio and statistical mapping'. *Incorporated Statistician*, 5, pp. 115–45.

Giaquinta, S. (1898). 'La difterite in Catania in quest'ultimo ventennio (1877–1896)'. *Giornale di Reale Società Italiana d'Igiene*, 20, pp. 345–69.

Gilbert (n. i.) (1896). 'Les causes de la fièvre typhoïde au Havre'. *Revue d'hygiène*, 18, pp. 377–98.

Glass, D. V. (1973). *Numbering the People: The Eighteenth-Century Population Controversy and the Development of Census and Vital Statistics in Britain*. Farnborough: D. C. Heath.

Gleason, W. (1990). 'Public health, politics, and cities in late imperial Russia'. *Journal of Urban History*, 16, pp. 341–65.

Goldberg, B. (1911). *Die Typhusbewegung auf der züricher medizinischen Klinik in den Jahren 1901–1909*. Zurich: G. Leeman & Co.

Goldschmidt, E., and Luxenburger, A. (1896). 'Zur Tuberculose-Mortalität und Morbidität in München'. *Münchener medizinische Wochenschrift*, 43, pp. 820–5.

Goodall, E. W., Greenwood, M., and Russell, W. T. (1929). *Scarlet Fever, Diphtheria, and Enteric Fever, 1895–1914: A Clinical Case Study*. Medical Research Council Special Report Series, No. 137. London: HMSO.

Gould, P. R. (1995). 'La géographie du Sida: étude des flux humains et expansion d'une épidémie'. *La recherche*, 280, pp. 36–7.

Grattan, H. W. (1910). 'A preliminary enquiry into the prevalence of paratyphoid fever in London, with remarks on blood culture in forty-eight cases of enteric fever'. *Journal of the Royal Army Medical Corps*, 14, pp. 385, 395.

Greene, J. C. (1977). 'The United States Public Health Service: a bicentennial report'. *Military Medicine*, 142, pp. 511–13.

Greenhalgh, D. (1986). 'Simple models for the control of epidemics'. *Mathematical Modelling*, 7, pp. 753–63.

Greenwood, M. (1935). *Epidemics and Crowd Diseases: An Introduction to the Study of Epidemiology*. New York: Macmillan.

Griffiths, D. A. (1973). 'The effect of measles vaccination on the incidence of measles in the community'. *Journal of the Royal Statistical Society A*, 136, pp. 441–9.

Grubler, A., and Nakicenovic, N. (1991). *Evolution of Transport Systems*. Vienna: IIASA Laxenburg.

Haggett, P. (1976). 'Hybridizing alternative models of an epidemic diffusion process'. *Economic Geography*, 52, pp. 136–46.

(1991). 'Some components of global environmental change'. In: Bannister, *Report of a Think Tank on the Potential Effects of Global Warming and Population Increase on the Epidemiology of Infectious Diseases*, pp. 5–14.

(1992). 'Sauer's "Origins and Dispersals": its implications for the geography of disease'. *Transactions of the Institute of British Geographers*, 17, pp. 387–98.

(1994). 'Geographical aspects of the emergence of infectious diseases'. *Geografiska Annaler*, 76B, pp. 91–104.

(1995). 'Some epidemiological implications of increased international travel'. In: *Proceedings, Review of International Response to Epidemics and Application of International Health Regulations*. Geneva: World Health Organization, WHO Document EMC/IHR/GEN/95.5.

Hamm, M. F. (ed.) (1986). *The City In Late Imperial Russia.* Bloomington: Indiana University Press.

Hand, D. J., and Taylor, C. C. (1987). *Multivariate Analysis of Variance and Repeated Measures.* London: Chapman and Hall.

Hansen, S. (1904). *Etude sur la répartition de la tuberculose à Copenhague.* Copenhagen: Gyldendal.

Harbitz, F. (1897). 'Aarsagsforholdene ved tyfusepidemien i Kristania høsten 1896'. *Norsk Magasin for Laegevidenskaben,* 12, pp. 894–937.

Harden, V. A. (1993). 'Typhus, epidemic'. In: Kiple, *Cambridge World History of Human Disease,* pp. 1080–4.

Hardy, A. (1993a). *The Epidemic Streets: Infectious Disease and the Rise of Preventive Medicine, 1856–1900.* Oxford: Clarendon Press.

(1993b). 'Scarlet fever'. In: Kiple, *Cambridge World History of Human Disease,* pp. 990–2.

(1993c). 'Whooping cough'. In: Kiple, *Cambridge World History of Human Disease,* pp. 1094–6.

Harman, H. H. (1960). *Modern Factor Analysis.* Chicago: University of Chicago Press.

Harrison, M. (1994). *Public Health in British India: Anglo-Indian Preventive Medicine, 1859–1914.* Cambridge: Cambridge University Press.

Heiberg, P. (1895). 'Er difteriens Intensitet i København under konstante ydre Forhold konstant eller varierende?' *Ugeskrift for Laeger,* 2, pp. 1101–9.

(1907). 'Om Varigheden af de dødelige Tilfaelde af Skarlagensfeber i den danske Bybefolkning urden for København: Aarene, 1885–1900'. *Ugeskrift for Laeger,* 14, pp. 241–8.

(1907–8). 'Über die Dauer der letalen Scharlachfieberfälle in der dänischen Stadtbevölkerung, Kopenhagen ausgenommen, in den Jahren 1885 bis 1900'. *Zeitschrift fur Hygiene und Infektionskrankheiten,* 58, pp. 79–84.

Henderson-Sellars, A., and Blong, R. J. (1989). *The Greenhouse Effect: Living in a Warmer Australia.* Kensington, Sydney: New South Wales University Press.

Henius (n. i.) (1904). 'Beiträge zur Diphtherie-Epidemie April–Mai 1903 zu Frankfurt a. M.'. *Berliner klinische Wochenschrift,* 41, p. 285.

Herlihy, P. (1978). 'Death in Odessa: a study of population movements in a nineteenth-century city'. *Journal of Urban History,* 4, pp. 417–42.

Higgs, R. (1979). 'Cycles and trends of mortality in eighteen large American cities, 1871–1900'. *Explorations in Economic History,* 16, pp. 381–408.

Hill, A. (1895–6). 'Remarks on the incidence of diphtheria in Birmingham'. *Public Health,* 8, pp. 342–4.

Hill, A. B. (1933). 'Some aspects of the mortality from whooping cough'. *Journal of the Royal Statistical Society,* 96, pp. 240–85.

Hilts, V. L. (1980). 'Epidemiology and the statistical movement'. In: A. M. Lilienfeld (ed.), *Times, Places, and Persons: Aspects of the History of Epidemiology.* Baltimore: Johns Hopkins University Press, pp. 43–55.

Hinman, A. R. (1966). *World Eradication of Infectious Diseases.* Springfield, IL: Thomas.

Hinman, A. R., Brandling-Bennett, A. D., Bernier, R. H., Kirby, C. D., and Eddins, D. L. (1980). 'Current features of measles in the United States: feasibility of measles elimination'. *Epidemiologic Reviews,* 2, pp. 153–70.

Hirsch, August (1883–6). *Handbook of Geographical and Historical Pathology* (3 vols.). London.

Hodgetts, C. A., and Amyot, J. A. (1905). 'Second report of the outbreak of enteric fever in London'. *Sanitary Journal of the Provincial Board of Health (Ontario)*, 24, pp. 148–51.

Hollingsworth, T. H. (1979). 'A preliminary suggestion for the measurement of mortality crises'. In: H. Charbonneau and A. Larose (eds.), *The Great Mortalities: Methodological Studies of Demographic Crises in the Past*. Liège: Ordina, pp. 21–8.

Holm, A. (1972). 'Copenhagen'. In: Robson and Regan, *Great Cities of the World, Volume I*, pp. 369–405.

Hope, E. W. (1931). *Health at the Gateway: Problems and International Obligations of a Seaport City*. Cambridge: Cambridge University Press.

Hopkins, D. R. (1983). *Princes and Peasants: Smallpox in History*. Chicago: University of Chicago Press.

Howard, W. T. (1903). 'A study of tuberculosis in Cleveland'. *Cleveland Medical Journal*, 2, pp. 59–61.

(1924). *Public Health Administration and the Natural History of Disease in Baltimore, Maryland, 1797–1920*. Washington, DC: Carnegie Institute of Washington.

Hunter, J. S. (1978). 'Public Health Reports' first century – a chronicle'. *Public Health Reports*, 98, pp. 591–9.

Hutchinson, J. F. (1990). *Politics and Public Health in Revolutionary Russia, 1890–1918*. Baltimore: Johns Hopkins University Press.

Intergovernmental Panel on Climatic Change (1990). *Scientific Assessment of Climate Change: Report Prepared for IPCC by Working Group 1*. Geneva: World Meteorological Organization.

Israel, R. A. (1990). 'The history of the International Classification of Diseases'. *Health Trends*, 22, pp. 43–4.

Jackson, J. M. (ed.) (1979). *The Third Statistical Account of Scotland: The City of Dundee*. Arbroath: Herald Press.

James, G., Cliff, A. D., Haggett, P., and Ord, J. K. (1970). 'Some discrete distributions for graphs with applications to regional transport networks'. *Geografiska Annaler B*, 52, pp. 14–21.

Jamieson, J. (1903). 'Typhoid in Hobart and Melbourne, and the influence of drainage on its prevalence'. *Australasian Medical Gazette*, 22, pp. 56–8.

Jannetta, A. B. (1987). *Epidemics and Mortality in Early Modern Japan*. Princeton: Princeton University Press.

Janney, O. E. (1903–4). 'The conditions producing typhoid fever with special reference to Baltimore city'. *American Medical Monthly*, 21, pp. 161–6.

Jenkins, G. M., and Watts, D. G. (1968). *Spectral Analysis and Its Applications*. San Francisco: Holden-Day.

Jephson, H. (1907). *The Sanitary Evolution of London*. London: T. Fisher Unwin.

Johnson, E. R. (1898). 'The early history of the United States Consular Service'. *Political Science Quarterly*, 13, pp. 19–40.

Johnston, W. D. (1993). 'Tuberculosis'. In: Kiple, *Cambridge World History of Human Disease*, pp. 1059–68.

Jones, J. (1894–5a). 'Contribution to the natural history and treatment of diphtheria in the United States, and more especially in New Orleans, La.'. *Virginia Medical Monthly*, 21, pp. 8–26.

(1894–5b). 'Personal experience with reference to diphtheria in New Orleans, La., 1868–1894; also progress of discovery with reference to nature and treatment of this disease during the past twenty-five years'. *Virginia Medical Monthly*, 21, pp. 135–43.

Jones, N. W. (1906). 'Some notes on the Chicago epidemic of typhoid of 1902'. *Medical Sentinel*, 14, pp. 579–87.

Jordan, E. O. (1927). *Epidemic Influenza*. Chicago: American Medical Association.

Karpat, K. H. (1985). *Ottoman Population, 1830–1914: Demographic and Social Characteristics*. Madison: University of Wisconsin Press.

Karve, D. G. (1955). 'Bombay'. In: W. Yust (ed.), *Encyclopaedia Britannica*, III, pp. 830–2.

Keely, C. B. (1979). *US Immigration: A Policy Analysis*. New York: The Population Council, Inc.

Keir, D. (ed.) (1966). *The Third Statistical Account of Scotland: The City of Edinburgh*. Glasgow: Collins.

Keltner, K. (1911). 'Typhoid fever epidemic in one street and its neighbourhood, in Prague, in November, 1910'. *Casopis lékaru ceskych*, 5, pp. 255–8.

Kendall, D. G. (1957). 'La propagation d'une épidémie au d'un bruit dans une population limitée'. *Publications de l'Institute de statistique de l'Université de Paris*, 6, pp. 307–11.

(1971). 'Construction of maps from odd bits of information'. *Nature*, 231, pp. 158–9.

(1975). 'The recovery of structure from fragmentary information'. *Philosophical Transactions of the Royal Society of London A*, 279, pp. 547–82.

Kennedy, C. S. (1990). *The American Consul: A History of the United States Consular Service, 1776–1914*. New York: Greenwood Press.

Kermack, W. O., and McKendrick, A. G. (1927). 'Contributions to the mathematical theory of epidemics'. *Proceedings of the Royal Society A*, 115, pp. 700–21.

Khlat, M., and Khoury, M. (1991). 'Inbreeding and diseases: demographic, genetic, and inbreeding perspectives'. *Epidemiological Reviews*, 13, pp. 28–41.

Khromov, S. S., Preobrazhensky, A. A., Promyslov, V. F., Roganov, A. M., and Sinitsyn, A. M. (1981). *History of Moscow: An Outline*. Moscow: Progress.

Kiple, K. F. (ed.) (1993). *The Cambridge World History of Human Disease*. Cambridge: Cambridge University Press.

Klein, I. (1973). 'Death in India, 1871–1921'. *Journal of Asian Studies*, 32, pp. 639–59.

(1986). 'Urban development and death: Bombay city, 1870–1914'. *Modern Asian Studies*, 20, pp. 725–74.

Kleinman, L. C. (1992). 'To end an epidemic: lessons from the history of diphtheria'. *New England Journal of Medicine*, 326, pp. 773–7.

Kober, G. M. (1897). 'Typhoid fever in the District of Columbia: frequency, causes, mortality, and prevention'. *National Medical Review*, 7, pp. 141–3.

Kosambi, M. (1986). *Bombay in Transition: The Growth and Social Ecology of a Colonial City, 1880–1980*. Stockholm: Almqvist & Wiksell.

Kozlova, N. A. (1973). 'Epidemiologic characteristics of pertussis in Leningrad (1850–1971)'. *Trudy Leningradskogo Instituta Epidemiologii i Mikrobiologii Imeni Pastera*, 39, pp. 13–24.

Kruskal, J. B. (1964a). 'Multidimensional scaling by optimizing goodness of fit to a nonmetric hypothesis'. *Psychometrika*, 29, pp. 1–27.

(1964b). 'Nonmetric multidimensional scaling: a numerical method'. *Psychometrika*, 29, pp. 115–29.

Kruskal, J. B., and Wish, M. (1978). *Multidimensional Scaling*. Beverly Hills: Sage.

Kuhn, H. W., and Kuenne, R. E. (1962). 'An efficient algorithm for the numerical solution of the generalised Weber problem in spatial economics'. *Journal of Regional Science*, 4, pp. 21–33.

Kunitz, S. J. (1986). 'Mortality since Malthus'. In: D. Coleman and R. Schofield (eds.), *The State of Population Theory*. Oxford: Blackwell.

(1991). 'The personal physician and the decline of mortality'. In: Schofield, Reher, and Bideau, *Decline of Mortality in Europe*, pp. 248–62.

La Berge, A. F. (1992). *Mission and Method: The Early Nineteenth-Century French Public Health Movement*. Cambridge: Cambridge University Press.

Laidler, P. W., and Gelfand, M. (1971). *South Africa: Its Medical History, 1652–1898. A Medical and Social Study*. Cape Town: C. Struik Ltd.

Lancaster, H. O. (1990). *Expectations of Life: A Study in the Demography, Statistics, and History of World Mortality*. Berlin: Springer-Verlag.

Lancreaux (n. i.) (1894). 'Etude comparative des épidémies de fièvre typhoïde observées dans Paris depuis l'année 1876'. *Union médicale*, 57, pp. 626–31.

Landers, J. (1993). *Death and the Metropolis: Studies in the Demographic History of London, 1670–1830*. Cambridge: Cambridge University Press.

League of Nations (1924a). *Kingdom of Belgium – Statistical Handbook No. 2*. Geneva: League of Nations Health Organisation.

(1924b). *Kingdom of Netherlands – Statistical Handbook No. 1*. Geneva: League of Nations Health Organisation.

(1925a). *Kingdom of Spain – Statistical Handbook No. 4*. Geneva: League of Nations Health Organisation.

(1925b). *Republic of Austria – Statistical Handbook No. 5*. Geneva: League of Nations Health Organisation.

(1926). *Scandinavian Countries and Baltic Republics – Statistical Handbook No. 6*. Geneva: League of Nations Health Organisation.

(1927). *French Republic – Statistical Handbook No. 9*. Geneva: League of Nations Health Organisation.

(1928). *Switzerland – Statistical Handbook No. 12*. Geneva: League of Nations Health Organisation.

(1929a). *Ireland – Statistical Handbook No. 11*. Geneva: League of Nations Health Organisation.

(1929b). *Scotland – Statistical Handbook No. 13*. Geneva: League of Nations Health Organisation.

LeBaron, C. W., and Taylor, D. W. (1993). 'Typhoid fever'. In: Kiple, *Cambridge World History of Human Disease*, pp. 1071–7.

Lebredo, G. (1904). *Contribucion al estudio de la escarlatina en la Habana*. Havana: n. p.

Lederberg, J., Shope, R. E., and Oaks, S. C. (eds.) (1992). *Emerging Infections: Microbial Threats to Health in the United States*. Washington, DC: National Academy Press.

Leemans, A. F. (1972). 'Amsterdam'. In: Robson and Regan, *Great Cities of the World, Volume I*, pp. 131–62.

Lemoine, G.-H. (1904). 'La fièvre typhoïde à Paris, en 1904'. *Revue d'hygiène*, 26, pp. 429–35.

Levine, R. M. (1978). *Pernambuco in the Brazilian Federation, 1889–1937*. Stanford: Stanford University Press.

Lindsay, J. A. (1898). 'Typhoid fever in Belfast'. *Lancet*, 1, p. 61.

Lingoes, J. C., and Roskam, E. E. (1973). 'A mathematical and empirical analysis of two multidimensional scaling algorithms'. *Psychometrika*, 38, monograph supplement.

Low, R. B. (1920). *The Progress and Diffusion of Plague, Cholera, and Yellow Fever Throughout the World, 1914–1917*. London: HMSO.

Luckin, B. (1984). 'Evaluating the sanitary revolution: typhus and typhoid in London, 1851–1900'. In: Woods and Woodward, *Urban Disease and Mortality*, pp. 102–19.

Luckin, W. (1980). 'Death and survival in the city'. *Urban History Yearbook*, pp. 53–62.

McCarthy, M. P. (1987). *Typhoid and the Politics of Public Health in Nineteenth-Century Philadelphia*. Philadelphia: American Philosophical Society.

McEvedy, C. (1988). 'The bubonic plague'. *Scientific American*, 254 (2), pp. 3–12.

MacGregor, A. (1967). *Public Health in Glasgow, 1905–1946*. Edinburgh: E. & S. Livingstone.

MacIntyre, D. (1926). 'The serum treatment of diphtheria'. *Lancet*, 1, pp. 855–8.

MacKellar, F. L. (1993). 'Early mortality data: sources and difficulties of interpretation'. In: Kiple, *Cambridge World History of Human Disease*, pp. 209–13.

McKendrick, A. G. (1912). 'On certain mathematical aspects of malaria'. *Proceedings of the Imperial Malaria Committee*, Bombay, 16–17 November 1911, pp. 54–66.

McKeown, T. (1976). *The Modern Rise of Population*. London: Edward Arnold.
   (1988). *The Origins of Human Disease*. Oxford: Blackwell.

McLain, D. H. (1974). 'Drawing contours from arbitrary data points'. *Computer Journal*, 17, pp. 318–24.

McLauthlin, H. W. (1896). 'The recent epidemic of typhoid fever at the County Hospital, Denver, with report of cases'. *Transactions of the Colorado Medical Society*, n. n., pp. 152–61.

McLeod, J. W. (1943). 'The types *mitis*, *intermedius*, and *gravis* of *Corynebacterium diphtheriae*: a review of observations during the past ten years'. *Bacteriological Review*, 7, pp. 1–56.

McNeill, W. H. (1977). *Plagues and Peoples*. Oxford: Basil Blackwell.

Madsen, T., and Madsen, S. (1956). 'Diphtheria in Denmark'. *Danish Medical Bulletin*, 3, pp. 112–15.

Makridakis, S., Wheelwright, S. C., and McGee, U. E. (1983). *Forecasting: Methods and Applications*. New York: Wiley.

Mair, L. W. D. (1909). 'The aetiology of enteric fever in Belfast in relation to water supply, sanitary circumstance, and shellfish'. *Proceedings of the Royal Society of Medicine (Epidemiology Section)*, 2, pp. 187–242.

Major, R. H. (1943). *War and Disease*. London: Hutchinsons.

Mansolas, A. (1867). *Renseignements statistiques sur l'Etat de la Grèce*. Athens: Imprimerie Nationale.

Mardia, K. V., Kent, J. T., and Bibby, J. M. (1979). *Multivariate Analysis*. London: Academic Press.

Marié-Davy, F. (1905). 'La mortalité par la tuberculose à Paris dans ses rapports avec la densité de la population et l'aération'. *Journale d'hygiène*, 30, p. 1.

Markowitz, L. E., and Nieburg, P. (1991). 'The burden of acute respiratory infection due to measles in developing countries and the potential impact of measles vaccine'. *Reviews of Infectious Diseases*, 13 (suppl. 6), pp. S555–61.

Marks, E., Seltzer, W., and Krotki, K. (1974). *Population Growth Estimation: A Handbook of Vital Statistics Measurement*. New York: United Nations.

Matthews, G. W., and Churchill, R. E. (1994). 'Public health surveillance and the law'. In: S. M. Teutsch and R. E. Churchill (eds.), *Principles and Practice of Public Health Surveillance*. New York: Oxford University Press, pp. 190–9.

Mattox, H. E. (1989). *The Twilight of Amateur Diplomacy: The American Foreign Service and Its Senior Officers in the 1890s*. Kent, OH: Kent State University Press.

Maxcy, K. F. (1973). 'Epidemiology'. *Encyclopaedia Britannica*, VIII, pp. 640–3.

Meeker, E. (1971–2). 'The improving health of the United States, 1850–1915'. *Explorations in Economic History*, 9, pp. 353–73.

Mehr, H. (1972). 'Stockholm'. In: Robson and Regan, *Great Cities of the World, Volume II*, pp. 873–901.

Miller, J. A. (1904). 'A study of the tuberculosis problem in New York City'. *Medical News*, 84, pp. 1014–21.

Mitchell, A. (1990). 'An inexact science: the statistics of tuberculosis in late nineteenth-century France'. *Social History and Medicine*, 3, pp. 387–403.

Mitchell, J. A. (1907). 'Enteric fever in Cape Colony: its public health aspects'. *South African Medical Record*, 5, pp. 177–83.

Mollison, D. (1991). 'Dependence of epidemic and population velocities on basic parameters'. *Mathematical Biosciences*, 107, pp. 255–87.

Montefusco, A. (1914). 'Note sur la diffusion du croup a Naples'. *Transactions of the International Congress of Medicine 1913, XVIII, Hygiene and Preventative Medicine* (pt. 2), p. 99.

Moorehouse, G. W. (1903). 'On the relation of age, sex, and conjugal condition to death from typhoid fever: based upon a study of the death reports of the city of Cleveland for thirteen years from 1890 to 1902, inclusive'. *Cleveland Medical Journal*, 2, pp. 215–28.

—— (1905). 'The typhoid mortality of Cleveland for the year 1904'. *Cleveland Medical Journal*, 4, pp. 134–8.

Morman, E. T. (1984). 'Clinical pathology in America, 1865–1915: Philadelphia as a test case'. *Bulletin of the History of Medicine*, 58, pp. 198–214.

Morse, S. S. (1993). 'Examining the origins of emerging viruses'. In S. S. Morse (ed.), *Emerging Viruses*. New York: Oxford University Press, pp. 10–28.

—— (1994). 'The viruses of the future? Emerging viruses and evolution'. In S. S. Morse (ed.), *The Evolutionary Biology of Viruses*. New York: Raven Press, pp. 325–35.

Musy, G. (1906). *Recherches statistiques sur la diphtérie à Lyon (1901–1905)*. Lyon: n. p.

Myrvik, Q. N., and Weiser, R. S. (1988). *Fundamentals of Medical Bacteriology and Mycology*. 2nd edn. Philadelphia: Lea & Febiger.

Neff, J. S. (1912). 'An epidemic of typhoid fever in Philadelphia'. *Journal of the American Medical Association*, 59, p. 1053.

Newsholme, A. (1923). *The Elements of Vital Statistics in Their Bearing on Social and Public Health Problems*. London: Allen & Unwin.

442   *References*

Niven, J. (1897). 'Typhoid fever in the city of Manchester'. *Journal of State Medicine*, 5, pp. 573–7.

Noah, N. D. (1989). 'Cyclical patterns and predictability in infection'. *Epidemiology and Infection*, 102, pp. 175–90.

Ord, J. K. (1972). *Families of Frequency Distributions*. London: Griffin.

Oslcr, W. (1894–5). 'Typhoid fever in Baltimore'. *Johns Hopkins Hospital Report*, 9, pp. 73–82.

Ostheimer, M. (1910). 'Measles and German measles: characteristics of the present outbreak in Philadelphia'. *Medical Record*, 78, p. 410.

Panum, P. L. (1847a). 'Beobachtungen über das Maserncontagium'. *Virchows Archiv für Pathologie und Medizin*, 1, pp. 492–512.

(1847b). 'Iagttagelser anstillede under maeslinge-epidemien paa Faeroerne i Aaret 1846'. *Bibliothek for Laeger*, 1, pp. 270–344.

(1940). *Observations Made During the Epidemic of Measles in the Faeroe Islands in the Year 1846*. New York: Delta Omega Society, American Public Health Association.

Parker, M. T. (1984). 'Enteric infections: typhoid and paratyphoid fever'. In: Topley and Wilson, *Topley and Wilson's 'Principles of Bacteriology, Virology, and Immunity' (7th Edition), Volume III*, pp. 407–33.

Parkes, L. C. (1898–9). 'Prevalence of diphtheria and scarlet fever in the various districts of western London from 1890 to 1897'. *Public Health*, 11, pp. 210–12.

Pascua, M. (1949). 'Evolution of mortality in Europe during the twentieth century'. *Epidemiological and Vital Statistics Report*, 2, pp. 64–80.

(1950). 'Evolution of mortality in Europe during the twentieth century'. *Epidemiological and Vital Statistics Report*, 3, pp. 30–62.

(1951). 'Evolution of mortality in Europe during the twentieth century'. *Epidemiological and Vital Statistics Report*, 4, pp. 36–137.

Patterson, K. D. (1986). *Pandemic Influenza, 1700–1900*. Totowa, NJ: Rowan and Littlefield.

(1993). 'Rabies'. In: Kiple, *Cambridge World History of Human Disease*, pp. 962–7.

Pennington, C. I. (1979). 'Morbidity and medical care in nineteenth-century Glasgow'. *Medical History*, 23, pp. 442–50.

(1982). 'Tuberculosis'. In: Checkland and Lamb, *Health Care as Social History*, pp. 86–99.

Perkins, R. G. (1911). 'Typhoid fever in Cleveland in relation to pollutions of Lake Erie'. *Cleveland Medical Journal*, 10, pp. 81–97.

Phillips, L. (1910). 'Typhoid and paratyphoid fever in Egypt'. *British Medical Journal*, 2, p. 969.

Pic, A. (1906). 'Contribution à l'étude de la mortalité hospitalière de la fièvre typhoïde: statistique d'un des services de l'Hôtel-Dieu de Lyon'. *Lyon médicale*, 107, pp. 709–14.

Pierce, B. L. (1970). 'Society and labor in an expanding city'. In: Wakstein, *Urbanization of America*, pp. 247–56.

Plischke, E. (1967). *Conduct of American Diplomacy (3rd Edition)*. Princeton: D. Van Nostrand Co., Inc.

Pooley, M. E., and Pooley, C. G. (1984). 'Health, society, and environment in Victorian Manchester'. In: Woods and Woodward, *Urban Disease and Mortality*, pp. 148–75.

Preston, S. H. (1976). *Mortality Patterns in National Populations with Special Reference to Recorded Causes of Death*. New York: Academic Press.

Preston, S. H., Keyfitz, N., and Schoen, R. (1972). *Causes of Death: Life Tables for National Populations*. New York: Seminar Press.

Preston, S. H., and Van de Walle, E. (1978). 'Urban French mortality in the nineteenth century'. *Population Studies*, 32, pp. 275–97.

Prinzing, F. (1916). *Epidemics Resulting from Wars*. Oxford: Clarendon Press.

Pyle, G. F. (1969). 'Diffusion of cholera in the United States'. *Geographical Analysis*, 1, pp. 59–75.

Quiroga, V. A. (1990). 'Diphtheria and medical therapy in late nineteenth-century New York City'. *New York Journal of Medicine*, 90, pp. 256–62.

Rakove, M. (1972). 'Chicago'. In: Robson and Regan, *Great Cities of the World, Volume I*, pp. 331–67.

Ramsay, A. M., and Emond, R. T. D. (1978). *Infectious Diseases*. London: William Heinemann.

Ransome, A. (1868). 'On epidemics, studied by means of statistics of disease'. *British Medical Journal*, n.n., pp. 386–8.

Rawlings, I. D. (1910). 'The campaign against diphtheria and scarlet fever in Chicago'. *Journal of the American Medical Association*, 55, pp. 570–5.

Regan, D. E. (1972). 'London'. In: Robson and Regan, *Great Cities of the World, Volume II*, pp. 503–72.

Rios, J. A. (1972). 'Rio de Janeiro'. In: Robson and Regan, *Great Cities of the World, Volume II*, pp. 821–51.

Risse, G. B. (1993). 'History of Western medicine from Hippocrates to germ theory'. In: Kiple, *Cambridge World History of Human Disease*, pp. 11–19.

Robson, W. A., and Regan, D. E. (eds.) (1972). *Great Cities of the World: Their Government, Politics, and Planning, Volumes I and II*. London: Allen & Unwin Ltd.

Rochard, J. (1894). 'Diminution de la fièvre typhoïde à Paris'. *Bulletin Académie de médecine (Paris)*, 31, pp. 120–4.

Roemer, M. I. (1993). 'Internationalism in medicine and public health'. In: W. F. Bynum and R. Porter (eds.), *Encyclopaedia of the History of Medicine, Volume II*. London: Routledge, pp. 1417–35.

Rogers, L. (1907). 'The incidence of typhoid fever on civilian Europeans and on natives in Calcutta and the importance of the anti-typhoid inoculation of all European immigrants to India'. *Indian Medical Gazette*, 42, pp. 291–3.

Rosenau, M. J., Lumsden, L. L., and Kastle, J. H. (1909). *Report No. 3 on the Origin and Prevalence of Typhoid Fever in the District of Columbia (1908)*. Washington, DC: Government Printing Office.

Rosqvist, R., Bolin, I., and Wolf-Watz, H. (1988). 'Increased virulence of Yersinia pseudotuberculosis by two independent mutations'. *Nature*, 334, pp. 522–4.

Ross, R. (1911). *The Prevention of Malaria (2nd Edition)*. London: John Murray.
  (1916). 'An application of the theory of probabilities to the study of *a priori* pathometry'. *Proceedings of the Royal Society A*, 92, pp. 204–30.

Royama, M. (1972). 'Tokyo and Osaka'. In: Robson and Regan, *Great Cities of the World, Volume II*, pp. 968–84.

Russel, J. B. (1895–6). 'The prevalence of diphtheria in Glasgow'. *Public Health*, 8, pp. 340–2.

Russell, W. T. (1943). *The Epidemiology of Diphtheria During the Last Forty Years*. Medical Research Council Special Report Series, No. 247. London: HMSO.

Rvachev, L. A., and Longini, I. M. (1985). 'A mathematical model for the global spread of influenza'. *Mathematical Biosciences*, 75, pp. 3–22.

Ryfkogel, H. A. (1907). 'Suggestions on methods of attacking typhoid fever in San Francisco'. *California State Journal of Medicine*, 5, pp. 204–6.

Sachs, T. B. (1904). 'Tuberculosis in the Jewish district of Chicago'. *Journal of the American Medical Association*, 43, pp. 390–5.

Sadik, T. (1991). *The State of World Population, 1991*. New York: United Nations Population Fund.

Sarda, A. (1907). *De la mort dans la coqueluche et de ses causes à l'Hospice de la charité de Lyon*. Lyon: n. p.

Sauer, L. W. (1955). 'Whooping cough'. *Encyclopaedia Britannica*, 23, pp. 587–8.

Sayre, W. S. (1972). 'New York'. In: Robson and Regan, *Great Cities of the World, Volume II*, pp. 689–729.

Schiffman, S. S., Reynolds, M. L., and Young, F. W. (1981). *Introduction to Multidimensional Scaling: Theory, Methods, and Applications*. New York: Academic Press.

Schmid, G. P. (1985). 'The global distribution of Lyme disease'. *Reviews of Infectious Diseases*, 7, pp. 41–50.

Schofield, R., and Reher, D. (1991). 'The decline of mortality in Europe'. In: Schofield, Reher, and Bideau, *Decline of Mortality in Europe*, pp. 1–17.

Schofield, R., Reher, D., and Bideau, A. (1991). *The Decline of Mortality in Europe*. Oxford: Clarendon Press.

Scott, H. H. (1934). *Some Notable Epidemics*. London: Edward Arnold.

Seber, G. A. F. (1984). *Multivariate Observations*. New York: Wiley.

Séchan, P. (1911). 'La diphtérie à Lyon, 1886–1910'. *Journal Prudhomme*, 49 (46 pp.).

Sedgwick, W. T. (1911). 'Notes on typhoid fever at Washington, DC'. *Journal of the New England Water Works Association*, 25, p. 470.

Seibert, A. (1904). 'Scarlet fever in New York and some of its therapeutic problems'. *New York Medical Journal*, 80, pp. 1153–9.

Sencer, D. J., Dull, H. B., and Langmuir, A. D. (1967). 'Epidemiological basis for the eradication of measles'. *Public Health Reports*, 82, pp. 253–6.

Serfling, R. E. (1963). 'Methods for current statistical analysis of excess pneumonia–influenza deaths'. *Public Health Report*, No. 78, Centers for Disease Control, US Department of Health, Education, and Welfare, Atlanta, pp. 494–506.

Serfling, R. E., Sherman, I. L., and Houseworth, W. J. (1967). 'Excess pneumonia–influenza mortality by age and sex in three major influenza A2 epidemics, United States, 1957–1958, 1960, and 1963'. *American Journal of Epidemiology*, 86, pp. 433–41.

Shepard, R. N. (1962). 'The analysis of proximities: multidimensional scaling with an unknown distance function'. *Psychometrika*, 27, pp. 125–40, 219–46.

Sherris, J. C. (ed.) (1990). *Medical Microbiology: An Introduction to Infectious Diseases*. 2nd edn. Amsterdam: Elsevier.

Shively, H. L. (1903). 'Immigration: a factor in the spread of tuberculosis in the city of New York'. *New York Medical Journal*, 77, pp. 222–6.

Showers, V. (1973). *The World in Figures*. New York: Wiley-Interscience.

Shryock, R. H. (1966). *Medicine in America: Historical Essays*. Baltimore: Johns Hopkins University Press.

Sibson, R. (1978). 'Studies in the robustness of multidimensional scaling: procrustes statistics'. *Journal of the Royal Statistical Society B*, 40, pp. 234–8.

—— (1979). 'Studies in the robustness of multidimensional scaling: perturbation analysis of classical scaling'. *Journal of the Royal Statistical Society B*, 41, pp. 217–29.

Skalicka, J. (1903). 'O pomerech brisniho tyfu v. Praze'. *Casopis lékaru ceskych*, 42, pp. 1050, 1076.

Skinner, F. W. (1986). 'Odessa and the problem of modern urbanization'. In: Hamm, *The City In Late Imperial Russia*, pp. 209–48.

Smallman-Raynor M., Cliff, A. D., and Haggett, P. (1992). *London International Atlas of AIDS*. Oxford: Blackwell Reference.

Smith, F. B. (1988). *The Retreat of Tuberculosis, 1850–1950*. London: Croom Helm.

Smith, H. B., and Tirpak, D. (eds.) (1989). *Potential Effects of Global Climatic Change on the United States, Volume G, Health*. Washington, DC: Government Printing Office (Environmental Protection Agency, EPA 230-05-89-057).

Smith, J. L., and Tennant, J. (1898). 'A study of the epidemic of typhoid fever in Belfast, 1898'. *British Medical Journal*, 1, pp. 193–7.

Smith, S. (1972). 'New York the unclean'. In: G. H. Brieger (ed.), *Medical America in the Nineteenth Century: Readings from the Literature*. Baltimore: Johns Hopkins University Press, pp. 263–77.

Smith, W. R. (1896). 'The prevalence of diphtheria in London and elsewhere'. *Journal of State Medicine*, 4, pp. 169–227.

Spear, A. H. (1970). 'The making of the black ghetto'. In: Wakstein, *Urbanization of America*, pp. 269–75.

Speck, R. S. (1993). 'Cholera'. In: Kiple, *Cambridge World History of Human Disease*, pp. 642–9.

Spink, W. W. (1978). *Infectious Diseases: Prevention and Treatment in the Nineteenth and Twentieth Centuries*. Folkestone: Dawson.

Springett, V. H. (1952). 'An interpretation of statistical trends in tuberculosis'. *Lancet*, 1, pp. 521–5.

Springthorpe, J. W. (1909). 'Recent Melbourne hospital typhoid statistics'. *Australasian Medical Congress Transactions*, 1, pp. 283–6.

Stallybrass, C. O. (1911–12). 'The causes of the reduction in typhoid fever in Liverpool during the last sixteen years'. *Public Health*, 25, pp. 427–33.

Stokes, W. R. (1908). 'The typhoid problem in Baltimore'. *Maryland Medical Journal*, 51, pp. 487–9.

Stone, A. K., and Wilson, A. M. (1905). 'The geographical distribution of tuberculosis in Boston in 1901–1903 as compared with the distribution in 1885–1890'. *Boston Medical and Scientific Journal*, 152, pp. 6–9.

Strong, C. J. (1910). 'Typhoid fever in Detroit'. *Journal of the American Medical Association*, 55, pp. 1284–7.

Stroup, D. F., Wharton, M., Kafadar, K., and Dean, A. G. (1993). 'An evaluation of a method for detecting aberrations in public health surveillance data'. *American Journal of Epidemiology*, 137, pp. 45–9.

Stuart, G. H. (1952). *American Diplomatic and Consular Practice*. New York: Appleton-Century-Crifts, Inc.

Subtelny, O. (1988). *Ukraine: A History*. Toronto: University of Toronto Press.

Swaisland, H. C. (1972). 'Birmingham'. In: Robson and Regan, *Great Cities of the World, Volume I*, pp. 199–237.

Sykes, J. F. J. (1893–4). 'The cause of the increase of mortality from diphtheria in London'. *Public Health*, 6, pp. 331–4.

—— (1894). 'On the increase of diphtheria mortality in London'. *Practitioner*, 53, pp. 137–48.

Szreter, S. (1988). 'The importance of social intervention in Britain's mortality decline, c. 1850–1914: a reinterpretation of the role of public health'. *Social History of Medicine*, 1, pp. 1–38.

'Tableau de la mortalité due à la fièvre typhoïde dans l'agglomération bruxelloise de 1893 à 1898 et de 1899 à 1906' (1907). *Mouvement hygiène*, 23, pp. 52–4.

Tait, H. P. (1974). *A Doctor and Two Policemen: The History of Edinburgh Health Department, 1862–1974*. Edinburgh: Edinburgh Health Department.

Talbott, J. H. (1970). *A Biographical History of Medicine: Excerpts and Essays on the Men and Their Work*. New York: Grune and Stratton.

Tan, N. (1991). 'Health and welfare'. In: E. C. T. Chew and E. Lee (eds.), *A History of Singapore*. Oxford: Oxford University Press, pp. 339–56.

Tawab, F. D. A. (1972). 'Cairo'. In: Robson and Regan, *Great Cities of the World, Volume I*, pp. 271–93.

Terrés, J. (1903). 'La tuberculosis en Distrito Federal'. *Gaceta médica*, 3, pp. 204–6.

Thacker, S. B., and Millar, J. D. (1991). 'Mathematical modeling and attempts to eliminate measles: a tribute to the late Professor George Macdonald'. *American Journal of Epidemiology*, 133, pp. 517–25.

Thoinot, L., and Dubief, H. (1896). 'Les eaux de la Vallée de la Vanne et la fièvre typhoïde à Paris en 1894'. *Annales d'hygiène*, 35, pp. 481–507.

The Times Atlas of the World (1986). 7th edn. London: Times Books Ltd.

Tinline, R. R. (1972). *A Simulation Study of the 1967–1968 Foot-and-Mouth Epizootic in Great Britain*. Unpublished PhD dissertation, Department of Geography, University of Bristol, England.

Topley, W. W. C., and Wilson, G. S. (1975). *Topley and Wilson's 'Principles of Bacteriology, Virology and Immunity' (7th Edition)*. London: Edward Arnold.

Torgerson, W. S. (1958). *Theory and Methods of Scaling*. New York: John Wiley.

Troconis Alcalá, L. (1906). 'Algunos datos sobre fiebre tifoidea en la Ciudad de México. Los baciliferos cróicos: su importancia desde el punto de vista de la higiene'. *Gaceta médica de México*, 1, pp. 380–90.

Tukey, J. W. (1977). *Exploratory Data Analysis*. Reading, MA: Addison-Wesley.

'Typhoid fever at Havre' (1894). *Lancet*, 2, p. 1052.

'Typhoid fever in Milwaukee and the water supply' (1910). *Journal of the American Medical Association*, 4, pp. 211–15.

UK, Medical Research Committee (1918). *An Investigation into the Epidemiology of Phthisis in Great Britain and Ireland*. Medical Research Committee Special Report Series, No. 18. London: HMSO.

University of Texas (1965a). *University of Texas International Population Census Bibliography, No. 1, Latin America and the Caribbean*. Austin: Bureau of Business Research, University of Texas.

—— (1965b). *University of Texas International Population Census Bibliography, No. 2, Africa*. Austin: Bureau of Business Research, University of Texas.

(1966). *University of Texas International Population Census Bibliography, No. 3, Oceania.* Austin: Bureau of Business Research, University of Texas.

(1967a). *University of Texas International Population Census Bibliography, No. 4, North America.* Austin: Bureau of Business Research, University of Texas.

(1967b). *University of Texas International Population Census Bibliography, No. 5, Asia.* Austin: Bureau of Business Research, University of Texas.

(1967c). *University of Texas International Population Census Bibliography, No. 6, Europe.* Austin: Bureau of Business Research, University of Texas.

Uruguay, Consejo Nacional de Higiene (1912). *Estadistica sanitaria de la fiebre tifoidea en el Uruguay y antecedentes sobre ejecución de las obras de saneamiento y provisión de agua portable en las ciudades y villas de la compaña.* Montevideo: G. V. Marino.

US Department of State (1880–1901). *Reports from the Consuls of the United States on the Commerce, Manufactures, Etc., of Their Consular District.* Washington, DC: Government Printing Office.

(1889). *Register of the Department of State Corrected to December 1, 1888.* Washington, DC: Government Printing Office.

(1893). *Register of the Department of State Corrected to July 1, 1893.* Washington, DC: Government Printing Office.

US Department of the Treasury (1875). *Cholera Epidemic of 1873 in the United States.* Washington, DC: Government Printing Office.

US Department of the Treasury, Bureau of Navigation (1901). *Annual Report of the Commissioner of Navigation for the Fiscal Year Ended June 30, 1901.* Washington, DC: Government Printing Office, Doc. 2245.

US Department of the Treasury, Bureau of Statistics (1850–1900). *The Foreign Commerce and Navigation of the United States.* Washington, DC: Government Printing Office.

(1890). *Annual Report and Statements of the Chief of the Bureau of Statistics on the Foreign Commerce and Navigation, Immigration, and Tonnage of the United States for the Fiscal Year Ending June 30, 1889.* Washington, DC: Government Printing Office.

(1891). *Report on the Internal Commerce of the United States for the Year 1890: Part II of Commerce and Navigation.* Washington, DC: Government Printing Office.

US House of Representatives (1856–1902). *Report on the Commercial Relations of the United States with All Foreign Nations.* Washington, DC: Government Printing Office.

US Marine Hospital Service (1883–94). *Annual Report of the Supervising Surgeon General of the Marine Hospital Service of the United States.* Washington, DC: Government Printing Office.

(1896). *Annual Report of the Supervising Surgeon General of the Marine Hospital Service of the United States for the Fiscal Year 1895.* Washington, DC: Government Printing Office.

(1901). *Annual Report of the Supervising Surgeon General of the Marine Hospital Service of the United States for the Fiscal Year 1899.* Washington, DC: Government Printing Office.

(1902). *Annual Report of the Supervising Surgeon General of the Marine Hospital Service of the United States for the Fiscal Year 1901.* Washington, DC: Government Printing Office.

(1914). *Annual Report of the Surgeon General of the Public Health Service of the United States, 1913*. Washington, DC: US Government Printing Office.

US National Archives and Records Service (1945–51). *Diplomatic Instructions of the Department of State, 1801–1906. Argentina, Jan. 6, 1872–Jan. 22, 1892*. Washington, DC: General Services Administration, National Archives and Records Service, Microfilm Series.

Vallin, E. (1894). 'L'épidémie de fièvre typhoïde à Paris et l'eau de la Vanne'. *Revue d'hygiène*, 16, pp. 284–95.

Vallin, J., and Meslé, F. (1988). *Les causes de décès en France de 1925 à 1978*. Paris: Colin.

van den Bosch, F., Metz, J. A. J., and Diekmann, O. (1990). 'The velocity of spatial population expansion'. *Journal of Mathematical Biology*, 28, pp. 529–65.

Van de Walle, E., and Preston, S. H. (1974). 'Mortalité de l'enfance au XIXe siècle a Paris dans le département de la Seine'. *Population*, 29, pp. 89–107.

Vigne, C., and Loir, A. (1911). 'Enquêtes sur la fièvre typhoïd au Havre en 1911: établissement de la statistique de mortalité par les Bureaux d'hygiène'. *Revue d'hygiène*, 33, pp. 1125–33.

Vögele, J. P. (1994). 'Urban infant mortality in imperial Germany'. *Social History of Medicine*, 7, pp. 401–25.

Waissenberger, R. (ed.) (1984). *Vienna, 1890–1920*. New York: Rizzoli.

Wakstein, A. M. (ed.) (1970). *The Urbanization of America: An Historical Anthology*. Boston: Houghton Mifflin Co.

Walford, E. (1898–9). 'Diphtheria in Cardiff'. *Public Health*, 22, pp. 89–101.

Welton, T. A. (1897). 'Local death-rates in England and Wales in the ten years 1881–1890'. *Journal of the Royal Statistical Society*, 60, pp. 33–75.

Welty, C. F. (1903). 'On the nativity of decedents from tuberculosis in Cleveland for the years 1895 to 1901'. *Cleveland Medical Journal*, 2, pp. 64–6.

Whipple, G. C. (1906). 'The Cleveland typhoid epidemic of 1903–1904'. *Journal of the New England Water Works Association*, 20, pp. 266–301.

White, B. (1929). 'Epidemic septic sore throat, I: historical review'. *New England Journal of Medicine*, 200, pp. 797–805.

Williams, B. (1989). 'Assessing the health impact of urbanization'. *World Health Statistics Quarterly*, 43, pp. 145–52.

Williams, R. C. (1951). *The United States Public Health Service, 1798–1950*. Washington, DC: Commissioned Officers of the United States Public Health Service.

Wilson, A. G. (1970). *Entropy in Urban and Regional Modelling*. London: Pion.

Wilson, G. S. (1984). 'General epidemiology'. In: Topley and Wilson, *Topley and Wilson's 'Principles of Bacteriology, Virology, and Immunity' (7th Edition), Volume III*, pp. 1–9.

Wilson, L. G. (1990). 'The historical decline of tuberculosis in Europe and America: its causes and significance'. *Journal of the History of Medicine and Allied Sciences*, 45, pp. 366–96.

Wolfe, R. J. (1982). 'Alaska's great sickness: an epidemic of measles and influenza in a virgin soil population'. *Proceedings of the American Philosophical Society*, 126, pp. 91–121.

Wolff, M. (1911). *La fièvre typhoïde à Lyon*. Lyon: A. Maloine.

Woods, H. M. (1933). *Epidemiological Study of Scarlet Fever in England and Wales Since 1900*. Medical Research Council Special Report Series, No. 180. London: HMSO.

Woods, R. (1978). 'Mortality and sanitary conditions in the "best governed city in the world" – Birmingham, 1870–1910'. *Journal of Historical Geography*, 4, pp. 35–56.

(1984). 'Mortality and sanitary conditions in late nineteenth-century Birmingham'. In: Woods and Woodward, *Urban Disease and Mortality*, pp. 176–207.

Woods, R., and Shelton, N. (1997). *An Atlas of Victorian Mortality*. Liverpool: Liverpool University Press.

Woods, R., and Woodward, J. (1984). 'Mortality, poverty, and the environment'. In: Woods and Woodward, *Urban Disease and Mortality*, pp. 19–36.

(1984) (eds.). *Urban Disease and Mortality in Nineteenth-Century England*. London: Batsford Academic.

World Health Organization (WHO) (1994). *World Health Statistics Annual 1993*. Geneva: World Health Organization.

(1995a). *International Travel and Health: Vaccination Requirements and Health Advice*. Geneva: World Health Organization.

(1995b). 'La poliomélite sera éradiquée'. Pamphlet. Geneva: World Health Organization, 7 April 1995.

(1995c). *The World Health Report 1995: Bridging the Gaps*. Geneva: World Health Organization.

World Health Organization, Global Programme for Vaccines and Immunization (1995). *Immunization Policy*. Geneva: World Health Organization.

Wrigley, E. A. (1969). *Population and History*. New York.

Wrigley, E. A., and Schofield, R. S. (1981). *The Population History of England, 1541–1871: A Reconstruction*. London: Edward Arnold.

(1989). *The Population History of England, 1541–1871: A Reconstruction*. 2nd edn. London: Edward Arnold.

Young, G. B. (1912). 'A measles outbreak in Chicago'. *American Journal of Public Health*, 2, pp. 791–3.

Zawadzki, S. (1972). 'Warsaw'. In: Robson and Regan, *Great Cities of the World, Volume II*, pp. 1039–75.

Ziegler, P. (1969). *The Black Death*. London: Collins.

Zinsser, H. (1935). *Rats, Lice, and History*. London: George Routledge and Sons.

Index

Cambridge Studies in Historical Geography

Titles marked with an asterisk* are available in paperback